Emergency and Primary Care of the Hand

Editors

Raymond G. Hart, MD, MPH, FACEP

Assistant Clinical Professor
Department of Emergency Medicine
University of Louisville School of Medicine
Attending Physician
Emergency Department
Veterans Administration Medical Center
Louisville, Kentucky

Dennis T. Uehara, MD, MSAM, FACEP

Clinical Professor of Surgery
Department of Surgery
University of Illinois College of Medicine at Rockford
Chairman
Department of Emergency Medicine
Rockford Memorial Hospital
Rockford, Illinois

Mary Jo Wagner, MD, FACEP

Program Director
Saginaw Cooperative Hospitals, Inc./Michigan State University
Emergency Medicine Residency Program
Saginaw, Michigan
Associate Professor
Program in Emergency Medicine
Michigan State University College of Human Medicine
East Lansing, Michigan

American College of
Emergency Physicians®

The American College of Emergency Physicians makes every effort to ensure that contributors to College-sponsored publications are knowledgeable authorities in their fields. Readers are nevertheless advised that the statements and opinions expressed in this book are provided as guidelines and should not be construed as College policy unless specifically referred to as such. The College disclaims any liability or responsibility for the consequences of any actions taken in reliance on those statements or opinions. The materials contained herein are not intended to establish policy, procedure, or a standard of care.

Additional copies of this publication can be ordered from ACEP, PO Box 619911, Dallas, TX 75261-9911; toll-free 800-798-1822, touch 6, or 972-550-0911; www.acep.org/bookstore.

Marta Foster, Senior Editor

Kaye Roberts, Editorial Assistant

Mike C. Goodwin, Graphic Design and Production Manager

Thomas S. Werlinich, Associate Executive Director, Educational and Professional Publications

Copyediting/proofreading: Allison Esposito, Red Oak, Texas

Illustrations: Steven K. Arendt, Louisville, Kentucky

Production: Carden Jennings Publishing Co., Ltd., Charlottesville, Virginia

Indexing: Sharon Hughes, Chicago, Illinois

Printing: The Covington Group, Kansas City, Missouri

Contributors

Brian N. Aldred, MD, FACEP, Clinical Assistant Professor of Surgery, Department of Surgery, University of Illinois College of Medicine at Rockford; Staff Physician, Department of Emergency Medicine, Rockford Memorial Hospital; Medical Director, Regional Emergency Acute Care Transport, Rockford Health System, Rockford, Illinois

Scott M. Benson, MD, Resident, Emergency Medicine Residency, West Virginia University, Morgantown, West Virginia

Todd H. Chaffin, MD, FACEP, Clinical Assistant Professor of Surgery, Department of Surgery, University of Illinois College of Medicine at Rockford; Staff Physician, Department of Emergency Medicine, Rockford Memorial Hospital, Rockford, Illinois

Harold W. Chin, MD, FACEP, Medical Director of Occupational Health, and Staff Physician, Department of Emergency Medicine, Lake Forest Hospital, Lake Forest, Illinois

Wendy C. Coates, MD, FACEP, Director, Medical Education, Department of Emergency Medicine, Harbor-UCLA Medical Center, Torrance, California; Associate Professor of Medicine, UCLA School of Medicine, Los Angeles, California

Paul J. Donovan, DO, FACEP, Director of Emergency Services, North Adams Regional Hospital, North Adams, Massachusetts; Assistant Professor of Emergency Medicine, University of Massachusetts Medical Center; Medical Director, Northern Berkshire Sports Medicine, Inc.; US Ski Team Physician

Wesley P. Eilbert, MD, FACEP, Clinical Assistant Professor, Department of Emergency Medicine, University of Illinois College of Medicine at Chicago; Director of Undergraduate Education, Department of Emergency Medicine, Mercy Hospital and Medical Center, Chicago, Illinois

Robert Escarza, MD, Clinical Instructor of Surgery, Department of Surgery, University of Illinois College of Medicine at Rockford; Staff Physician, Department of Emergency Medicine, Rockford Memorial Hospital, Rockford, Illinois

Madonna Fernández-Frackelton, MD, Assistant Professor of Medicine, Department of Emergency Medicine, Harbor-UCLA Medical Center, Torrance, California

Lance K. Freeman, MD, FACEP, Staff Physician, Covenant Health Care Emergency Department, Saginaw Cooperative Hospitals, Inc./Michigan State University Emergency Medicine Residency Program, Saginaw, Michigan; Assistant Clinical Professor, Michigan State University College of Human Medicine, East Lansing, Michigan

Raymond G. Hart, MD, MPH, FACEP, Assistant Clinical Professor, Department of Emergency Medicine, University of Louisville School of Medicine; Attending Physician, Emergency Department, Veterans Administration Medical Center, Louisville, Kentucky

Thomas Harter, MD, Kleinert Kutz and Associates; Clinical Assistant Professor of Plastic Surgery, University of Louisville School of Medicine, Louisville, Kentucky

Gregory C. Hoskins, MD, Department of Emergency Medicine, University of Arkansas for Medical Sciences, Little Rock, Arkansas

Stephen McCabe, MD, Kleinert Kutz and Associates; Clinical Assistant Professor of Plastic Surgery, University of Louisville School of Medicine, Louisville, Kentucky

Charles F. Pattavina, MD, FACEP, Assistant Professor, Department of Medicine, Division of Emergency Medicine, Brown University; Attending Physician, Emergency Medicine, Miriam Hospital, Providence, Rhode Island

Arthur F. Proust, MD, FACEP, Clinical Assistant Professor of Surgery, Department of Surgery, University of Illinois College of Medicine at Rockford; Associate Director, Department of Emergency Medicine, Rockford Memorial Hospital, Rockford, Illinois

Kevin G. Rodgers, MD, Associate Program Director, and Associate Clinical Professor of Emergency Medicine, Indiana University Emergency Medicine Residency, Indianapolis, Indiana

John P. Rudzinski, MD, FACEP, Clinical Professor of Surgery, Department of Surgery, and Clinical Professor of Medicine, Department of Medicine, University of Illinois College of Medicine at Rockford; Vice Chairman, Department of Emergency Medicine, Rockford Memorial Hospital, Rockford, Illinois

Robert C. Satonik, MD, FACEP, Assistant Residency Director, Saginaw Cooperative Hospitals, Inc./Michigan State University Emergency Medicine Residency Program, Saginaw, Michigan; Staff Physician, Covenant Health Care Emergency Department; Assistant Clinical Professor, Program in Emergency Medicine, Michigan State University College of Human Medicine, East Lansing, Michigan

Russell Shatford, MD, Kleinert Kutz and Associates; Assistant Professor of Hand Surgery, University of Louisville School of Medicine, Louisville, Kentucky

Jonathan I. Singer, MD, FACEP, Professor, Emergency Medicine and Pediatrics, Wright State University School of Medicine, Dayton, Ohio

Brian T. Stubitsch, MD, Clinical Instructor of Surgery, Department of Surgery, University of Illinois College of Medicine at Rockford; Staff Physician, Department of Emergency Medicine, Rockford Memorial Hospital, Rockford, Illinois

James H. Sullivan, MD, FACEP, Clinical Assistant Professor of Surgery, Department of Surgery, University of Illinois College of Medicine at Rockford; Staff Physician, Department of Emergency Medicine, Rockford Memorial Hospital, Rockford, Illinois

George D. Tsonis, MD, Clinical Instructor of Surgery, Department of Surgery, University of Illinois College of Medicine at Rockford; Staff Physician, Department of Emergency Medicine, Rockford Memorial Hospital, Rockford, Illinois

Mary Jo Wagner, MD, FACEP, Program Director, Saginaw Cooperative Hospitals, Inc./Michigan State University Emergency Medicine Residency Program, Saginaw, Michigan; Associate Professor, Program in Emergency Medicine, Michigan State University College of Human Medicine, East Lansing, Michigan

Jason M. White, MD, FACEP, Attending Physician, Department of Emergency Medicine, Saint Mary's, Saginaw Cooperative Hospitals, Inc./Michigan State University Emergency Medicine Residency Program, Saginaw, Michigan; Associate Clinical Professor, Program in Emergency Medicine, Michigan State University College of Human Medicine, East Lansing, Michigan

Janet M. Williams, MD, FACEP, Professor, Department of Emergency Medicine, and Director, Center for Rural Emergency Medicine, West Virginia University, Morgantown, West Virginia

Dean E. Wolanyk, MD, FACEP, FACP, Clinical Associate Professor of Surgery, Department of Surgery, and Clinical Associate Professor of Medicine, Department of Medicine, University of Illinois College of Medicine at Rockford; Staff Physician, Department of Emergency Medicine, Rockford Memorial Hospital, Rockford, Illinois; Director, Department of Emergency Medicine, Harvard Memorial Hospital, Harvard, Illinois

Robert W. Wolford, MD, FACEP, Co-Residency Director, Saginaw Cooperative Hospitals, Inc./Michigan State University Emergency Medicine Residency Program, Saginaw, Michigan; Associate Professor and Vice Chair, Program in Emergency Medicine, Michigan State University College of Human Medicine, East Lansing

Table of Contents

Section II: Fractures and Dislocations

Section III: Specific Injuries

Acknowledgments

The editors thank everyone who participated in this textbook. Although impossible to list all, many deserve special mention.

- First, thanks to Tom Werlinich and the American College of Emergency Physicians for their vision and unwavering support of this project.
- We also thank Angel Farris, Ron Meadors, and Melinda Wardin for their administrative assistance and manuscript preparation.
- A special thanks to our illustrator, Kip Arendt, who provided timely and valuable contributions to this book.
- Our medical editor, Marta Foster, from the American College of Emergency Physicians, deserves praise. Her devotion and calm leadership directed this entire project to completion.
- Finally, but most especially, thanks to the individual authors for their time, energy, and expertise.

Raymond G. Hart, MD, MPH, FACEP
Dennis T. Uehara, MD, MSAM, FACEP
Mary Jo Wagner, MD, FACEP
Editors

Dedication

To Harold E. Kleinert, MD, and Joseph E. Kutz, MD, two heroic pioneers in the field of hand surgery who demonstrate leadership, creativity, the value of hard work, and the joy of a tireless search for knowledge.
RGH

To my wife, Jane, and my children, Julie, Lisa, and Kevin, for their love and unwavering support.
DTU

To Glenn C. Hamilton, MD, and Raymond P. Ten Eyck, MD, who first supported my efforts at writing and academic emergency medicine.
MJW

Preface

This textbook is a testimony to the maturation of the specialty of emergency medicine. As the editors, we developed and designed it to define and expand on the present body of knowledge on emergency hand care, and to enhance our working relationship with our esteemed colleagues, the hand surgeons. The invaluable support we received from the American College of Emergency Physicians and the insightful contributions of the emergency physician authors give this book its shape and scope.

We three editors represent three distinct eras in emergency medicine. Dennis T. Uehara, MD, MSAM, FACEP, is one of the original emergency medicine educators on hand injuries and continues to provide leadership through his teaching, writing, and clinical expertise. Dr. Uehara's mentoring and guidance led to a working relationship and friendship with Raymond G. Hart, MD, MPH, FACEP, that began in the early 1980s. Dr. Hart was initiated to the care of hand injuries in the late 1970s while working in the surgical suites of Dr. Kleinert and Dr. Kutz prior to medical school. Dr. Hart was residency director at the University of Illinois at Chicago from 1993 to 1996 and during that time developed a professional relationship with Mary Jo Wagner, MD, FACEP. Dr. Wagner is part of the new generation of dynamic emergency medicine educators and leaders. As a residency director, Dr. Wagner ensures that the knowledge and experience gained by her generation are passed on to the next. We three worked together to develop a thorough but concise textbook that covers all aspects of emergency hand care and gives depth and validity to its study.

This book is for the hand-injured patients in our emergency departments. Our goal is to educate each other and the emergency medicine community so that we can provide patients with the best care possible.

RGH
DTU
MJW

CHAPTER 1

Anatomy and Terminology

Raymond G. Hart, MD, MPH, FACEP

The human hand provides the opportunity and ability for creativity and precision through its mobility and sensation. It also is vulnerable to injury; an estimated 5% of emergency department visits are for evaluation and treatment of hand injuries.[1]

Emergency assessment of the injured hand must begin with a complete evaluation of the patient for other possible injuries. This initial assessment and the stabilization of other conditions must focus on life and limb preservation. Then, when the patient is deemed stable, the hand injury can be evaluated.

A thorough and careful evaluation includes a detailed history and physical examination, the foundation of which is an understanding of the detailed anatomy of the hand. This basic anatomic knowledge is vital to understanding normal hand function, determining loss of function, and comprehending possible mechanisms of injury. Only by having this information can the physician develop an accurate evaluation and treatment plan.

Another key to conducting an accurate and complete emergency department evaluation is knowledge of formal hand terminology. This evaluation must be complemented with an appropriate description. Anatomic landmarks as well as sensory and functional motor descriptions must be related clearly between the physician who evaluates the injury initially and the physician who provides definitive or followup care. The result will be the correct and safest treatment plan.

The scope and design of this book preclude a lengthy outline of anatomy in this chapter. Instead, separate chapters are devoted to each specific hand structure, and each chapter includes detailed discussions with illustrations.

Surface Anatomy and Terminology

The detailed anatomy of the hand is intricate, but much can be learned through observation and superficial palpation of the injured hand. In fact, physicians can learn a great deal about hand anatomy by palpating and examining their own hands, learning to identify structures and understand their normal movement.

This process begins with an understanding of the landmarks of the hand and their terminology (Figure 1-1). The hand has a **volar**, or **palmar**, surface and the opposite **dorsal** surface. The digits are identified as **thumb** and **index**, **middle**, **ring**, and **little** fingers. There is a **radial** and an **ulnar** border, or **aspect**, in reference to the hand and its individual digits.

Each finger has a **distal phalanx**, a **middle phalanx**, and a **proximal phalanx**; the thumb has only a distal and a proximal phalanx. The joints are referred to as the **distal interphalangeal** (DIP), the **proximal inter-**

Figure 1-1.

Palmar (volar) surface anatomy.

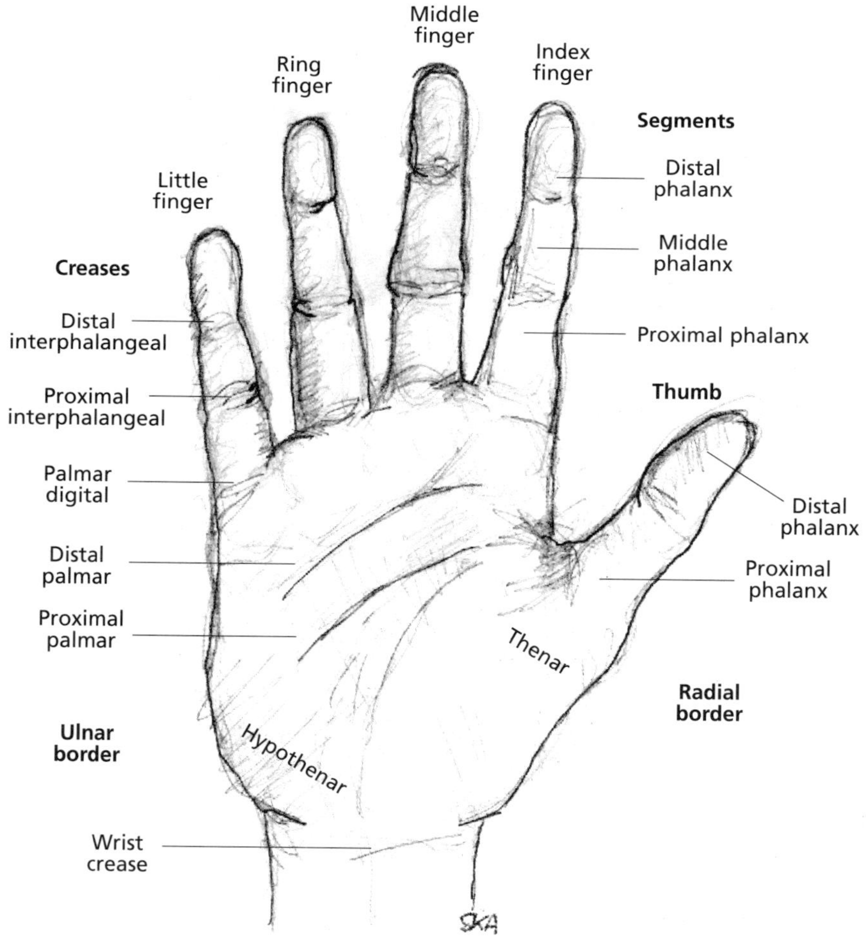

phalangeal (PIP), the **metacarpophalangeal** (MCP), and the **carpometacarpal** (CMC).

The **thenar eminence** is visualized and palpable at the base of the thumb. The **hypothenar eminence** is the opposite prominence of the palm at the base of the little finger. The **digital**, **palmar**, and **wrist creases** are readily identifiable landmarks.

The surface anatomy of the hand also can be learned through self-inspection. Structures identifiable on the volar surface of the wrist progressing from the radial to the ulnar border include the easily palpable **radial artery**, the powerful **flexor carpi radialis**, and, when present, the **palmaris longus**. The palmaris longus is best identified by firmly opposing the thumb to the little finger and flexing the wrist to approximately 15 degrees. When present, the palmaris longus becomes prominent and palpable. It is a valuable and critical landmark for evaluation of wrist lacerations because it lies ulnar to the flexor carpi radialis and superficial to the **median nerve**. The insertion of the **flexor carpi ulnaris** is palpable with firm flexion of the ulnar wrist area. The **ulnar neurovascular bundle** lies radial to this tendon.

Inspection of the dorsal surface of the hand reveals the **nail plates**, the **creases** of the interphalangeal joints, and the prominent superficial

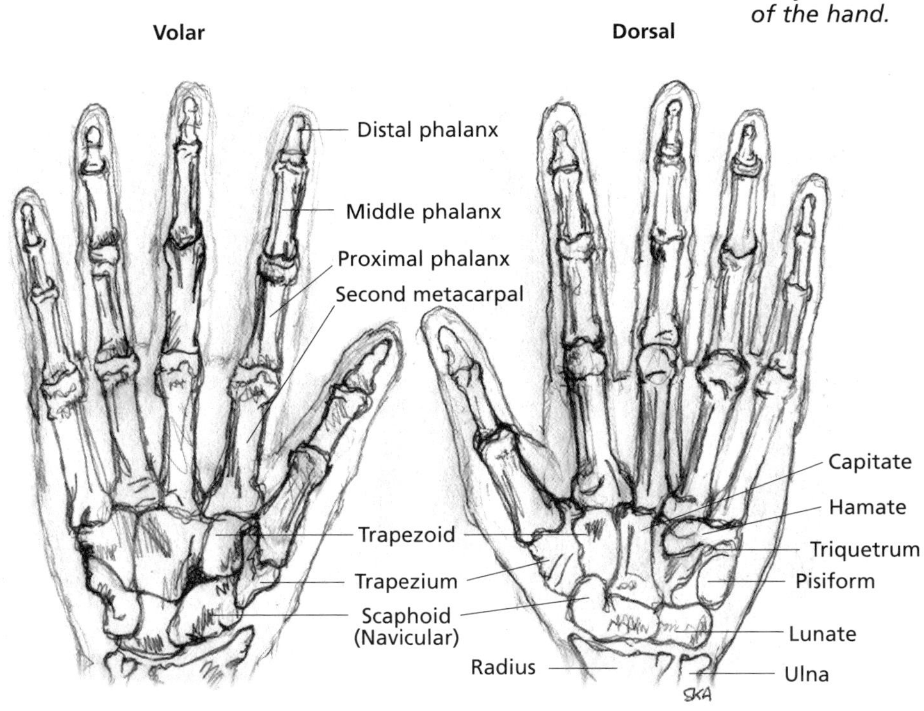

Figure 1-2.

Bony structures of the hand.

extensor tendons. The **metacarpals** are palpable, as is the **ulnar styloid** at the wrist.

Figure 1-2 illustrates the bony structures of the hand. The distal, middle, and proximal phalanges of the fingers and the proximal and distal phalanges of the thumb are easy to identify. The **metacarpals** are identified by number beginning with the thumb as the **first metacarpal**. The eight bones of the wrist are the **carpal bones**. The four distal carpal bones, from the radial to the ulnar border, are the **trapezium**, **trapezoid**, **capitate**, and **hamate**. The four proximal carpal bones, from radial to ulnar, are the **scaphoid** (or **navicular**), **lunate**, **triquetrum**, and **pisiform**. The distal **radius** and **ulna** also can be visualized.

Figure 1-3 illustrates the bony structure of the joints. The finger joints are, again, the distal interphalangeal (DIP), the proximal interphalangeal (PIP), the metacarpophalangeal (MCP), and the carpometacarpal (CMC). The thumb has the **interphalangeal** (IP), the metacarpophalangeal (MCP), and the carpometacarpal (CMC) (or **basilar**, or **saddle**) joints.

Attitude of the Hand

The framework of the hand is established by the delicate and precise balance of opposing flexion and extension forces. The skeleton supported by the joints moves gracefully, balancing these opposing actions. At rest, the hand assumes a natural position, or **attitude**, with the digits in gradually increasing flexion from the index finger to the little finger.

Figure 1-3.

Joint terminology.

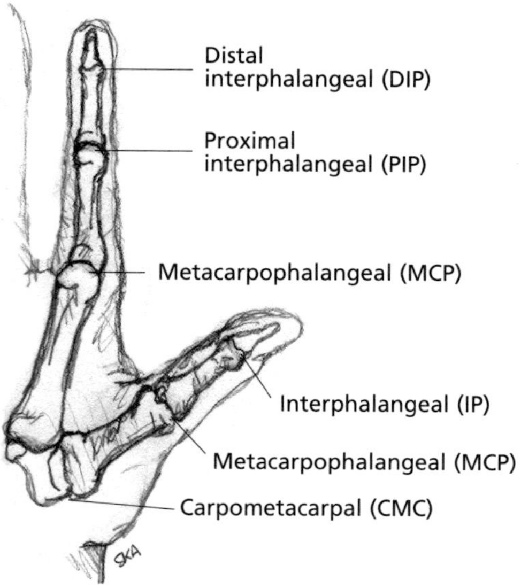

Figure 1-4.

Hand position.

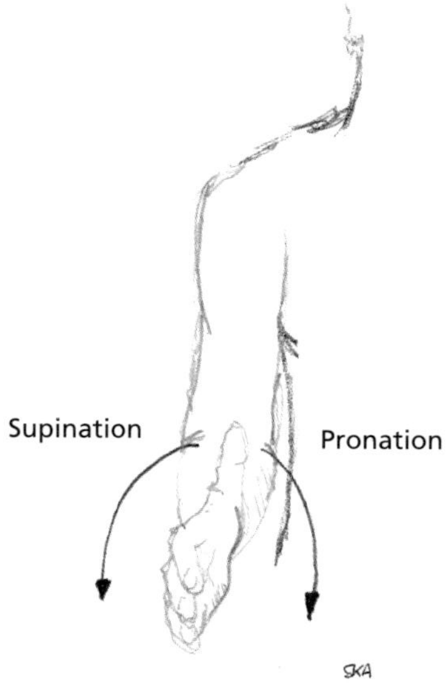

There is a corresponding tendency for all nail beds to point toward the scaphoid. This natural pose is important in the initial assessment of hand injuries, most notably tendon lacerations. A deviation is highly suggestive of significant injury and should raise the physician's index of suspicion.

Skin

The hand has two distinctly different skin surfaces. The dorsal surface is exposed, and the skin is mobile to allow ease of movement. This skin is thin compared to the volar surface and is hair bearing. It swells easily as a result of trauma or infection.

The volar surface skin is thick, keratinized, and stable. This stability results from the fibrous connections to the deeper surfaces and dermal insertions to the palmar fascia. Strong, tight fibrous septa in the fat pad of the distal phalanx anchor to the underlying periosteum.

Epithelial ridges of dermis arranged on the volar surfaces, particularly in areas for gripping at the tips of each digit, form a pattern that is unique to every person—the **fingerprints**. The grasping function is assisted by sweat glands in this skin, which promote a stickiness.

The skin of the hand has a rich blood supply that promotes effective healing. It also has an abundance of sensory receptors, including encapsulated mechanoreceptors and free nerve endings, that provide excellent protective and functional sensation.

The **fingernail** is a refined feature of the dorsal skin. It protects the

Figure 1-5.

Movements at the wrist.

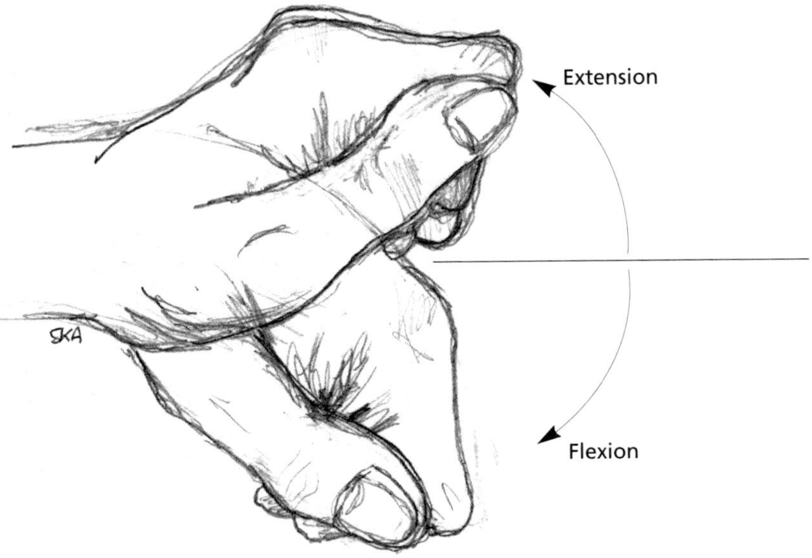

end of the finger and supports it for maximal precision. The **nail bed** and **germinal matrix** must be repaired carefully to maintain the function of this dorsal external skeleton.

Hand and Digit Motion

The hand can assume a position of **supination** or **pronation** (Figure 1-4). This movement is initiated at the elbow by the radial head. In the supinated position, the palm faces up, as if holding a bowl of soup. In the pronated position, the palm faces down.

Movements about the wrist include **flexion** and **extension** (Figure 1-5). Flexion at the wrist is powerful and generated primarily by the flexor carpi radialis and the flexor carpi ulnaris. Extension of the wrist is dependent on an intact radial nerve and is a good test for this nerve function. Wrist movements that move the hand laterally are called **radial deviation** and **ulnar deviation** (Figure 1-6).

The digits also have identified movements. The movement of a digit away from the midline is **abduction**; movement toward the midline is **adduction** (Figure 1-7). The digits also move in flexion, extension, and **hyperextension** (Figure 1-8).

The thumb has its own unique and identified movements. It moves in flexion and extension (Figure 1-9); when it moves across the palm to touch the tip of the small digit, the movement is termed **opposition** (Figure 1-10). The thumb also can perform abduction and adduction. Movement of the thumb at a 90-degree angle away from the palm is **palmar abduction** (Figure 1-11). This is an excellent test for the motor

Figure 1-6.

Lateral movements at the wrist.

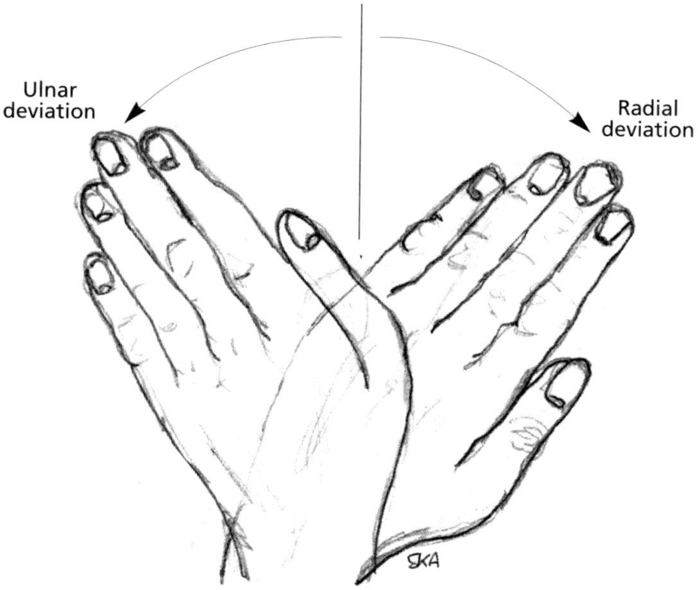

integrity of the median nerve. Movement of the thumb in the same plane as but away from the palm is **radial abduction** (Figure 1-12).

Injury Terms and Definitions

Transverse fracture. A fracture line that is perpendicular to the long axis of the bone. This fracture generally is caused by direct trauma and usually is stable.

Oblique fracture. A fracture line that is oblique to the long axis of the bone. Generally caused by indirect trauma.

Spiral fracture. A fracture line that spirals around the long axis of the bone. Usually caused by torsional or rotational force.

Pathologic fracture. A fracture that occurs in bone that is vulnerable and weakened by disease, typically tumors, infection, or osteoporosis. Because the strength of the bone has been compromised, even minor trauma can cause the fracture.

Avulsion fracture. A bony fragment that has been detached secondary to the powerful force or traction of ligament or tendon insertion. The avulsion of bone at the insertion of the extensor tendon to the dorsal base of the distal phalanx results in mallet finger. Gamekeeper thumb may involve an avulsion fracture when there is a rupture of the ulnar collateral ligament with an attached bony fragment.

Tapping fracture. A transverse fracture that results from a small, localized force. The bone absorbs the bulk of the energy, and there is minimal soft tissue damage.

Angulation fracture. When a transverse fracture occurs and one end of the bone is under tension and the other is under compression, the result is an angulation fracture. This fracture occurs initially in the area under tension. A measurement of the angle between the longitudinal axes of the fracture fragments must be determined. Fractures with clinically significant angulation must be reduced to prevent compromised function. A Colles fracture is an example of an angulated fracture at the distal radius that results in dorsal angulation of the distal fragment, a description of the relationship of the bone distal to the fracture with respect to the proximal bone.

Rotational fracture. A fracture that occurs under a combination of horizontal and vertical stresses. The fracture line will occur at 45 degrees to the long axis

Figure 1-7.

Finger movements.

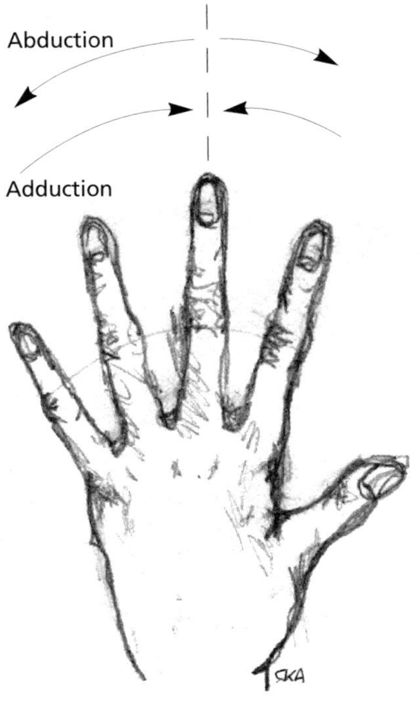

of the bone. This fracture occurs in the hand, primarily in metacarpal fractures. It can displace or shorten and may lead to significant problems.

Crush injury. An injury that results from a large force that causes fracture and extensive soft tissue injury. For example, a person whose hand gets caught in a cornpicker will likely sustain a crush injury with devastating fractures. The soft tissue injury makes the healing process more tenuous.

Penetrating injury. An injury that results from a high-impact force that breaks the skin, for example, a gunshot wound. Extensive soft tissue and bony injury may result. The evaluation of a penetrating injury to the hand must include a careful search for intact and injured structures because they are in such close proximity to each other.

Named Fractures of the Hand and Wrist

Bennett fracture. A thumb fracture in which an oblique fracture of the first metacarpal base separates a small triangular fragment of the volar lip. The resultant instability causes the metacarpal shaft to displace proximally.

Boxer fracture. A fracture of the fourth or fifth metacarpal neck with volar displacement of the metacarpal head.

Chauffeur fracture (or **Hutchinson fracture**). An oblique fracture of the radial styloid. Originally described as resulting from misfire of the starting crank of an engine.

Colles fracture. A fracture of the distal radius with dorsal displacement, with or without an accompanying fracture of the ulnar styloid. Originally had a more precise description but now a more general term.

Die-punch fracture. An intra-articular fracture of the distal radius with resulting impaction of the dorsal aspect of the lunate fossa.

Figure 1-8.

Finger movements.

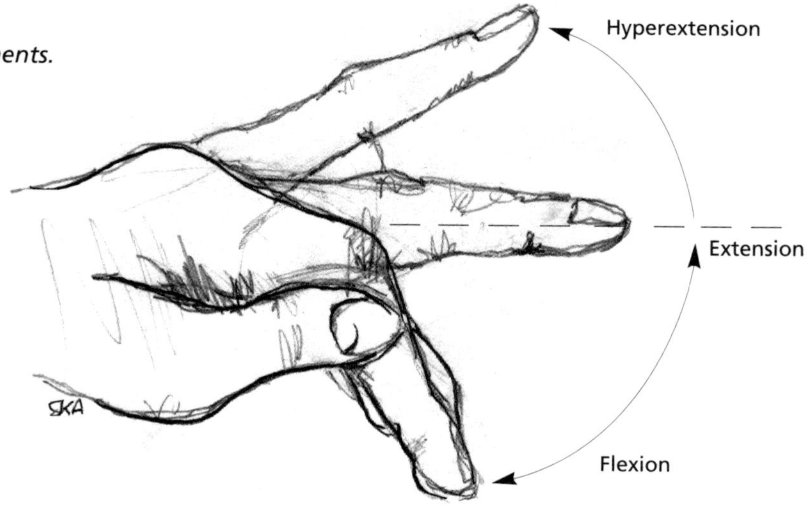

Mallet finger. A flexion deformity at the DIP joint that occurs when the extensor tendon insertion at the dorsal distal phalanx has been damaged. The damage may be to the extensor tendon itself or an avulsion fracture at the distal phalanx.

Rolando fracture. A Y-shaped intra-articular fracture of the base of the thumb metacarpal at the CMC joint. This is an unstable fracture.

Smith fracture. A fracture of the distal radius that results in palmar displacement of the distal fragment. Also known as a reverse Colles fracture.

Tuft fracture. A fracture of the distal phalanx, usually comminuted, that generally involves an associated nail bed injury.

Specific Named Hand Problems

de Quervain disease (tenosynovitis). An inflammatory condition of the abductor pollicis longus and extensor pollicis brevis tendons, usually as a result of overuse. Patients complain of severe pain over the radial styloid exacerbated by thumb movement.

Dupuytren contractures. A disease of the palmar and digital fasciae. The involved fascia becomes increasingly thick and causes finger flexion at the MCP joint.

Gamekeeper thumb (or **skier thumb**). A disruption of the ulnar collateral ligament at the MCP joint of the thumb. Occurs secondary to trauma and results in instability at the thumb MCP joint.

Ganglion cyst. A common benign tumor of the hand that develops from synovial fluid leaking from an adjacent tendon sheath.

Lunate dislocation. A wrist dislocation of the carpal lunate bone. It is diagnosed on a lateral radiograph with the lunate pushed off the radius and toward the palm, the **spilled teacup sign**.

Perilunate dislocation. Another wrist dislocation. It is diagnosed on a lateral radiograph that reveals that the lunate is maintaining contact with the radius and the capitate is positioned posterior to the lunate.

Terry Thomas sign. A radiographic finding consistent with scapholunate dissociation, an abnormal widening of the space between the two bones. Named for the English actor with the famed gap-toothed grin.

Trigger finger. A condition that results from a mass or nodule on the flexor tendon that continually gets caught in the proximal pulley, causing the finger to catch or lock.

Figure 1-9.
Thumb movements.

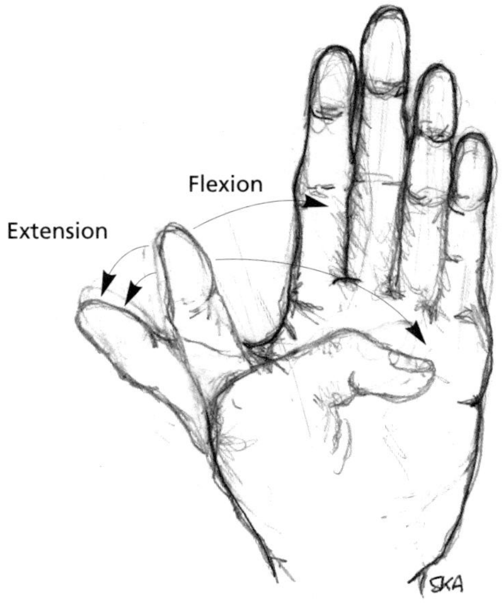

Joint and Soft Tissue Terms

Dislocation. A condition that results from the loss of congruity of the articulating surfaces of a joint. It is described by the joint involved and the position of the distal bone. A dislocation of the PIP joint of a digit usually is a dorsal dislocation because of the relative integrity of the volar plate.

Subluxation. A partial dislocation. There is still contact between the bone surfaces.

Fracture-dislocation. A dislocation complicated by a fracture through one of the intra-articular surfaces of the bones of the joint.

Sprain. A condition that results from a tear or disruption of the ligaments that stabilize a joint. Graded from minor to complete ligament disruption and instability.

Strain. An injury to the musculotendinous unit that results from excessive stretch or contraction of the muscle. Graded from minor to severe, which involves a complete disruption of the musculotendinous unit.

Tendonitis. A painful condition of the tendon with inflammation usually secondary to overuse.

Tenosynovitis. A synovial space infection or inflammation that usually involves the flexor tendon sheath. Described by **Kanavel's four cardinal signs**: uniform swelling of the digit, semiflexed resting position of the digit, tenderness along the entire course of the sheath, and pain along the entire sheath with passive extension of the digit.

Figure 1-10.
Opposition.

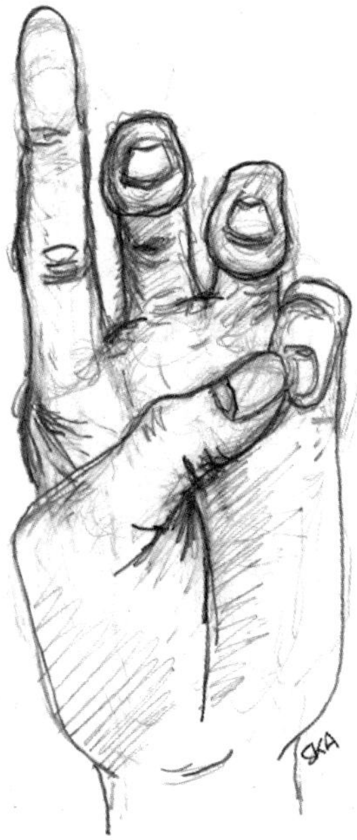

Reference

1. Uehara DT, ed. The hand in emergency medicine. *Emerg Med Clin North Am.* 1993;11:557-583, 585-600.

Additional Reading

American Society for Surgery of the Hand. *The Hand, Examination and Diagnosis.* 3rd ed. Philadelphia, Pa: Churchill-Livingstone; 1990.

American Society for Surgery of the Hand. *The Hand, Primary Care and Common Problems.* 2nd ed. Philadelphia, Pa: Churchill-Livingstone; 1990.

Hart RG, Rittenberry TJ, Uehara DT, eds. *Handbook of Orthopedic Emergencies.* Philadelphia, Pa: Lippincott-Raven; 1999.

Mercier LR. *Practical Orthopedics.* 4th ed. St Louis, Mo: Mosby; 1995.

Ruiz E, Cicero JJ. *Emergency Management of Skeletal Injuries.* St Louis, Mo: Mosby; 1995.

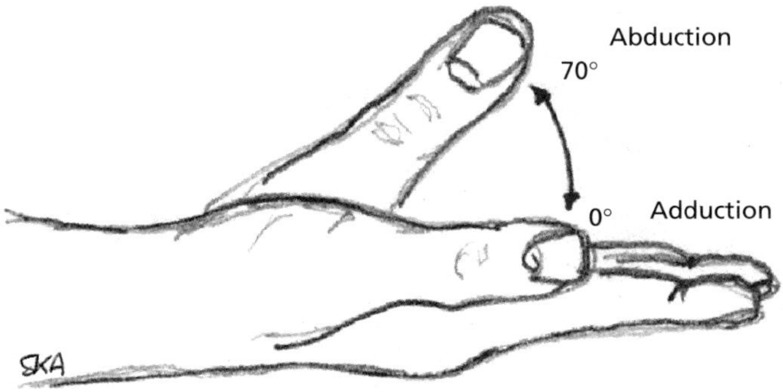

Figure 1-11.
Palmar abduction.

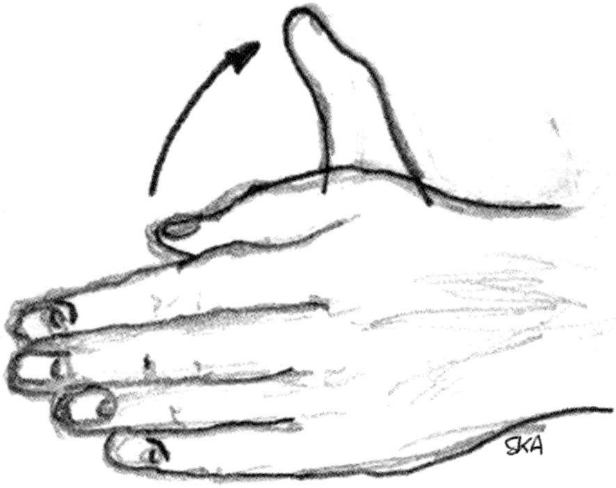

Figure 1-12.
Radial abduction.

CHAPTER 2

History and Physical Examination

Raymond G. Hart, MD, MPH, FACEP

History

Thorough history-taking is important in the evaluation of all emergency department patients, and those with hand injuries are no exception. The gathering of historical information must be concise and focused yet complete. The history must be properly directed depending on the source, site, and extent of the injury.

Demographic Data

Age

Knowing the patient's age can help the emergency physician determine the potential injury, guide the treatment plan, and influence the outcome. A particular mechanism of injury or type of fall can cause different injuries depending on the patient's age. For example, an elderly person who falls on an outstretched hand is likely to sustain a Colles fracture, but the same fall in a pediatric patient is more likely to result in a buckle fracture of the distal radius. An injured elderly patient with osteoporosis is more apt to have a fracture than is a middle-aged patient with solid bone density. A fracture in a pediatric patient must be evaluated carefully for injury to the growth plate. Fingertip and soft tissue injuries in children heal nicely secondary to healthy, young tissue and excellent blood flow. Younger patients are much more tolerant of immobilization after injury; elderly patients are more likely to experience stiffness, weakness, and relatively poor healing. Complications from similar injuries also vary significantly between the pediatric and geriatric age groups.

Sex

The most important difference in hand injuries between men and women is most likely to be related to occupation or avocation. Football injuries, hammer strikes to the fingertips, and sawblade lacerations are seen as more traditionally male injuries, although those differences are less significant in many jobs and households today. Elderly women have less bone density and a greater propensity for fractures. Women also have comparatively smaller hands, although that has no clinical significance.

Occupation

It is difficult to think of an occupation in which hand use is not important, but some jobs are virtually impossible to perform without two fully functional hands. A telephone operator, for example, might be able to use a headset and continue to work with one functioning hand, but a professional violinist so afflicted would be precluded from work. Certain surgical repairs may be undertaken with this information considered in the decision.

Certain occupations expose workers to a higher risk of hand-related injuries. Carpal tunnel syndrome and other overuse syndromes are prevalent among office personnel who use computers routinely and for long periods. A sawmill is more likely to be the site of a finger, hand, or arm amputation. Builders and construction workers have a higher incidence of assorted hand-related injuries. A detailed history of a work-related injury should prompt a search and recommendations for a safer work environment.

Hand Dominance

Knowing which of the patient's hands is dominant may provide clues to the mechanism of injury. A hammer strike is most likely to be performed with the dominant hand and result in injury to the opposite hand. Theoretically, at least, the repair of a dominant hand injury may be undertaken in preference to a similar repair of the opposite injured hand. A hand injury must always be repaired so that the patient (and the hand) can return to his or her highest (and, as close as possible, original) level of function regardless of hand dominance.

History of Present Illness

Mechanism of Injury

Critical information about an injury must be obtained to ensure accurate diagnosis and treatment. Most patients with hand injuries are in the emergency department soon after the injury occurs, but it is still important to ascertain the time of injury accurately. A laceration that is a couple of hours old can be closed primarily, but one that is 24 hours old is more prone to poor healing and infection. The decision to start antibiotic prophylaxis is guided by historical information and by time elapsed from injury to treatment.

The cause of a laceration, with or without associated blunt trauma, has an impact on both treatment and recuperation. Knowing whether the object was blunt or sharp, clean or dirty, determines what type of repair is appropriate and whether antibiotics are needed. A history of a foreign body in the wound influences imaging decisions and triggers a foreign body search.

The force or angle of a fall also may provide clues to the possible injury. Knowing the position of the hand at the time of injury can be helpful and may greatly influence treatment. Treatment of a boxer fracture may seem routine, but if the patient also has a laceration at the MCP joint, a human bite must be considered, and the treatment plan becomes admission, surgical exploration, and irrigation with intravenous antibiotics. A search for other associated injuries must always be considered.

Injury Sequelae

The patient should be asked to describe any changes or findings that occurred at the time of or soon after the injury. A distinct pop followed by the inability to flex the distal phalanx suggests the rupture of a profundus tendon insertion or a delayed tendon rupture. A snap followed by sharp, localized pain suggests a fracture. A patient who has an unstable fracture of the hand will complain of pain and instability. The history of a dislocation usually is distinctive, including a possible history of spontaneous reduction or reduction of the dislocation prior to emergency department arrival. Localized pain and tenderness, swelling, and discoloration are all clues to potential injuries. Patient complaints of motor or sensory changes in the hand with a mechanism consistent with nerve damage will lead a search to the most accurate diagnosis.

Treatment in the Field

Obtaining a history of treatment administered before arrival in the emergency department, for example, a dislocation that was reduced before arrival, may yield important information. An amputated finger that has been properly prepared and placed on ice has a higher probability of successful replantation. Witnesses and EMS personnel should be actively questioned. Their accurate descriptions of the mechanism of injury and details of the treatment provided are valuable.

Past Medical History

A history of previous medical illnesses can significantly influence the outcome of a patient's hand injury. History of bleeding diatheses, peripheral vascular disease, and insulin-dependent diabetes mellitus can affect treatment and outcome. Metabolic disorders, cancer, renal disease, and immunocompromised states must all be evaluated and treatment options considered. A history of juvenile rheumatoid arthritis or some other connective tissue disease has obvious importance in hand-related injuries. A history of hypertension or heart or liver disease may also affect surgical and anesthesia options.

Past Surgical History

A complete surgical history is indicated, but most notably surgical procedures to the affected hand or arm. It is important to determine if the patient has had a previous injury to the affected hand, particularly with a resultant deficit. Scars on the arm and hand may indicate previous significant injuries or surgeries.

Tetanus

Tetanus immunization status must be determined and appropriately updated for all lacerations and open wounds.

Last Meal

It is always advisable to determine when the patient last ate if general anesthesia is a consideration.

Medications

A patient's medication list often is the best information source for determining an accurate past medical history. Sedatives, pain medications, and muscle relaxers can affect patient cooperation and the physician's ability to determine pain levels and deficits. Anticoagulant use is common and may affect treatment options. Potential drug interactions must be determined before administering medications in the emergency department. This is critical for outpatient treatment as well, particularly for sedation, pain control, and prophylaxis.

Allergies

It also is important to review the patient's history of medication allergies. When indicated, alternative medications must be chosen carefully, particularly antibiotics.

Family History

A family history of arthritides or connective tissue disease must be noted, as well as insulin-dependent diabetes mellitus, bleeding disorder, or peripheral vascular disease. Cancer and metabolic or immunocompromise diseases may be significant.

Social History

A history of alcohol or tobacco use must be determined, as well as

Figure 2-1.

Patient positioned for hand examination.

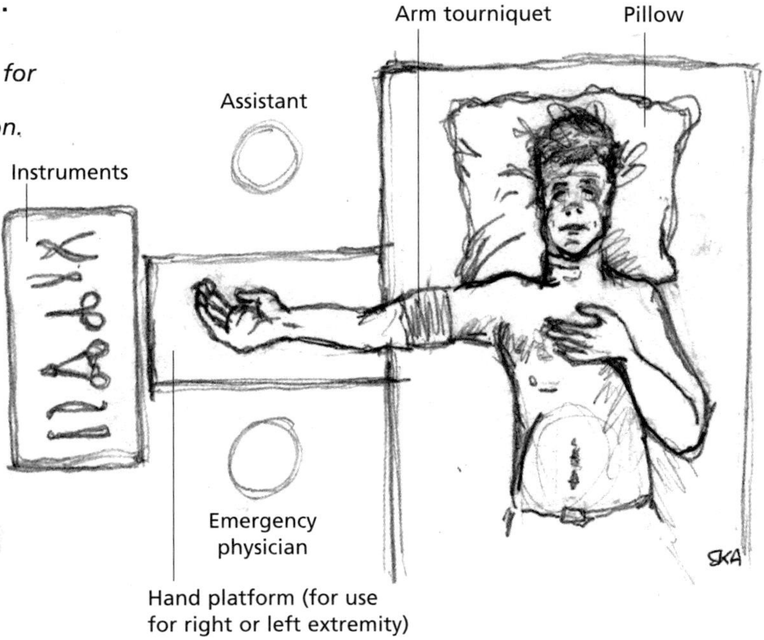

illicit drug use. The patient's occupational history and hobbies such as music and woodworking are important historical considerations.

Review of Systems

A complete review of systems may uncover essential information relevant to the patient's care. Nausea and vomiting may indicate a gastrointestinal illness and preclude the use of oral medications. Fever and chills may suggest a viral or systemic infectious condition. Chest pain, syncope, and other medical conditions may suggest a cause of a fall or injury and have ominous implications. They must be addressed and attended to promptly.

Physical Examination

Emergency department patients with hand injuries must undergo a complete yet focused physical examination. The tendency is to place a hand-injured emergency department patient in a chair or in an examination area that is inadequate for an appropriate evaluation. This must be judiciously avoided. The initial evaluation must address the threats to life and limb as well as the ABCs. Assuming these have been excluded, the patient must then be examined to determine any lesser obvious sites of injury.

The patient should change into a gown, be placed in a supine position, and ideally, rest the injured hand on a bedside hand examination table (Figure 2-1). All jewelry and watches must be removed. Good lighting, adequate exposure, and a bloodless field are essential. The physician must avoid focusing entirely on the obvious injury site. Instead, the hand injury should be approached systematically from the shoulder, down the arm, toward the hand, and finally, to the point of injury.

When documenting a hand injury, it is essential to accurately note whether the right or left hand is involved. When possible, a hand-drawn, labeled illustration of the injury site should be produced. Unfortunately, an appropriate and professionally completed history and physical examination can be negated by inadequate or incomplete chart documentation.

Inspection

The proper inspection of a hand injury demands patience and astute observation. The physician should begin by examining the entire patient, then move to the upper extremity, then the forearm, wrist, hand, and last, the spe-

Figure 2-2.

Normal attitude of the hand.

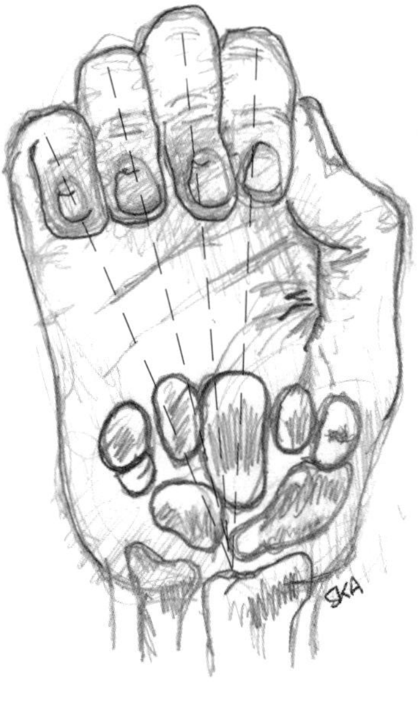

cific injury site. The neurovascular and musculoskeletal implications of every injury must be considered and the entire upper extremity inspected with these in mind. Inspecting the opposite hand and upper extremity for asymmetry and comparison purposes is a good idea. The physician should examine for obvious and subtle deformities, note swelling or erythema, and carefully inspect the skin for lesions, lacerations, bites, ecchymoses, and abrasions. Small, seemingly innocuous wounds can mask significant damage. The attitude of the hand must be determined (Figure 2-2). Abnormal hand positions can indicate fractures, dislocations, angulation, rotation, and tendon lacerations.

Palpation

Palpation is universally more successful when done calmly, gently, and systematically. A patient will become increasingly uncooperative if the physician grabs the hand at its maximal point of tenderness. Instead, the physician should begin with the opposite, uninjured extremity to gain patient confidence and comparative information, moving to the affected extremity proximally, at the shoulder, then gradually but purposefully toward the hand and the specific site of injury. Palpation may reveal instability, crepitus, a point of maximal tenderness, or temperature variability. It is advisable to stabilize an obvious or unstable fracture and obtain radiographs before palpation.

Range of Motion

Range of motion testing should be performed at the wrist, fingers, and thumb of the injured hand. This is best performed using both active and passive techniques. Active range of motion testing is performed when the patient actively initiates the movement evaluated. With passive range of motion testing, the examiner performs the test on the patient. This testing will determine the extent of pain and any lost or decreased motor function. It is most effectively evaluated compared to the opposite, uninjured hand. Normal values for range of motion of the wrist, fingers, and thumb are listed in Table 2-1. The use of a goniometer is helpful in measuring range of motion. At a baseline 0 degrees, the joint is extended in anatomic position (Figure 2-3).

Table 2-1.

Normal values for range of motion of joints of the wrist and hand.

Joint	Motion (degrees)
Wrist	
Flexion	80
Extension	70
Ulnar deviation	30
Radial deviation	20
Fingers	
Abduction	20
Adduction	0
MCP flexion	90
MCP extension	30
PIP flexion	100
PIP extension	0
DIP flexion	90
DIP extension	10
Thumb	
Abduction	70
Adduction	0
MCP flexion	50
MCP extension	0
IP flexion	90
IP extension	20

Strength

Joint movement, primary muscles, peripheral nerves, and nerve roots are listed in Table 2-2. Strength testing determines the integrity of the motor pathway from the cerebral cortex through the spinal cord, into the peripheral nerves, and to the musculature. A baseline should be determined from the contralateral, uninjured hand; the physician should keep in mind that strength testing can be greatly influenced by poor patient cooperation, pain, and fear. Motor strength to the hand is evaluated by testing for the radial, median, and ulnar nerves. The radial nerve is tested by extending the wrist against resistance. This isolates testing of the wrist extensors. The median nerve is best tested by placing the patient's hand in a supine position and having the patient move the thumb in palmar abduction (lifting the thumb away from the palm) against resistance. This isolates testing of the abductor pollicis brevis. The ulnar nerve is tested by asking the patient to spread the fingers apart against resistance. This isolates for testing of the intrinsics, including the lumbricals. More isolated muscle testing may be performed as suspicion warrants. Figure 2-4 is a muscle strength grading scale.

Sensation

Sensation must be tested in all hand injuries and specifically evaluated in potential nerve injuries. It must be tested accurately and documented distal to the injury site. Two-point discrimination is most accurate for digital nerve testing and is best tested with a paper clip, with the two blunt ends folded as makeshift calipers (Figure 2-5). The intact digital nerve should allow discrimination between one and two points to a distance of 5 mm. Light touch and pinprick also should be tested in each area.

Potential digital nerve lacerations should be evaluated at the distal tip on the volar surface at both the radial and ulnar aspects of each digit.

Radial nerve sensation is tested in the area of the anatomic snuffbox on the dorsal surface of the hand between the thumb and the index finger. The median nerve is best tested at the distal tip on the volar surface of the index finger. The ulnar nerve is tested at the distal tip on the volar surface of the little finger.

Vascular Integrity

Vascular status can best be checked by palpating peripheral pulses and capillary refill testing. Skin color and temperature also are valuable clues. Arterial lacerations usually are self-evident, with vast amounts of pulsatile bright red blood spurting from the injury site. Use of a handheld Doppler can enhance arterial flow evaluation. ***Vascular compromise to an extremity is a true emergency.***

Figure 2-3. *Baseline 0 degrees for range of motion measurements.*

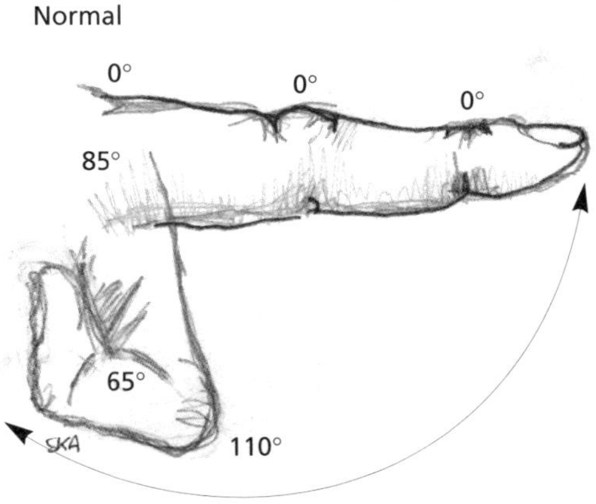

A significant laceration to an artery at the wrist or in the hand is rarely isolated, so any related injured structures must be identified. Keeping in mind the anatomy of the digital neurovascular bundle, the physician must remember that a laceration to a digital artery generally involves the digital nerve as well.

Specific Approach to Multisystem Trauma

History

In a hand trauma case, the history must be obtained rapidly and simultaneously with resuscitation efforts. It is tempting to rush to the obvious site of the severe hand injury, but the focus must remain on salvaging life and limb. The physician should determine the mechanism of injury, keeping in mind the possibility of a medical illness as a con-

Table 2-2.

Innervation of the primary muscles of movement for the wrist and hand.

Joint Movement	Primary Muscles	Peripheral Nerves	Nerve Root
Wrist			
Flexion	Flexor carpi radialis	Median	C7
	Flexor carpi ulnaris	Ulnar	C8
Extension	Extensor carpi radialis longus	Radial	C6
	Extensor carpi radialis brevis	Radial	C6
	Extensor carpi ulnaris	Radial (posterior interosseous)	C7
Fingers			
Abduction	Dorsal interossei	Ulnar	C8-T1
	Abductor digiti minimi	Ulnar	C8-T1
Adduction	Palmar interossei	Ulnar	C8-T1
MCP flexion	Lumbricals: medial 2	Ulnar	C8
	lateral 2	Median	C7
PIP flexion	Flexor digitorum superficialis	Median	C7-T1
DIP flexion	Flexor digitorum profundus	Ulnar, median (anterior interosseous)	C8-T1
Finger extension	Extensor digitorum communis	Radial (posterior interosseous)	C7
	Extensor indicis	Radial (posterior interosseous)	C7
	Extensor digiti minimi	Radial (posterior interosseous)	C7
Thumb			
Abduction	Abductor pollicis longus	Radial (posterior interosseous)	C7
	Abductor pollicis brevis	Median	C6-7
Adduction	Adductor pollicis	Ulnar	C8
MCP flexion	Flexor pollicis brevis, medial portion	Ulnar	C8
	lateral portion	Median	C6-7
IP flexion	Flexor pollicis longus	Median (anterior interosseous)	C8-T1
MCP extension	Extensor pollicis brevis	Radial (posterior interosseous)	C7
IP extension	Extensor pollicis longus	Radial (posterior interosseous)	C7
Opposition	Opponens pollicis	Median	C8-T1
	Opponens digiti minimi	Ulnar	C8

tributing factor. Heart disease, neurologic disease, and metabolic illnesses may contribute to falls. Domestic violence and suicide attempt also must be considered.

The time elapsed since the injury must be ascertained, as must any source of contamination. A dirty wound can result from a dirty weapon or environment. Bite wounds also must be considered. Tetanus immunization status and rabies risk must be investigated. A more detailed history must be taken at a later time.

Initial Assessment and Resuscitation

In the setting of multisystem trauma, the physician must first address the ABCs. The patient must be undressed and a thorough and complete search for other sites of trauma conducted. Intravenous fluids and oxygen must be administered and cardiac monitoring started. Vital signs must be monitored closely and any abnormalities addressed. Evaluating the hand injury may be less important until the patient is resuscitated and stabilized.

Hemorrhage Control

A severe hand laceration that is bleeding heavily usually will have been addressed prior to the patient's arrival. Direct pressure and elevation initiated in the field is also the preferred method of control in the emergency department. ***The physician should not blindly clamp vessels in a bleeding hand wound.*** Tearing or crushing a vessel makes subsequent repair more difficult, and clamping may damage other vital structures, including nerves, tendons, and other adjacent vessels. Judicious use of a tourniquet may be beneficial.

Life-threatening hemorrhage from an upper extremity wound is rare. Injuries that threaten function or even survival of the injured part are more common.

Neurovascular and Tendon Function

A careful evaluation of the neurologic status of the hand is indicated, and a motor and sensory examination must be performed as previously discussed. Vascular status and tendon function must be determined as well.

Anesthesia

The patient may need anesthesia to tolerate a complete examination. The physician should choose the safest, most effective method of anesthesia to facilitate patient comfort and cooperation for a direct, detailed wound examination. Once intact nerve status has been documented, adequate anesthesia is indicated.

Direct Wound Inspection

Direct inspection of the wound is best carried out with the patient in a supine position and the injured hand

Figure 2-4.

Grading scale for muscle strength.

5	Movement against gravity with full resistance
4	Movement against gravity with some resistance
3	Movement against gravity
2	Movement with gravity eliminated
1	Slight muscle contraction, no movement
0	No contraction detected

placed in a supine position on a hand examination table. The examiner should be comfortably seated with good lighting on the wound. The field should be sterile and bloodless. An arm tourniquet may be used for large or more proximal injuries (Figure 2-6). A standard-sized blood pressure cuff with a protective layer of Webril cotton undercast padding (The Kendall Company, Mansfield, Mass) between the cuff and skin may be safely inflated. The cuff can become increasingly uncomfortable, so patient desires will make each minute precious. Initially the hand should be elevated, then exsanguinated from distal to proximal with a 4-inch Ace wrap. The cuff can be inflated to approximately 150 mm Hg and locked but for no longer than 20 minutes. Then, the Ace wrap is unwound from distal to proximal to expose the exsanguinated hand.

The most effective finger tourniquet is a 0.5-inch Penrose drain (Figure 2-7). The digit should be elevated and, beginning at the distal tip, the Penrose wrapped from distal to proximal to exsanguinate the digit. Then, the Penrose can be unwound to one layer at the base of the digit. A mosquito clamp can be used to hold it safely in place. The Penrose ***must not be allowed*** to bunch or become too narrowly constricting. Other finger tourniquet methods are available, but the Penrose provides variability and less constriction.

The wound should be irrigated copiously with normal saline solution, after which a careful, direct wound examination can be performed. All intact and injured structures should be identified.

Ultimately, restoring function to the injured part depends on a systematic repair performed in the operating room. An intact vascular system with adequate skin cover and proper bone alignment are of utmost importance. Joint, tendon, and nerve function also must be restored to the highest level possible.

Figure 2-5.

Paper clip calipers for sensory examination, two-point discrimination.

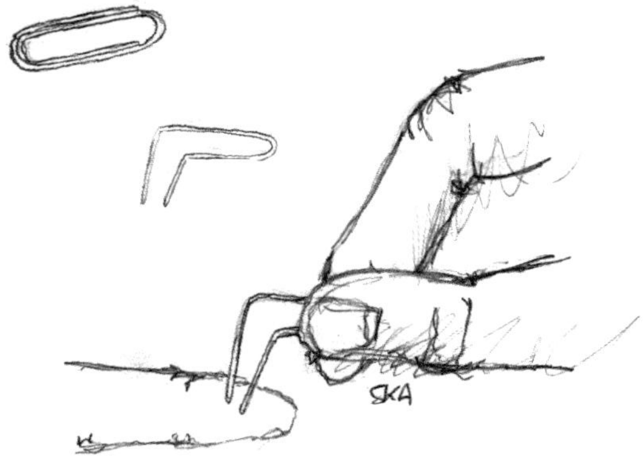

Specific Named Tests

Flexor Digitorum Profundus Test

This test is performed to determine if the **flexor digitorum profundus (FDP) tendon** is intact. The patient is instructed to extend all digits and place the hand in a supine position on a flat surface. The examiner then presses firmly on the middle and proximal phalanges at the PIP joint of the finger being evaluated. The patient is instructed to flex the distal tip of the digit, which will cause flexion at the DIP joint. This isolates flexion of the FDP tendon. An inability to flex the distal phalanx suggests a complete laceration or rupture of the FDP tendon. This test must be performed against resistance by applying firm pressure to the flexed tip. If the patient can flex the distal phalanx but complains of weakness or pain or is easily overcome with resistance, a partial FDP tendon laceration is likely.

Flexor Digitorum Superficialis Test

This test is performed to determine if the **flexor digitorum superficialis (FDS) tendon** is intact. The patient is instructed to place the hand in a supine position on a flat surface and extend all digits. The examiner then holds all the digits in extension except the one to be tested. The patient is instructed to flex the specific digit, which will cause flexion at the PIP joint. This isolates flexion of the FDS tendon. An inability to flex the middle phalanx at the PIP joint suggests a laceration of the FDS tendon. This test must be performed against resistance to search for a partial FDS tendon laceration. If the patient complains of weakness or pain or the examiner can easily overcome the flexion, a partial FDS tendon laceration is likely.

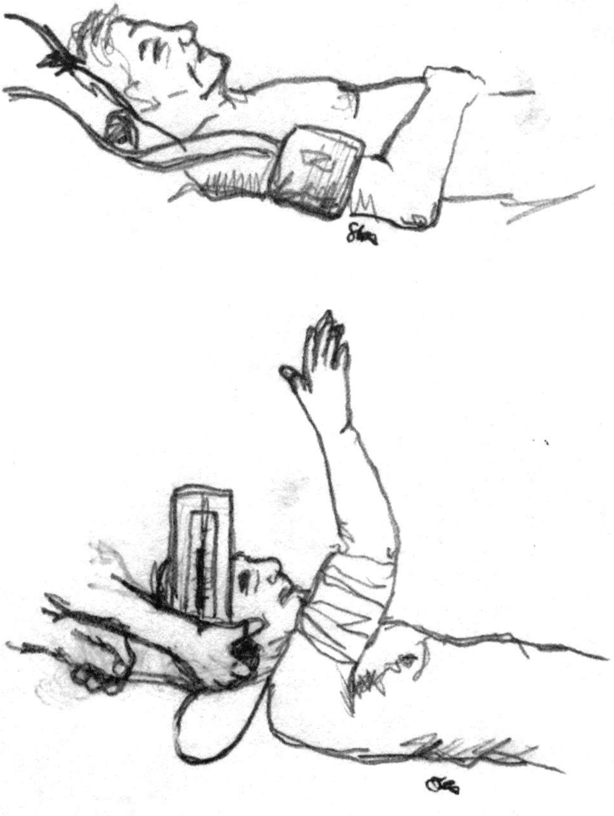

Figure 2-6.
Arm tourniquet.

Allen Test

This test is performed to determine if the radial and ulnar arteries are intact. The patient is instructed to place the hand comfortably in a supine position on a flat surface. The examiner should then identify the radial and ulnar arteries and instruct the patient to make a fist repeatedly by opening and tightly closing the hand. The patient should hold the fist closed, then the examiner should apply pressure to occlude the radial and ulnar arteries at the wrist. This temporarily exsanguinates the hand. After several seconds, the patient should be instructed to open the hand slowly; the hand will be pale in the palm and digits. The examiner releases pressure on one of the arteries while maintaining pressure on the other. If the hand does not immediately flush, a partial or complete arterial occlusion should be suspected. The test should be repeated, releasing the opposite artery. It is advisable to compare the injured hand with the contralateral, uninjured hand. This test also can be performed at the level of the digital arteries.

Phalen Test

This test is performed to determine whether a patient has carpal tunnel syndrome. The patient is instructed to flex both wrists maximally and hold them in this position for approximately 1 minute. If the patient develops paresthesias in the distribution of the median nerve in this time period, the test is positive for carpal tunnel syndrome.

Tinel Test

This test also is performed to determine whether a patient has carpal tunnel syndrome. The patient is instructed to rest the elbow and proximal forearm on a firm surface with the hand resting freely in a supine position. The examiner should then lightly but repeatedly use finger percussion over the transverse carpal ligament at the wrist. If the patient develops paresthesias in the distribution of the median nerve, the test is positive for carpal tunnel syndrome.

Figure 2-7.

Penrose finger tourniquet.

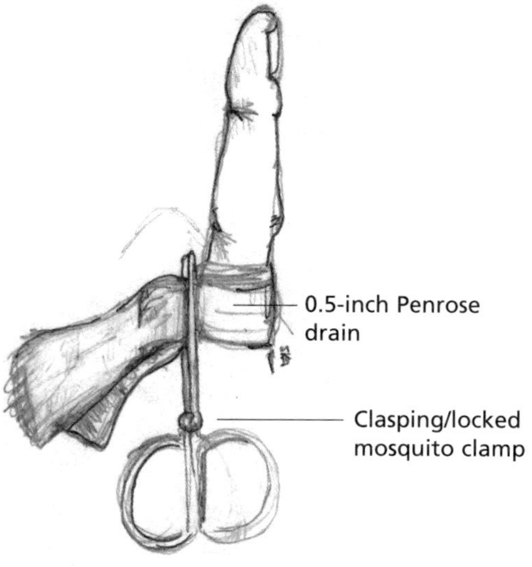

Summary

Hand injuries are common emergency department presentations, and concise yet complete histories must be obtained on all these patients. Valuable diagnostic information may be obtained through careful attention to the mechanism of injury. The physical examination must be performed systematically to determine all potentially injured structures. An accurate history and thorough physical examination, combined with a solid working knowledge of hand anatomy, are paramount for making the proper diagnosis. Every effort must be made to return an injured hand to its highest level of function.

Additional Reading

American Society for Surgery of the Hand. *The Hand, Examination and Diagnosis.* 3rd ed. Philadelphia, Pa: Churchill-Livingstone; 1990.

American Society for Surgery of the Hand. *The Hand, Primary Care and Common Problems.* 2nd ed. Philadelphia, Pa: Churchill-Livingstone; 1990.

Hart RG, Rittenberry TJ, Uehara DT, eds. *Handbook of Orthopedic Emergencies.* Philadelphia, Pa: Lippincott-Raven; 1999.

Mercier LR. *Practical Orthopedics.* 4th ed. St Louis, Mo: Mosby; 1995.

Ruiz E, Cicero JJ. *Emergency Management of Skeletal Injuries.* St Louis, Mo: Mosby; 1995.

Uehara DT, ed. The hand in emergency medicine. *Emerg Med Clin North Am.* 1993;11:585-600.

CHAPTER 3

Diagnostic Imaging

Charles F. Pattavina, MD, FACEP

Well-chosen imaging is the cornerstone of diagnosis for many injuries. The most commonly used technique is plain radiography, or x-ray imaging, a category of ionizing radiation in the form of photon-emitted electromagnetic energy. Plain radiography may not be appropriate for every acute hand problem, but it is widely used and universally available. Newer imaging modalities such as nuclear medicine, ultrasonography, computed tomography (CT, a computerized variation on x-ray), and magnetic resonance imaging (MRI) are replacing procedures such as conventional tomography. Improvements in each technique provide for more and better images.

Emergency physicians are called on at all hours to read a wide variety of diagnostic imaging studies in the emergency department. In most cases, an emergency physician's reading is the only timely interpretation that affects a patient's care while he or she is in the emergency department. For this reason, emergency physicians must continue to develop and improve their skills, especially for interpreting plain radiographs and performing ultrasonography.

Viewing Films in the Emergency Department

Films that are evaluated in the emergency department (plain radiographs, CT scans) usually are placed against a view box that is backlit by fluorescent bulbs. Typical luminance is 2000 to 2500 nt, but some boxes may be 3500 nt or even higher. Good intensity makes use of the "hot light" less of a necessity. As opposed to the film in a typical 35-mm camera, conventional x-ray film has emulsion on both sides. This allows an enhanced image by lifting the film off the board to view it obliquely (at a 45-degree angle instead of perpendicularly).

Characteristics of Acutely Broken Bones

Adult. A cortical break usually is seen as a complete break and is diagnostic of a fracture.

Pediatric. Possibilities include a partial cortical break (greenstick fracture), a one-sided buckling of the cortex (torus fracture), or bending with no cortical defect (plastic fracture).

Impacted fracture. The only finding may be an increased area of bone density, but usually there is some disruption of the cortex.

Fracture margins are sharp and not corticated, as opposed to sesamoid bones or accessory ossification centers (or old fractures), which are well corticated and smoother.

Associated soft tissue signs of acute fracture are absent in an old fracture or nonfracture.

Orthopedic texts and atlases of normal radiographic anatomy and normal variants should be available and referred to in order to describe fractures accurately. They are most helpful for determining when an unusual finding is not a fracture.

Plain Radiography

Radiographic Bone Anatomy

See Figure 3-1.

Articular cartilage is not evident on plain radiographs. It is radiolucent.

The **epiphysis** is the bone's primary growth center. It contributes to the growth of bone length.

The **physis** is a radiolucent band between the epiphysis and the metaphysis.

The **metaphysis** is the funnel-shaped area of the bone.

The **diaphysis** is the long, tubular segment of the bone. It has the central medullary cavity, spongiosa, and the dense cortex.

An **apophysis** is an accessory ossification center that does not contribute to bone growth. There are several apophyses throughout the skeletal system. The greater trochanter of the femur is an apophysis.

Definitions

Ray. An individual finger, composed of a metacarpal and its three phalanges: distal, middle, and proximal.

Syndactyly. A fusion of two or more of the distal rays.

Polydactyly. A duplicative anomaly in which there is an additional ray beyond the normal five.

Arachnodactyly. The abnormally long, thin fingers frequently associated with **Marfan syndrome**.

Sesamoid bone. An accessory bone, frequently found in the foot but in the hand and wrist as well. Occasionally fractured in the foot but rarely in the hand or wrist. May be mistaken for a fracture.

Degenerative osteoarthritis. Inflammatory condition characterized by joint space narrowing, irregular articular margins, hypertrophic spurs, and subarticular sclerosis. Common in adults by age 40, with signs frequently noted in the DIP joints. **Heberden nodes** are a clinically palpable finding.

Rheumatoid arthritis. An arthritis with characteristic joint changes noted on plain radiographs. Early signs include periarticular soft tissue swelling followed by widened joint spaces and demineralization. These result from inflammatory hyperemia of the intra-articular fluid and synovial thickening. Eventually there is joint space narrowing and the classic finding of ulnar subluxation. There is no evidence of spur formation.

Radiographic Analysis

The physician should always view the entire radiograph and avoid focusing on an obvious injury. Focusing on an obvious fracture, for example, may lead to missing an associated dislocation. Bone density, architecture, trabecular pattern, joints, and soft tissue should be evaluated separately.

A radiograph should always be viewed with the assumption that an

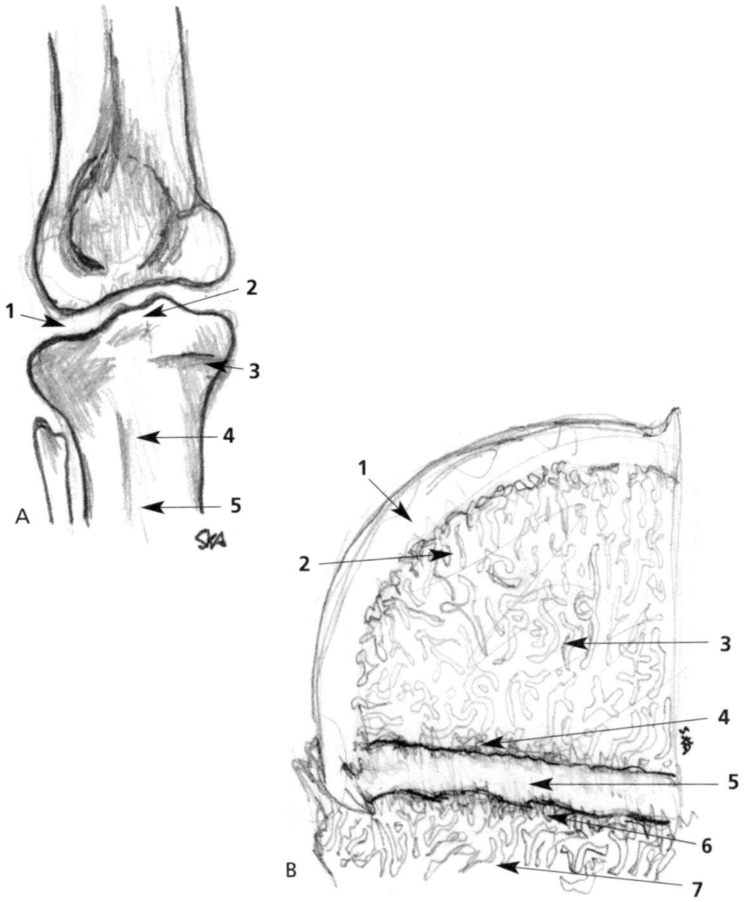

Figure 3-1.

Bone anatomy. **A)** *Radiologic terms:* **1)** *articular cartilage does not show in the film;* **2)** *epiphysis;* **3)** *epiphyseal line;* **4)** *metaphysis, including both calcified cartilage and newly formed bone;* **5)** *diaphysis or shaft.* **B)** *Histologic terms:* **1)** *articular cartilage;* **2)** *compact bone of subarticular margin;* **3)** *epiphysis, spongy bone;* **4)** *terminal plate;* **5)** *physis;* **6)** *metaphysis;* **7)** *spongy bone of diaphysis.*

abnormal finding is present. A systematic search should continue until the entire radiograph is proved normal.

Standard Views

It is essential to obtain correct views that show the areas of interest adequately. These views usually include an anteroposterior (AP), a lateral (at a 90-degree angle to the AP), and, for some body parts, one or more oblique films. As a general rule, films of long bones should show at least the adjacent joint on either side. There are special views for every area imaged, and unconventional views can be improvised when needed.

In any unusual circumstance, it is critical to communicate directly with the technician concerning the area and extent of interest to reduce the likelihood that a patient has to go back for additional views. Sending a patient back to the radiology suite may be unavoidable if the views are inadequate.

The key to ordering the correct films is to examine the patient thoroughly first. The areas for imaging should be identified precisely, and images should be requested of only those areas. Abnormalities such as fractures may be missed if the wrong areas are radiographed (hand versus wrist), when the images do not include enough of the affected area, or when the angles are not correct.

The body's bilateral symmetry facilitates the imaging of a contralateral normal for comparison, which is especially useful in pediatric cases. However, ordering a comparison view before viewing the films of the affected side usually is not necessary. And if there is an obvious fracture or dislocation, comparison views generally are not necessary. If there is a questionable finding on only one or two views, comparison films can be limited to the one or two corresponding views. Comparison views may be needed in selected pediatric cases because growth rates vary, as does the appearance of growth plates.

Figure 3-2.

Significant anterior and posterior fat pad signs of joint effusion secondary to probable radial head fracture.

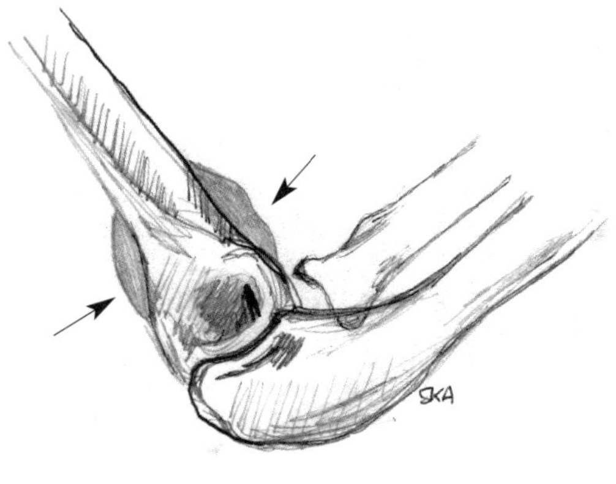

Added Views

Additional views usually are needed when a suspected fracture is not seen on standard views. A nondisplaced fracture can be difficult to see on a radiograph performed the day of injury. Occasionally *indirect* evidence of a fracture is apparent on the initial set of films. For example, the **fat pad sign** in the elbow caused by fluid or blood in the joint might be the *only* manifestation of a radial head fracture in an adult. Soft tissue swelling, usually noted as swelling and/or obliteration of normal fascial planes, may be associated with an underlying fracture (Figure 3-2).

Special additional views of such bones as the scaphoid (carpal navicular views) can be ordered when indicated by point tenderness. Other modalities such as CT may be added as necessary.

Postreduction Views

Postreduction views should always be obtained after a dislocation is reduced to allow for identification of associated fractures and to document improvement.

Repeat Views

Clinically suspected fractures that are not evident using any of these approaches should be splinted (treated as fractures), and repeat views should be taken in 7 to 10 days. It is far better to find a fracture by signs of proper healing 1 week after initial treatment than to not treat the injury at all.

Other Imaging Modalities

Computed Tomography

Since its initial development, CT imaging has been improved and refined and is now used either primarily or to prove or disprove a fracture when plain films are equivocal. It has additional value for examining soft tissues and demonstrating complex joint fractures.

Arteriography

Plain films and/or fluoroscopy with injected contrast medium may be needed to evaluate a dislocated joint or penetrating injury for associated vascular injury.

Nuclear Medicine

Although generally not helpful on the day of injury, a bone scan can identify occult fractures that have begun to heal, as well as osteomyelitis and metastases that are causing bone pain. Bone scans detect areas of rapid bone turnover. Generally, about 2 to 5 days postinjury fracture demonstration is optimal. A bone scan is effective for identifying and monitoring the progress of osteomyelitis and demonstrating response to therapy.

Ultrasonography

This noninvasive modality is used in emergency hand care primarily to locate foreign bodies. Even when a foreign body is evident on plain radiography, an ultrasound examination can facilitate its removal. Ultrasonography cannot image bone but is excellent for evaluating soft tissue, particularly muscle. It also is a valuable adjunct to biopsies of tumors and abscesses.

Magnetic Resonance Imaging

This relatively new technique represents a significant advance in the imaging of soft tissues, although it sometimes is inferior to CT for identifying fractures. Its usefulness in the acute setting is limited because placing an immobilized trauma victim into a narrow tube for a long period of time is difficult. This technique is best for imaging soft tissue injuries of joints, osteomyelitis, avascular necrosis, and suspected bone tumors.

Imaging Specific Areas

Forearm

Except for torus fractures and the nightstick fracture, forearm fractures include at least two breaks or one break and one dislocation (**Monteggia fracture**). The standard views on plain radiography, as with all long bones, are the AP and the lateral to include both the elbow and the proximal wrist. Various fractures and fracture-dislocations occur in the radius/ulna ring structure.

Wrist

This group includes distal forearm fractures and wrist joint injuries. A few infrequently described congenital anomalies affect the carpal bones, including agenesis, hypoplasia, fusion anomalies, and synostosis. Accessory bones and bone islands do occur but not commonly. The wrist is frequently injured, especially by falls on an outstretched hand. There also are patterns of injury that correspond to the patient's age (Colles fractures tend to occur in older patients).

Plain Films

Standard views (four) include posteroanterior (PA), lateral, and oblique (two). The PA view allows identification of the carpal bones and the three arcs they form, as follows:

- The proximal articular margins of the proximal row
- The distal articular margins of the proximal row
- The proximal articular margins of the distal row (capitate and hamate)

Normally, the cortical integrity of these bones should be intact, and the intercarpal joint spaces should all be about 2 mm. The hook of the hamate should be seen en face on the PA view. A true lateral view evaluates carpal dislocations and fracture displacements (lunate, perilunate). A true lateral must include the radius, lunate, capitate, and third metacarpal, which should all be coaxial. Dorsal chip fractures, usually from the triquetrum, are seen on the lateral, and small dorsal bony flakes may be seen in a simple sprain.

Navicular views elongate the profile of the scaphoid (carpal navicular) and may elucidate an acute fracture. Such a fracture sustained in a fall on an outstretched hand may not be visible until healing is noted by callus formation in 7 to 10 days. It should be preemptively diagnosed and treated on clinical evidence.

Stress views or **radial and ulnar deviation views** can be used to demonstrate scapholunate dissociation, which may be characterized by an abnormal widening of the space between the two bones (Terry Thomas sign). Normal intercarpal joint spaces are about 2 mm.

A **supinated oblique view** may help reveal a fracture of the hook of the hamate. This also may be seen on a **carpal tunnel view**, but the latter is generally difficult to obtain in an acutely injured wrist and provides little other information.

Fluoroscopy

Fluoroscopy can be helpful in diagnosing wrist instability.

Computed Tomography

Computed tomography can be helpful for diagnosing scaphoid fractures and distal radioulnar dislocations.

Magnetic Resonance Imaging

Magnetic resonance imaging is useful for diagnosing avascular necrosis, which occurs most frequently following injury to the scaphoid or lunate bones.

Hand

Plain Films

Plain radiography usually is adequate for diagnosing acute hand injuries other than those involving nonradiopaque foreign bodies.

Standard views include AP and oblique views of the hand. Lateral views of the digits as well as AP and lateral views of the thumb may be ordered as well. An AP view of the hand prominently shows normal nutrient artery canals on the phalanges. These may be confused with fractures; however, they usually appear on more than one digit or on both hands. Tuft fractures of the distal phalanges are well seen, as are midshaft fractures.

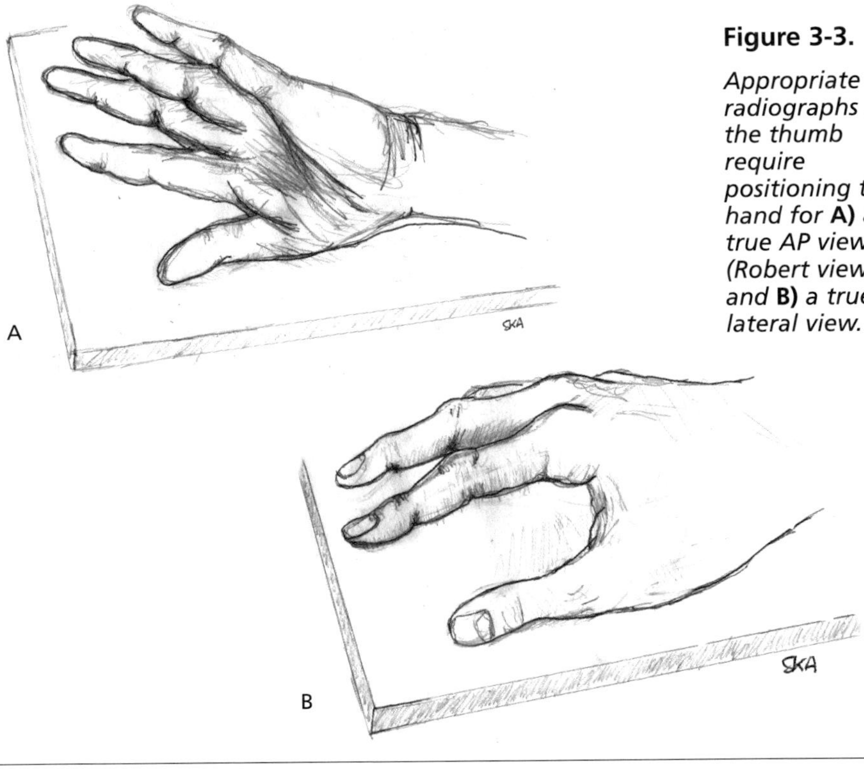

Figure 3-3.

Appropriate radiographs of the thumb require positioning the hand for **A)** *a true AP view (Robert view) and* **B)** *a true lateral view.*

The oblique view of the hand is used, in exception to the general rule of two views at a 90-degree angle, because the hand lateral view superimposes at least four metacarpal bones. It is useful for the CMC joint area and fingers when they are properly positioned. For the oblique view, the fingers must be spread apart, or fanned, to prevent overlap.

Lateral views of the digits should be obtained by tightly flexing all the uninvolved fingers or positioning each finger in a different degree of flexion (index finger only slightly flexed, with each more ulnar finger more flexed and the little finger in the greatest flexion). The lateral best demonstrates tuft and avulsion fractures.

Thumb AP and lateral views are required when a thumb injury is suspected because none of the above positions allows either the true frontal or the lateral aspect to be seen (Figure 3-3A-B).

Special views. The **reversed oblique view** is added to identify occult avulsion fractures, usually at tendon insertions, and to assess the position of radiopaque foreign bodies. Other oblique angles can be helpful. Stress views may be useful in identifying a volar or lateral avulsion, such as gamekeeper thumb (AP view). A tear of the ulnar collateral ligament of the MCP joint of the thumb demonstrates joint widening with abduction stress (Figure 3-4). Comparison stress views might be needed.

A **carpometacarpal PA** view for suspected dislocations is taken with the hand and fingers flat on the cassette. Normal CMC joint spaces have a consistent width, and the opposing articular surfaces are parallel and in a zig-zag pattern.

Magnetic Resonance Imaging

Magnetic resonance imaging can be useful for identifying tendon retraction and positioning. However, it is rarely needed in the emergency department management of hand injuries.

Figure 3-4.

Abduction stress testing of thumb ulnar collateral ligament for gamekeeper thumb.

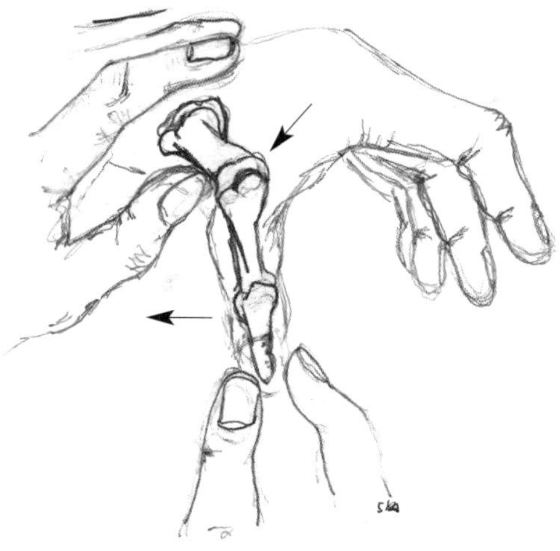

Additional Reading

Harris JH, Harris WH. *The Radiology of Emergency Medicine.* 2nd ed. Baltimore, Md: Williams & Wilkins; 1981.

Hart RG, Rittenberry TJ, Uehara DT, eds. *Handbook of Orthopedic Emergencies.* Philadelphia, Pa: Lippincott-Raven; 1999.

Manaster BJ. *Handbook of Skeletal Radiology.* 2nd ed. St Louis, Mo: Mosby-Yearbook; 1997.

Mercier LR. *Practical Orthopedics.* 4th ed. St Louis, Mo: Mosby; 1995.

Ruiz E, Cicero JJ. *Emergency Management of Skeletal Injuries.* St Louis, Mo: Mosby; 1995.

Squire LF. *Fundamentals of Radiology.* 3rd ed. Cambridge, Mass: Harvard University Press; 1982.

Wiest PW, Roth PG. *Fundamentals of Emergency Radiology.* Philadelphia, Pa: WB Saunders; 1996.

CHAPTER 4

Anesthesia

Mary Jo Wagner, MD, FACEP

Pain control is a vital component in the proper examination and treatment of acute hand injuries. Local anesthesia can be provided before close inspection, cleansing, and manipulation or repair of a wound or injury. For an extensive area of injury, a regional block can provide adequate anesthesia. If relaxation and systemic pain control are needed to care for a patient's injury, conscious sedation may be best. A firm grasp of the basic principles of analgesia and proficiency with specific anesthetic techniques give the physician the capability to care for the injured hand appropriately.

Local Anesthesia and Regional Blocks

The use of local anesthesia was first documented in the 1880s, when physicians found that cocaine could be administered topically or locally for pain control. Procaine, the first synthesized anesthesia, was produced in 1905; it remains the basis of many present anesthetic agents. In the mid-1900s, lidocaine, an amine, was synthesized as an alternative to the more antigenic procaine-based ester anesthetic agents. The search for a perfect anesthetic agent has continued, with many compounds now available.

Properties of Pharmacologic Agents

The ideal anesthetic agent would have a short time of onset, a predictable duration of action, no toxicity to local structures, and a low systemic toxicity, and it would allow painless application. Local anesthetic agents have some of these qualities, and the thoughtful use of anesthetic agents can achieve most of the remaining properties. When choosing an anesthetic agent, familiarity with its properties makes it possible to use the most appropriate agent for each situation. For example, most of the agents have an onset of action of 2 to 10 minutes. Agents with a shorter onset of action often have a shorter duration of action. A comparison of the most common agents and their properties is given in Table 4-1.

Unlike cocaine, synthesized anesthetic agents cause vasodilatation, so epinephrine is added to lidocaine or bupivacaine. The vasoconstriction properties of epinephrine increase the duration of the local anesthetic agent and decrease local bleeding. Traditionally, it was taught that epinephrine should never be used in the hand because of the significant constriction of the end arterioles in this area. However, current plastic surgery and podiatry literature now suggest that, with careful screening to avoid patients who have complicating disease processes such as peripheral vascular disease or pheochromocytoma, epinephrine may be used in the hands and feet, including in digital blocks, on a limited basis.[1] Two studies have shown that the adjunctive use of epinephrine (at 1:100,000 to 1:200,000 concentration) with lidocaine causes vasoconstriction three times that of plain lidocaine, with perfusion levels returning to baseline at 1 hour after the injection.[2,3] Epinephrine should be safer than a tourniquet because the solution does not completely occlude the vascular supply (as occurs with the use of tourniquets). Although the standard of care in most emergency departments remains to avoid the use of epinephrine in the digits, cautious use on the palm or dorsal surface of the hand is not contraindicated.

Allergic and Adverse Reactions

The allergic reactions most commonly reported by patients do not occur in response to the local anesthetic agents. Tachycardia, diaphoresis, and prolonged anesthesia are often reported with the use of local anesthetic agents, especially during dental procedures, but they are thought

Table 4-1.

Comparison of commonly used local and regional anesthetic agents.

Pharmacologic Agent	Pharmacologic Class	Normal Concentration for Peripheral Nerve Block	Duration of Action	Maximum Dose	Time to Onset
Procaine	Ester	1%	60-90 min	7 mg/kg	2-5 min
Tetracaine	Ester	Only used cutaneously	30-60 min	0.75 mg/kg	3-8 min
Lidocaine	Amide	1-2%	1-2 h	5 mg/kg	2-5 min
Bupivacaine	Amide	0.25-0.5%	4-8 h	2 mg/kg	2-10 min
Mepivacaine	Amide	1-2%	2-3 h	6 mg/kg	3-5 min
Diphenhydramine	Antihistamine	1-2%	30-60 min	2 mg/kg	2-5 min

From Wagner MJ. Principles of anesthesia for orthopaedic procedures. In: Hart RG, Rittenberry TJ, Uehara DT, eds. *Handbook of Orthopaedic Emergencies*. Philadelphia, Pa: Lippincott-Raven; 1998:49. Copyright Lippincott Williams & Wilkins. Adapted with permission.

to be more likely vagal reactions or to be due to intra-arterial injection. Some patients are allergic to the additive (methylparaben) in the anesthetic agent; additive-free lidocaine, such as the formulation used for cardiac arrhythmias, is available for these patients. The ester-based anesthetic agents (procaine and tetracaine) have a higher incidence of true IgE–mediated allergies, and there does not seem to be a crossover to the amine-based anesthetic agents. When a patient has a true allergic reaction, local injection of diphenhydramine has had acceptable results.[4] There is a risk of local irritation and even necrosis when diphenhydramine is administered into the fingertips, so its use in areas supplied by the end arteries, such as the fingers, should be avoided.

Reactions to local anesthetic agents are most likely systemic toxic effects. Toxic reactions are generally dose related or associated with inadvertent intra-arterial administration. The common toxicity symptoms for lidocaine and procaine derivatives are tinnitus, dizziness, disorientation, hypotension, respiratory depression, tonic-clonic seizures, and cardiac dysrhythmias. Serious toxic effects can best be avoided through careful dose calculation to avoid high levels. Although the typical dose for an adult with a hand injury may not approach dangerous levels, in a small child, the same dose could rapidly be toxic. For example, with 2% lidocaine (20 mg/mL), the maximum dose at 5 mg/kg for a 10-kg child is 2.5 mL, an amount easily needed for a moderate-sized wound. (Maximum dosage recommendations are given in Table 4-1.) Care also must be taken to avoid intra-arterial injection, which has been reported to result in cardiovascular collapse in some patients. Bupivacaine, in particular, has serious myocardial depression effects, so special care must be taken to avoid toxic doses or inadvertent intravascular injection of this agent.

Indications and Contraindications

Local or regional anesthesia commonly is necessary for pain control before the thorough evaluation and treatment of a hand injury. A brief examination that includes neurovascular status must be performed before the use of anesthesia, but most complete examinations of the deep structures, including tendon function, cannot be performed until pain is controlled.

Contraindications for the use of local anesthesia include a true allergy to the medication or an inability to achieve adequate anesthesia without exceeding the toxic range of the drug. If local use of the solution would distort the wound margins enough to make repair difficult, another method of anesthesia such as digital or regional block should be considered.

History and Physical Examination

The patient's history must be obtained before local or regional anesthetic agents are administered. This history must include details of the mechanism or injury, the time the injury occurred, and a description of treatment provided. History-taking also must elicit information on the patient's tetanus immunization status, allergies, and previous reactions.

Physical examination should include careful inspection of the injured hand, including its resting position and any signs of vascular compromise. A specific sensory examination should include two-point discrimination and light touch testing. The motor examination, including tendon strength, can be attempted and should be documented. This portion of the examination may be accomplished more easily after appropriate pain control is achieved. Abnormalities in any part of the motor examination should be noted but do not preclude the use of anesthesia. Specific motor and sensory examinations are described in Chapter 2.

Local Anesthesia

For local pain control, a local anesthetic agent must be applied in some manner to the skin near the wound site. Recently significant research has been devoted to evaluating the least painful method of obtaining local anesthesia. Several researchers have studied the use of plain lidocaine applied topically to a wound before injection but have found that it did not decrease patients' perception of pain.[5] In one recent study of the topical solution LET (4% lidocaine, 1:1,000 epinephrine, and 0.5% tetracaine), application for 20 to 30 minutes before wound manipulation resulted in adequate anesthesia in more than half of the patients and decreased pain for the remaining patients.[6] Half of the patients had this solution used on their hand injuries without complications resulting from vasoconstriction.[6]

An anesthetic agent such as lidocaine is injected locally after brief cleansing of the wound. Several techniques make injection less painful for the patient (Figure 4-1); the region and technique of injection are critical. Injection inside the cut wound edge decreases the discomfort of injection compared with injection through intact skin.[7] The use of a small (27- to 30-gauge) needle and a slow rate of injection also can alleviate some of the pain.

The use of warm (40°C), buffered anesthetic agents also makes the injection significantly less painful.[8,9] To make a buffered solution, sodium bicarbonate (44 mEq/50 mL) is added to lidocaine in a 1:10 ratio (1 mL of bicarbonate is added to 9 mL of lidocaine).

Regional Blocks

The use of a regional block has several advantages in the evaluation and repair of hand injuries. Anesthetizing nerves proximal to the injury prevents distortion of the wound by the solution that would otherwise have to be infiltrated locally. A proximal regional nerve block often is less painful than an injection into the distal fingertips, where the sensory fibers are more numerous. For larger wounds, less anesthetic agent and, often, fewer injection sites are needed to achieve complete pain control. The use of a specific type of

Figure 4-1.

Methods for decreasing the pain of achieving local anesthesia.

- Buffer solution with bicarbonate
- Inject warm solution (40°C)
- Apply topical LET solution
- Use a small needle (27 to 30 gauge)
- Inject into wound edge, not intact skin
- Inject slowly

block should be based on the need for a particular anatomic region of anesthesia.

With all blocks, the intact skin through which the needle is to be inserted must be carefully cleansed with an antibacterial solution. A small (27- to 30-gauge) needle should be used for all injections. If a patient feels significant paresthesias when the needle is being positioned, the needle must be withdrawn 1 to 2 mm to avoid direct intraneural injection. Injection into the nerve itself may cause either local irritation or ischemia of the nerve that results in permanent dysesthesia. Before the anesthetic agent is injected, the syringe should be aspirated to look for blood return, which indicates possible intravascular injection. If this occurs, repositioning of the needle is necessary.

Digital Block

Almost any wound on a finger should be repaired using a digital or metacarpal block to avoid injecting along the sensitive finger and to prevent distortion of the wound in this area of tightly bound tissue. The volar and dorsal nerves of the finger run along the medial and lateral edges of the phalanges on their respective sides. The consistency with which they are found here allows easy access for anesthesia.

First, the unbroken skin at the base of the affected finger should be cleansed carefully. Then, a small needle is used to puncture the skin on the dorsal surface of the finger, at the distal web space, along the side of the bony phalanx (Figure 4-2). The dorsal nerve runs under the skin, so after aspiration to avoid intravascular injection, 0.5 to 1 mL of the local anesthetic agent is deposited here. Without withdrawing, the needle is advanced through the soft tissue to the volar side of the bony phalanx. The volar nerves run here, and another 0.5 to 1 mL of the anesthetic agent is injected here. This procedure is repeated on the opposite side to anesthetize all four nerves that innervate the finger. The volume of anesthetic agent used must not cause significant tension around the phalangeal skin; if it does, it can cause compression of the vasculature and nerves, resulting in complications. In children, the volume may have to be decreased even more to avoid constriction around the digit.

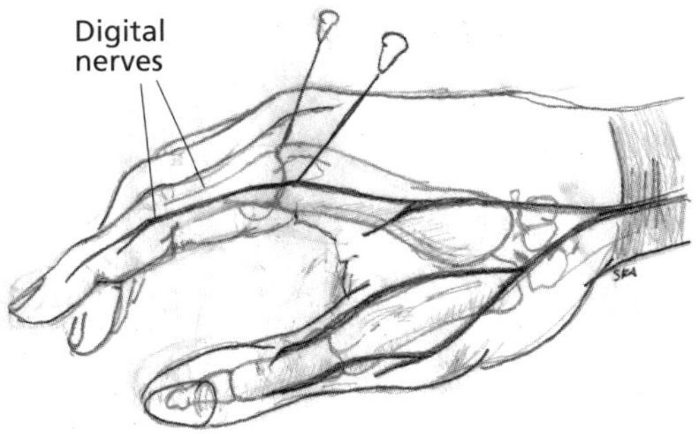

Figure 4-2. *Digital block.*

Metacarpal Block

Some physicians advocate the use of metacarpal blocks instead of digital blocks based on the theory that there is a decreased likelihood of vascular compromise by injecting in an area proximal to the end arteries. Most practitioners use the digital block instead of the metacarpal block, however, without complications.

The traditional technique (after cleansing the skin) is to insert the needle into the palmar surface directly over the metacarpal head of the digit to be anesthetized (Figure 4-3A). Once the needle is subcutaneous, it is directed to one side of the bony metacarpal and advanced approximately 1 cm, at which point 3 mL of the anesthetic agent is injected (after the syringe is aspirated to ensure the needle is not in a vessel). The needle is withdrawn most of the way, then redirected to the opposite side of the same metacarpal, and the procedure is repeated. Although the initial placement of the needle on the palmar surface is considered more painful, it is done only once to anesthetize both nerves. If this technique does not anesthetize the distal dorsal fingertips, a subcutaneous wheal may be needed on the dorsal surface distal to the MCP joint if this area is involved.

According to some,[10] a dorsal approach to a metacarpal block decreases the pain of the palmar injection (Figure 4-3B). The dorsal approach begins with placement of the needle 1 cm proximal to the MCP joint on the dorsal surface of the hand in the web space. The needle is advanced to the volar edge of the metacarpal or just until the palmar aponeurosis is felt, and then approximately 2 mL of anesthetic agent is injected. As the needle is withdrawn, another 1 mL is placed along the track. The procedure is repeated on the dorsal surface of the opposite side of the same metacarpal. However, this technique was rated as painful as a digital block, and the digital block had a more rapid onset and provided adequate anesthesia more consistently.[10]

Wrist Block

The three nerves that innervate the hand are the radial, median, and ulnar nerves (Figure 4-4). If anesthesia is needed in only the dermatome area of one nerve, this isolated block can be performed. If complete anesthesia of the entire hand is desired, a wrist block that involves all three nerves must be performed.

Figure 4-3.

Metacarpal block. **A)** *Palmar technique.* **B)** *Dorsal technique.*

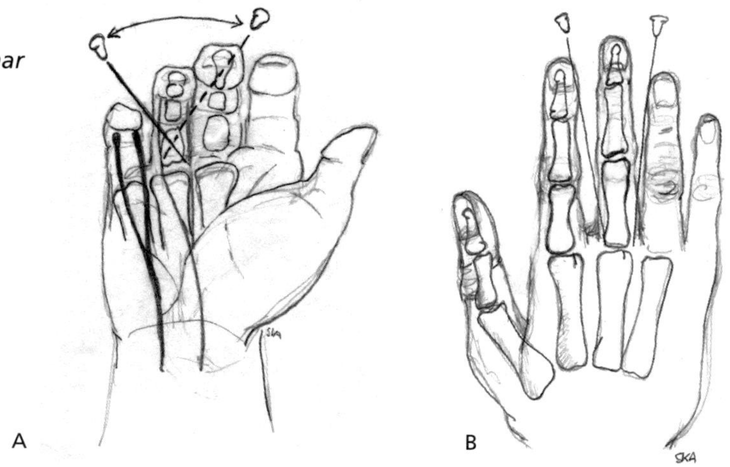

Radial nerve block. The radial nerve innervates the dorsum of the hand on the radial side and most of the thumb. This nerve lies just lateral to the radial artery (Figure 4-5). After cleansing, a small needle is placed lateral to the palpable radial pulse at the wrist crease and aspirated to ensure that the needle is not in the artery, then 2 to 5 mL of the anesthetic agent is injected slowly. Some of the nerve fibers originate from the proximal arm, so a field block must be performed with the specific nerve block to anesthetize all of this area. The field block should consist of up to 5 mL of anesthetic agent injected subcutaneously to create a wheal from the radial nerve back to the midline of the hand along the dorsal wrist crease.

Median nerve block. The median nerve primarily innervates the palmar surface of the first three digits of the hand and is useful for procedures that involve this location (Figure 4-6A). The median nerve is located 1 cm toward the ulna from the flexor carpi radialis, between this tendon and the palmaris longus if it is present. The small needle should be placed just proximal to the proximal wrist crease over this nerve and advanced until it enters the flexor retinaculum. A pop may be felt, and the patient may complain of paresthesias when the needle is in this area. The needle should be withdrawn a few millimeters to avoid intraneural injection and then 3 to 5 mL of anesthetic agent is injected. Because the solution is injected into the constricting retinaculum, this procedure may be contraindicated in patients with carpal tunnel syndrome.

Ulnar nerve block. The ulnar nerve provides sensation to the volar and dorsal surface of the last two digits of the hand and the associated palm. To perform a complete wrist block, this nerve also must be anes-

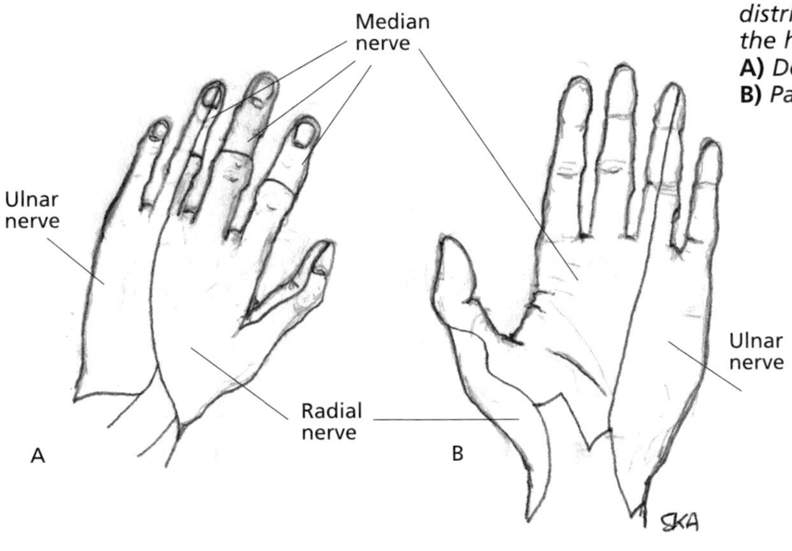

Figure 4-4.

Sensory distribution of the hand.
A) *Dorsal.*
B) *Palmar.*

thetized. The ulnar nerve follows the ulnar artery under the flexor carpi ulnaris, which is easily palpated on the volar wrist next to the ulnar styloid (Figure 4-6B). To perform this block, a small needle is advanced 1 cm between the ulnar artery and the flexor carpi ulnaris tendon. If the patient notes paresthesias, the needle is withdrawn a few millimeters and aspirated to avoid intra-arterial injection, then 5 mL of anesthetic agent is deposited. If the dorsal surfaces of the fourth and fifth digits require anesthesia, the superficial branch of the ulnar nerve is found just distal to the ulnar styloid and a superficial wheal of anesthetic agent is placed in that subcutaneous tissue.

Hematoma Block

If a fracture must be reduced, one option for pain relief is a hematoma block. Contamination of the fracture must be prevented by carefully cleansing the skin before introducing a needle into the area of the fracture. To achieve this block, a small needle is advanced into the hematoma that surrounds the fracture. Approximately 5 to 10 mL of the anesthetic agent (usually 2% lidocaine) is injected into the area. Care must be taken to avoid placing the needle with the anesthetic agent into an epiphyseal fracture, into any open fracture, or through contaminated skin.

Bier Block

An alternative to the wrist block is the use of intravenous regional anesthesia, commonly called a Bier block. Modifications of the original dosing regimen have made this method of anesthesia relatively safe and effective.[11] This block might be used in a patient with a finger or wrist dislocation or if significant débridement is needed for a large area of the hand. Lidocaine is the anesthetic agent of choice for this technique; there are some case reports of cardiac instability associated with the use of bupivacaine.[12]

An intravenous line must be started in the affected hand; it has been found that the more distal the line, the more efficacious the block. A pneumatic cuff is placed around the patient's arm with padding under it. The hand is elevated for a few minutes to allow for limb exsanguination, and then the cuff is inflated rapidly to 50 mm Hg above the patient's systolic blood pressure. A solution of 1% lidocaine is diluted 1:1 with normal saline, and then 1.5 mg/kg of the solution is injected into the line. A maximum of 100 mg is used initially for adults (the solution would contain 10 mL of normal saline and 10 mL of lidocaine). Adequate anesthesia should be achieved within 15 minutes, although the patient may still have some intact sensation. If acceptable anesthesia

Figure 4-5.

Radial nerve block.

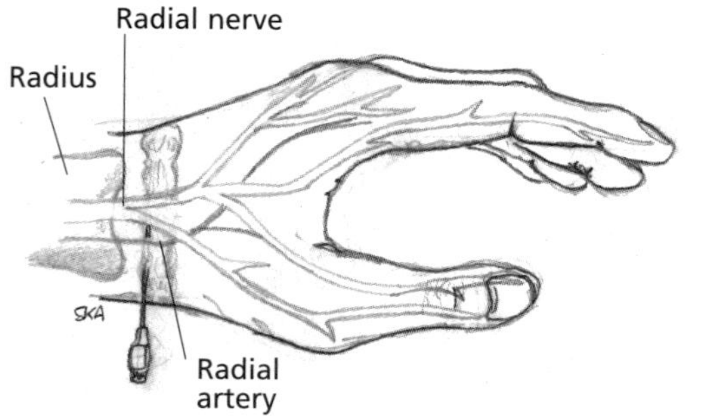

is not achieved, an additional 0.5 mL/kg of the diluted lidocaine solution may be used. When a sufficient level of anesthesia has been reached, a reduction or another procedure can be performed. The cuff can be released slowly to prevent a systemic vascular bolus of the lidocaine that has not been absorbed by the tissues. The cuff should be left in place for a minimum of 20 minutes to avoid rapid systemic infusion of the lidocaine. The cuff should not remain on the arm for more than 90 minutes because ischemia of the distal extremity may occur.

Care must be taken when performing this procedure because a rapid release of this dose of lidocaine can cause toxic reactions. Even though the initial dosage is the same as that recommended for cardiac dysrhythmias, hypotension and other side effects can occur. For this reason, some physicians perform this regional intravenous procedure with an additional line established in the opposite arm to allow rapid access if any serious side effects occur.

Complications

Complications associated with local anesthesia are those that might occur with any injection into the skin, including bleeding, wound infection, toxic reactions, and increased pain. Prolonged numbness is uncommon but possible, especially if the anesthetic agent was injected directly into larger nerve roots.

A common complication of regional anesthesia is chemical irritation or ischemia as a result of direct injection of the local anesthetic agent into the nerve, which can cause prolonged anesthesia. This can be avoided by redirecting the needle if the patient describes an acute paresthesia during the injection process. Direct compression of the vessel can be caused by a hematoma, resulting in prolonged pain, vasoconstriction, or

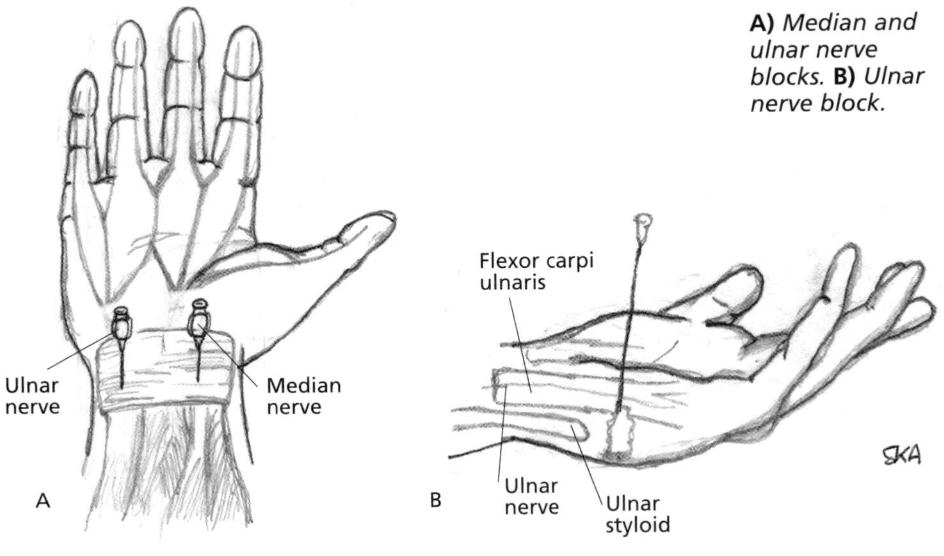

Figure 4-6.

A) *Median and ulnar nerve blocks.* **B)** *Ulnar nerve block.*

further tissue damage. This complication can be avoided by aspirating the syringe before injecting the agent to ensure there is no blood return.

Dose-related toxic reactions are more likely to occur with regional anesthesia than with local anesthesia. These can be avoided by calculating dosages carefully before administration. Avoiding direct intra-arterial injection also limits the risk of an acute toxic complication.

Disposition

General wound care discharge instructions must be given to all patients with hand injuries, along with detailed instructions for their specific injuries. The use of local anesthesia in these wounds does not necessitate additional instructions unless a long-acting agent was used. In the case of continued anesthesia from a regional block, the patient must be warned about causing further injury to the insensate digit or hand before the anesthetic agent wears off. Suggestions for pain control after the anesthesia can include keeping the injured hand elevated or applying ice to decrease swelling, as well as any pharmaceutical agent that the patient should take.

Conscious Sedation

Systemic analgesia or amnestic agents have been used for 150 years to reduce the pain and anxiety associated with a painful procedure. Loosely defined, conscious sedation is the use of pharmacologic agents to decrease a patient's perception of pain or anxiety while allowing the patient to maintain all protective respiratory reflexes. In patients with hand injuries, regional blocks can reduce the need for systemic sedation. In children with hand injuries, however, in whom adequate pain control may still not ensure adequate cooperation, conscious sedation is quite useful.

Pharmacologic Agents

Inhalants

In the emergency department, the only commonly found inhalant is nitrous oxide. This agent provides some sedative and dissociative effects and has a short onset of action and a short half-life. Nitrous oxide usually is available in the emergency department in a 50% mixture with oxygen. Self-administration is preferred; sedated patients hold the mask themselves, releasing it spontaneously when drowsy.

Analgesics

For pain control, narcotic analgesics provide the most dependable and quickest response. Common agents and usual dosages are listed in Table 4-2. The most reliable means of administering these agents is the intravenous route. Most of these medications can be administered intramuscularly, but this method prevents easy titration. Although several of these medications cause somnolence or sedation, that is not their primary action.

The most commonly used analgesic agents are divided into two classes: the **narcotics** (fentanyl, meperidine, and morphine) and the **narcotic agonist-antagonists** (nalbuphine and butorphanol), which are purported to cause less respiratory depression. All of these agents have vasodilatory effects that result in hypotension. Both of these reactions are dose related and usually can be eliminated by slow administration and careful titration.

Providers may have an arbitrary maximum dosage for narcotic medication, but the patient's response to these agents should be the only limit. If a patient in pain remains alert, normotensive, and without respiratory effects, then the dosage is not sufficient.

Sedatives and Amnestic Agents

For patients who require relaxation or relief from anxiety and for whom another form of analgesia is used, such as with laceration repair, a sedative may be a more appropriate agent. Sedatives and amnestic agents are used in conscious sedation to decrease a patient's awareness of the surroundings without significantly altering his or her protective airway reflex or respiratory effort. These agents also provide some muscle relaxation and thus are useful in the reduction of fractures. As with the analgesic agents, titration of the medications is most easily controlled through intravenous administration. Also, when medications are administered intravenously, the onset of action is quite rapid, usually within 3 minutes. Table 4-3 reviews frequently used sedative and amnestic agents and provides therapeutic doses.

Table 4-2.

General analgesic agents.

Pharmacologic Agent	Dose for IV Use	Duration of Action	Time to Onset	Comments
Narcotics				
Fentanyl (Sublimaze)	0.5-1 μg/kg	30-60 min	1-3 min	May lead to muscle rigidity
Meperidine (Demerol)	1-2 mg/kg	2-4 h	5-15 min	Do not use in patients on MAO inhibitors; use with caution in renal failure
Morphine	0.1 mg/kg	1-2 h	2-3 min	
Narcotic Agonist-Antagonists				
Butorphanol (Stadol)	0.015-0.02 mg/kg	2-4 h	2-5 min	1 mg intranasally in adults
Nalbuphine (Nubain)	0.1-0.2 mg/kg	3-6 h	2-3 min	

From Wagner MJ. Principles of anesthesia for orthopaedic procedures. In: Hart RG, Rittenberry TJ, Uehara DT, eds. *Handbook of Orthopaedic Emergencies*. Philadelphia, Pa: Lippincott-Raven; 1998:61. Copyright Lippincott Williams & Wilkins. Adapted with permission.

Two of these agents should be discussed in detail. **Ketamine** is a dissociative anesthetic agent that provides sedation, amnesia, and analgesia. It causes lacrimation and salivation, so many practitioners use atropine or glycopyrrolate in conjunction with ketamine to minimize secretions. It also can cause an increased gag response or, very rarely, laryngospasm. For this reason, ketamine must be used cautiously in children with upper respiratory infections or airway anomalies and in very young children (younger than 6 months). The well-publicized **emergence phenomenon** (hallucinations, nightmares) does not seem to be very common in children, and the addition of a benzodiazepine seems to nearly eliminate this effect in adults. (If another agent such as midazolam is added to ketamine, the dose of ketamine may have to be decreased slightly.)

Midazolam, a benzodiazepine, can be administered using a variety of routes and usually is quite effective. This medication alone is often sufficient when sedation is sought in children with hand injuries whose pain is controlled with local anesthetic agents. The oral route has been quite suc-

Table 4-3.

Sedative and amnestic agents.

Pharmacologic Agent	Dose for IV Use	Duration of Action	Time to Onset	Other Available Routes	Comments
Chloral hydrate (Noctec)	—	1-4 h	20-60 min	Oral (only): 50 mg/kg	Slow onset
Diazepam (Valium)	0.04-0.2 mg/kg	2-4 h	3-10 min	Rectal: 0.5 mg/kg	
Lorazepam (Ativan)	0.02-0.1 mg/kg	2-6 h	5-10 min	IM: Same as IV	
Midazolam (Versed)	0.03-0.05 mg/kg	1-2 h	3-5 min	IM: 0.05-0.1 mg/kg Intranasal: 0.2-0.4 mg/kg Oral: 0.5-0.7 mg/kg	
Ketamine	1-2 mg/kg	30-120 min	1-3 min	IM: 4 mg/kg	Add atropine at 0.01 mg/kg (minimum 0.1 mg, maximum 0.5 mg)
Propofol	0.5-2 mg/kg	15-30 min	1-2 min		Use drip for continued sedation: 25-130 mg/kg/min

From Wagner MJ. Principles of anesthesia for orthopaedic procedures. In: Hart RG, Rittenberry TJ, Uehara DT, eds. *Handbook of Orthopaedic Emergencies*. Philadelphia, Pa: Lippincott-Raven; 1998:62. Copyright Lippincott Williams & Wilkins. Adapted with permission.

cessful for this purpose. Very few children have paradoxical reactions to midazolam, but if this occurs, another method of sedation may be needed.

Indications and Contraindications

For most patients who need conscious sedation, a combination of analgesic and sedative agents is useful. A true allergy to the medication is the only absolute contraindication. However, several situations merit consideration of the risks compared with the benefits.

Respiratory depression is the most common reaction, so any patient with **respiratory problems** (chronic obstructive pulmonary disease or sleep apnea) should be screened carefully. Even patients with minor upper respiratory infections can have increased hypoxia when given these agents. If a patient has an obvious anatomic airway deformity that might make bag ventilation or even intubation difficult, other solutions to anesthesia should be considered.

Hypotension is another common side effect, and patients with any **hemodynamic instability** should be given these medications only under close supervision. Any patient with a significant history of cardiac or vascular problems should be monitored carefully.

History and Physical Examination

Any time conscious sedation is being considered, the patient's complete medical history should be elicited. Special attention should be paid to any recent history of upper respiratory infection, chronic obstructive pulmonary disease, or other respiratory problems. A history of an allergic or adverse reaction to narcotic or sedative medications also is significant. The patient also should be asked about current or recent medication use, with special attention to narcotics, tricyclic antidepressants, benzodiazepines, or other sedatives. Although having recently eaten a large meal is not a contraindication for sedation, the timing may indicate the risk of aspiration if there is any respiratory compromise.

The physical examination should include careful examination of the upper airway, lungs, and heart, as well as the obvious hand injury. Any abnormalities should be investigated before the use of conscious sedation. The ease of obtaining intravenous access should be assessed if another route of administration is planned.

Technique

Any patient who is given an agent that may alter respiratory or hemodynamic stability must be monitored closely. Oxygen saturation should be monitored continuously with pulse oximetry; a nasal cannula should either be in place or be ready to use. Heart rate and blood pressure should be monitored according to age-appropriate standards. An assistant who is not involved with the procedure must be present to monitor the patient's respiratory status and level of consciousness. A flow sheet should be used to document the patient's status.

Proper supportive equipment must be readily available in the room in which the procedure is taking place. This equipment should include an appropriate-sized bag and mask, suction device, and intravenous fluid.

Reversal agents that might be used also should be available at the bedside.

Many combinations of these medications produce successful results. Examples of typical dosages for conscious sedation are as follows:

- For one-dose intramuscular administration in children, combined in the same syringe: 0.01 mg/kg atropine (minimum 0.1 mg, maximum 0.5 mg); 0.1 mg/kg midazolam; and 3 mg/kg ketamine (may repeat 2 mg/kg ketamine in 10 minutes if the desired effect is not achieved initially)
- For intravenous administration in adults or children: 0.02 to 0.04 mg/kg midazolam (repeat every 2 minutes until desired sedation is achieved) and 0.5 to 1 µg/kg fentanyl over 30 to 60 seconds (may repeat every 2 to 3 minutes to achieve desired results)

After the medication is administered, a qualified medical staff person must be present at the bedside until the patient is no longer significantly sedated. The patient should be monitored for a minimum of 1 hour after the procedure is complete. The patient should be arousable, without any respiratory effects.

Complications

The physician must be prepared for any possible complication and have the technical and clinical skills to provide reversal or supportive therapeutics for reactions to these agents, to obtain vascular access, and to manage the airway.

The most common complication of conscious sedation is depressed respiratory effort. This is dose dependent; slow, careful titration of the medications helps prevent this problem. Reversal agents such as naloxone and flumazenil can be used, but the provider must be familiar with their dosages, indications, and contraindications.

Naloxone is a narcotic antagonist that reverses the respiratory depression and hypotensive effects. It is recommended that the usual dose (0.4 to 2 mg IV) be administered in diluted aliquots to prevent rapid reversal.

Flumazenil is a benzodiazepine antagonist that reverses the respiratory depression but has little effect on the hypotension. This agent may cause prolonged seizures in patients who are on long-term benzodiazepine or tricyclic antidepressant therapy and thus is contraindicated in

Figure 4-7.

Discharge instructions for patients who receive conscious sedation.

A responsible adult should watch the patient for the next 8 hours.

The patient should be awakened every 2 hours and checked for appropriate behavior.

The patient should not drive, operate heavy equipment, or use equipment that requires coordination (bicycle) for the next 12 hours.

No eating or drinking for the first 2 hours after discharge if still sleepy. No drinking of alcohol for the next 24 hours after discharge.

The patient should return to the emergency department if he or she cannot be awakened; has slow, shallow, or difficulty breathing; has vomiting that will not stop; or has any sign of an allergic reaction, such as rash, itching, throat swelling, or wheezing.

this group. Reversal of the respiratory depression also results in reversal of the analgesia and sedation, so cautious use of these agents is recommended. It is recommended that the usual dose (0.2 mg IV) be administered over 15 to 30 seconds, with repeat doses of 0.1 mg/min IV (to a total maximum of 1 mg IV) until an effect is seen.

The other common complication is hypotension, which generally is related to the rate of administration of the medication. Patients generally respond quickly to cessation of the medication and to the infusion of intravenous fluids.

Disposition

The routine instructions for wound care must be given to all patients with hand injuries, including detailed directions for care of the specific injury. Patients who have received conscious sedation should not be released from the emergency department or clinic until they are able to ambulate without assistance and can follow verbal instructions. Sleepiness without other symptoms does not necessitate keeping the patient for further observation. Any patient who receives conscious sedation must be discharged in the care of a competent adult who will watch the patient for the next 8 hours.

Additional instructions for these patients include reviewing the normal reactions as well as common side effects for the medications. The caregiver should be counseled regarding specific reactions (amnesia or nausea). An example of typical discharge instructions is given in Figure 4-7.

References

1. Wilhelm BJ, Blackwell SJ, Miller J, et al. Epinephrine in digital blocks: revisited. *Ann Plast Surg.* 1998;41:410-414.
2. Green D, Walter J, Heden R, et al. The effects of local anesthetics containing epinephrine on digital blood perfusion. *J Am Podiatr Med Assoc.* 1992;82:98-110.
3. Scarlet JJ, Walter JH, Bachmann RJ. Digital blood perfusion following injection of plain lidocaine and lidocaine with epinephrine: a comparison. *J Am Podiatr Med Assoc.* 1978;68:339-346.
4. Green SM, Rothrock SG, Gorchynski J. Validation of diphenhydramine as a dermal local anesthetic. *Ann Emerg Med.* 1994;23:1284-1289.
5. Stewart GM, Simpson P, Rosenberg NM. Use of topical lidocaine in pediatric laceration repair: a review of topical anesthetics. *Pediatr Emerg Care.* 1998;14:419-423.
6. Adler AJ, Dubinisky I, Eisen J. Does the use of topical lidocaine, epinephrine, and tetracaine solution provide sufficient anesthesia for laceration repair? *Acad Emerg Med.* 1998;5:108-112.
7. Bartfield JM, Sokaris SJ, Raccio-Robak N. Local anesthesia for lacerations: pain of infiltration inside vs outside the wound. *Acad Emerg Med.* 1998;5:100-105.
8. Mader TJ, Playe SJ, Garb JL. Reducing the pain of local anesthetic infiltration: warming and buffering have a synergistic effect. *Ann Emerg Med.* 1994;23:550-554.
9. Brogan GX, Giarrusso E, Hollander JE, et al. Comparison of plain, warm, and buffered lidocaine for anesthesia of traumatic wounds. *Ann Emerg Med.* 1995;26:121-125.
10. Knoop K, Trott A, Syverud S. Comparison of digital versus metacarpal blocks for repair of finger injuries. *Ann Emerg Med.* 1994;23:1296-1300.
11. Farrell RG, Swanson SL, Walter JR. Safe and effective IV regional anesthesia for use in the emergency department. *Ann Emerg Med.* 1985;14:288-292.
12. Rosenberg PH, Kalso EA, Tuominen MK, et al. Acute bupivacaine toxicity as a result of venous leakage under the tourniquet cuff during a Bier block. *Anesthesiology.* 1983;58:95-98.

CHAPTER 5

Laceration and Wound Care

Wendy C. Coates, MD, FACEP

Lacerations to the hand are common. Blunt trauma often results in crush injuries, which produce significant tissue edema and may introduce foreign material. Hand lacerations frequently result from penetrating trauma caused by knife wounds, broken glass, bites, or industrial accidents. Impeccable wound care technique is critical because the hand is one of the most functionally and cosmetically important areas of the body. In general, standard wound care principles are applicable to hand lacerations.[1,2]

History and Physical Examination

Knowledge of the mechanism of injury can direct the workup. The patient should be asked about the circumstances surrounding the event, including the mechanism of injury, time since injury, position of the hand at the time the laceration occurred, current sensorimotor function of the affected part, and tetanus immunization status[3,4] (Table 5-1).

A complete physical examination should be performed (see Chapter 2), with special attention to the underlying structure and function of the affected areas. The distal sensorimotor examination should take place before anesthesia, and focused exploration should occur after appropriate local or regional anesthesia (see Chapter 4). Extreme care should be taken to protect partially damaged structures such as tendons, vessels, and nerves that may be under the laceration; vigorous probing or range of motion exercises may further injure already damaged structures.

Radiographic imaging of all wounds caused by broken glass is imperative to look for retained foreign bodies. Visual inspection and the use of ultrasonography may reveal the presence of foreign bodies that do not show up on standard radiography.[5]

Treatment

Local Wound Care

The most important preventive measure against wound infection is the reduction in bacteria and foreign material (metal, wood, dirt) in the wound to a level of less than 10^5 organisms/mm^2. Cleansing can begin at the sink; an ambulatory patient can be instructed simply to wash his or her hands, which is effective for removing gross debris and grease before irrigation. The cleansing process is most effective after the patient has received adequate anesthesia. Irrigation with 200 mL of normal saline under 15 psi of continuous pressure effectively cleans a simple wound. This can be achieved with a 30-mL syringe and an 18-gauge angiocatheter or splash shield. Wounds that appear to be dirty should be irrigated with sufficient saline until they appear to be clean and then with an additional 200 mL of saline. Iodine-containing compounds such as povidone-iodine solution should not be introduced into open wounds because they are toxic to fibroblasts. These products can be applied to the surrounding intact skin before suturing, if desired.

Most wounds can be closed primarily within 12 hours after injury. Older wounds or those that appear to be infected or are likely to become

Table 5-1.

Tetanus prophylaxis summary.

History of Adsorbed Tetanus Toxoid (doses)	Clean, Minor Wounds		All Other Wounds*	
	Td†	TIG	Td†	TIG
Unknown or less than three	Yes	No	Yes	Yes
Three or more‡	No§	No	No¶	No

*Includes but is not limited to wounds contaminated with dirt, feces, soil, and saliva; puncture wounds; avulsions; and wounds that result from missiles, crushing, burns, and frostbite.

†For children younger than 7 years, DTP (DT if pertussis vaccine is contraindicated) is preferred to tetanus toxoid alone. For persons 7 years old or older, Td is preferred to tetanus toxoid alone.

‡If only three doses of fluid toxoid have been received, then a fourth dose of toxoid, preferably an adsorbed toxoid, should be administered.

§Yes, if more than 10 years since the last dose.

¶Yes, if more than 5 years since the last dose. (More frequent boosters are not needed and can accentuate side effects.)

Reprinted from Diphtheria, tetanus, and pertussis: recommendations for vaccine use and other preventive measures. Recommendations of the Immunization Practices Advisory Committee (ACIP). *MMWR Morb Mortal Wkly Rep.* 1991;40(RR 10):1-28.

infected may be considered for the delayed primary closure technique described later in this chapter.

Débridement

Before suturing occurs, wound edges should appear healthy. Minimal débridement may be necessary to achieve viability and to ensure adequate wound healing. Every effort should be made to minimize tissue loss, and débridement should be performed sparingly.

Materials and Equipment

The instruments and suture materials necessary for repair of hand lacerations are summarized in Figure 5-1. Most hand lacerations can be repaired with 5-0 synthetic monofilament suture (nylon). Selected clean lacerations can be repaired with a 5-0 rapidly absorbing suture (Vicryl Rapide [polyglactin 910], Ethicon, Inc, Somerville, NJ), which is applied as an external suture and does not require subsequent removal. Examples of such suture use include nail bed lacerations, lacerations in children *if at low risk for infection*, and lacerations in selected adults who are unlikely to return for suture removal. Wounds without any appreciable tension and with negligible risk of infection can be closed with tissue adhesive. Wounds that are under significant tension may require a deep layer of absorbable suture. Patients who are known to be prone to keloid formation may benefit from deep sutures to anchor the dermis and tissue adhesive to approximate the epidermis. Standard wound preparation, including irrigation, is as important in wounds repaired with tissue adhesive as it is in sutured lacerations.

Figure 5-1.

Equipment for hand laceration repair.

Instruments
- Adson toothed forceps
- Needle holder
- Iris scissors
- Suture scissors

Suture Material for Deep Layer
- 4-0, 5-0* absorbable (Vicryl, Dexon, Monocryl)

Suture Material for Superficial Layer
- 4-0, 5-0* nylon
- 4-0, 5-0* polypropylene-coated nylon
- 4-0, 5-0* rapidly absorbing (Vicryl Rapide)
- Wound adhesive strips and tincture of benzoin
- Tissue adhesive

Dressings
- Petroleum jelly gauze
- Antibiotic ointment
- Sterile 4 × 4 pads
- Adhesive strips
- Kerlix
- Splinting materials
- Adhesive tape

*Most commonly recommended suture size for hand indications.

Suture Techniques

Most hand lacerations can be closed using the **simple interrupted stitch** (Figure 5-2). The suture width across the wound (2×) is twice the distance between subsequent stitches (×) (Figure 5-2A). The needle should enter the skin at a 90-degree angle, and the curvature of the needle should be followed to allow for a smooth, symmetric stitch and to prevent the needle from bending. Adson toothed forceps can be used to assist in visualization by reflecting back the skin and facilitating the 90-degree angle entry (Figure 5-2B-C). Underlying structures such as tendons, nerves, and vessels must be visualized at all times to prevent accidental damage by the needle or constriction by the tied stitch. In many cases, this means that the stitch must be completed in two stages rather than blindly passing the needle directly from one side of the wound to the other. Knots should be tied and moved to one side of the wound. Care should be taken to tie the stitches so the wound edges are just approximated. Stitches that are tied too tightly may cause increased scarring from the inevitable tissue edema that results during wound healing.

Palm Lacerations

Palmar surface skin is difficult to approximate in the usual manner. To avoid the frustration of sutures that pull and tear through this area, palm lacerations can be repaired with the horizontal mattress suture, which enables the tension to be spread over a greater surface area and minimizes skin tearing.

The **horizontal mattress stitch** is performed by first applying a simple interrupted-type stitch. Instead of cutting and tying this stitch, a second stitch is applied from the *second* side of the laceration back to the first. It is then tied parallel to the wound on the *first* side. Spacing of the

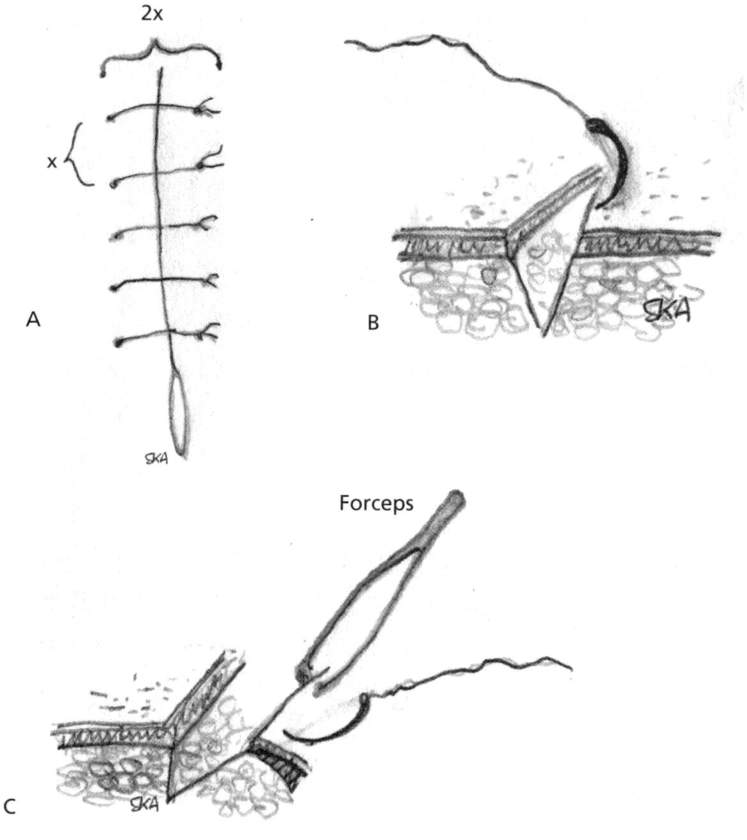

Figure 5-2.

Simple interrupted stitch. **A)** *The distance between stitches is related to the width of the stitch. Knots should be aligned on one side of the laceration.* **B)** *The needle should enter the skin at a 90-degree angle.* **C)** *Adson forceps can be used to move the skin to a position that facilitates entry and maximizes visibility of underlying structures.*

horizontal mattress stitch follows the same guidelines as the simple interrupted stitch (Figure 5-3). Careful attention must be paid to avoiding the underlying flexor tendons while repairing palm lacerations.

V-Shaped Lacerations

Many hand lacerations are irregularly shaped. V-Shaped lacerations on the dorsal surface of the hand can be repaired with the **half-buried mattress stitch,** or **corner stitch**. The initial stitch should enter distal to the tip of the flap and exit the skin in the middermis. The needle is then passed through the dermis of the tip of the flap *at the same depth* as the initial stitch. To complete the stitch, the needle enters the anchoring skin at the same dermal depth and is tied. Care should be taken not to tie the stitch over the flap itself (Figure 5-4). Use of the corner stitch alone is not effective in V-shaped lacerations that are under significant tension.

Joint Lacerations

Lacerations over joints in the hand can be sutured in the usual manner after ensuring that the joint space has not been violated. This can be determined through visual inspection or by noting air in the joint space on radiographic evaluation. If necessary, a small amount of sterile saline to which a couple drops of fluorescein have been added can be injected into the unaffected side of the joint and the laceration viewed using a Wood's lamp. Fluorescent effluent from the laceration site indicates that the joint space may have been violated.[6] Consultation with a specialist is then indicated to determine whether the patient should be admitted for surgical washing of the joint or whether routine wound management is sufficient. Antibiotics should be administered parenterally for admitted patients and as a prescription for outpatient use. A single intramus-

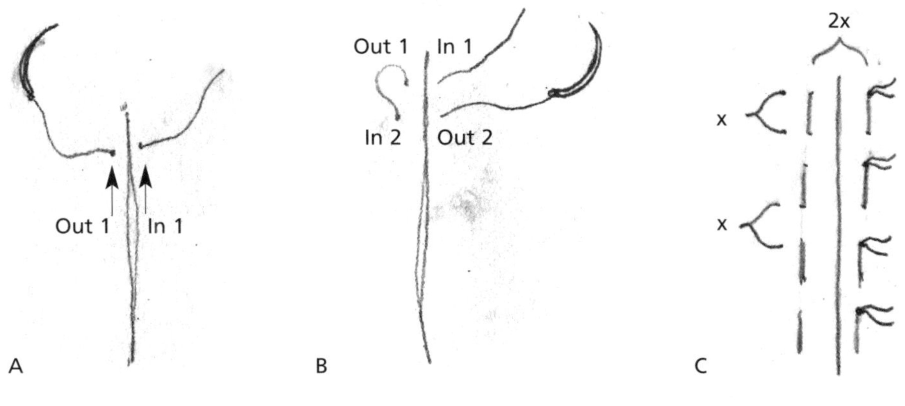

Figure 5-3.
Horizontal mattress stitch.

cular dose of an antibiotic is sometimes administered before discharge from the emergency department to begin the outpatient course of therapy. If a laceration over a joint is sutured, a splint should be applied to prevent movement of the joint during the healing process. Sutures are often left in for 10 days (for fingers) to 2 weeks (for the wrist).

Bite Wounds

Wounds caused by human or animal bites are at high risk for infection. Traumatic wounds of the knuckles that occur after an altercation often are the result of contact with human teeth (fight bite) and should be treated as a bite wound. Standard wound care is essential. Patients should be discharged with a course of antibiotics to cover the usual oral flora (including *Pasteurella*, especially in animal bites). In most cases, amoxicillin/clavulanate or an equivalent is a good choice. Special circumstances such as marine organism bites may require broader coverage to include *Vibrio* species. Many of these lacerations can be repaired using the delayed primary closure technique.

Tissue Adhesives

Tissue adhesives may be used to repair lacerations that are not at risk for infection and are under no appreciable tension. Use on carefully selected wounds, especially on the dorsal surface of the hand, may be appropriate. Elderly persons who have very thin skin may benefit from this method of wound repair. Care should be taken to irrigate the

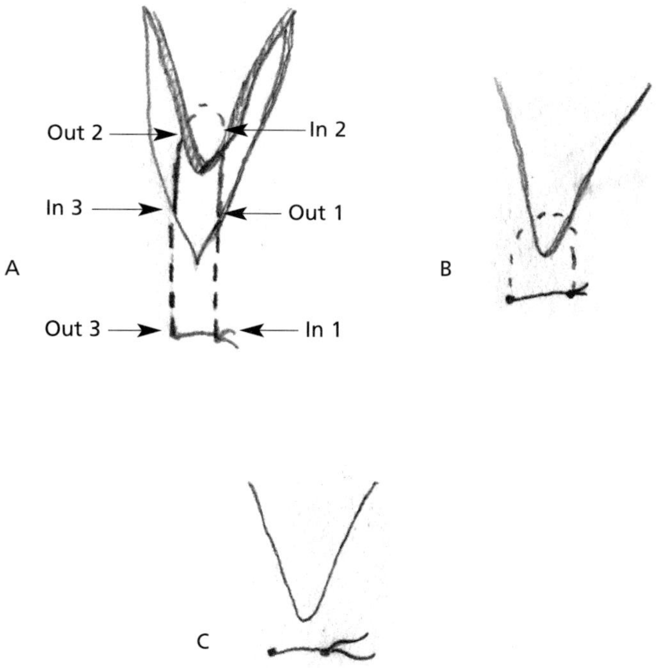

Figure 5-4.

Half-buried mattress stitch, or corner stitch. **A)** *and* **B)** *All aspects of the stitch should take place at the same depth of the dermis. Dashed lines represent the suture material that is not visible externally. Solid lines represent the suture material that is visible during repair.* **C)** *Correct appearance of finished stitch. Do not tie stitch over the flap.*

wound properly before applying the tissue adhesive. Petroleum-based ointments should be avoided. Tissue adhesives serve as their own dressings and do not have to be removed.

Delayed Primary Closure

Infected wounds or wounds that are older than 12 hours can be considered for delayed primary closure. On the day of injury (or on initial presentation to the emergency department), the wound should be anesthetized, explored, and irrigated to physically sterilize it in the usual manner. A nonadherent gauze is placed between the wound edges and a sterile dressing applied. The patient should begin taking the appropriate antibiotics (cephalexin) to chemically sterilize the wound and return on the third day for closure. At that time, the dressing is removed and the wound reinspected, anesthetized, and irrigated again. If the edges appear healthy and there are no signs of infection, the wound is closed primarily and the patient is instructed to continue the antibiotic for a total course of 5 to 7 days.

If the wound does not meet the criteria for delayed closure, it must heal by secondary intention. Future scar revision by a hand specialist may be necessary.

Referral Guidelines

Most hand lacerations can be repaired safely in the emergency department. If the physician is not comfortable performing the procedure, consultation, referral, or both are appropriate. Patients with lacerations that involve flexor tendons, nerves, or vessels should always be referred to a hand specialist for definitive management. Wounds that violate the joint capsule should be managed in conjunction with a specialist. If immediate repair by a specialist is not possible, it is appropriate to close some wounds temporarily in the emergency department and refer the patient to a specialist. In such a case, the wound should be anesthetized, irrigated, sutured, and splinted. Prompt followup with the hand specialist should be arranged by the emergency physician.

Dressings

Dressings provide appropriate protection for a healing wound. They should be applied carefully to ensure a moist environment and to maintain cleanliness. In some cases, dressings should apply pressure to prevent rebleeding.

A standard dressing should provide a nonadherent surface that is placed next to the wound. A small strip of petroleum jelly gauze usually is effective. Excessive gauze may result in a wet wound that will become macerated and impair healing. The next layer should provide a wick that can absorb discharge. The outer layer should have a neat appearance; this layer is visible to the patient and should appear to have been applied professionally. The dressing may be as simple as an adhesive strip. Specialized fingertip bandages are available. In addition, aluminum splints may provide extra protection against accidental bumping, especially on lacerations near the fingertip. Dressings used for young children should be bulky and prevent access to the wound. In most cases, this can be achieved with Kerlix bandage roll (Kendall Healthcare Company, Tyco International, Mansfield, Mass) wrapped around the standard dressing.

Pressure dressings consist of the same layers, but additional layers of gauze often are applied. Taping should begin in the center of the dressing and proceed outward in a lenticular manner so that the ends of each subsequent piece of tape point toward the ends of the initial piece of tape. This serves to lend support at the central portion of the wound. In most cases, these dressings can be converted to standard dressings after 24 hours.

Wounds repaired with tissue adhesives do not require additional dressing, except as noted for children to protect the wound. Petroleum products should never be applied to these wounds because these compounds dissolve the tissue adhesive.

Discharge Guidelines

Most patients with simple hand lacerations can be discharged from the emergency department after the repair. Patients with infections such as cellulitis, tenosynovitis, or osteomyelitis often must be hospitalized for intravenous antibiotic therapy. Patients with lacerations that involve underlying structures such as flexor tendons, bones, nerves, or joints may be admitted for definitive repair or have their lacerations sutured in the emergency department with appropriate specialty followup care.

Suture Removal

For most hand lacerations, sutures can be removed in 1 week. Exceptions include sutures in lacerations over joints, which usually are splinted and removed in 10 days (for fingers) to 2 weeks (for the wrist); tissue adhesive, which dissolves in 5 to 10 days; and wound adhesive strips, which fall off in 5 to 10 days. Absorbing Vicryl Rapide sutures usually dissolve in about 1 week.

Patient Instructions

Patients should be instructed to keep their injured hands elevated to prevent swelling and to keep the wounds clean at all times and dry for 24 hours. After 24 hours, sutured lacerations can be safely exposed to running water (shower, routine handwashing) but not to stagnant water (swimming pool, bathtub, dishwashing in sink). Over-the-counter analgesics usually are sufficient for pain relief, although some patients may require stronger medication such as prescription-strength nonsteroidal anti-inflammatory drugs (NSAIDs) or narcotics for 1 or 2 days.

Patients should be advised to return immediately if there is pus in the wound, extreme pain, bleeding, loss of sensation or change in color of the fingers distal to the laceration, fever, or lymphangitic streaking up the arm. Wounds repaired with tissue adhesive manifest infection by developing blisters filled with pus. In this event, the layer of adhesive may be lifted with forceps and the wound infection treated in the usual manner.

Routine wound checks are unnecessary except when a patient is unable to recognize complications or the physician wants to check a wound at high risk for infection or complication. In this case, the wound check should occur at least 48 hours after the repair to allow sufficient time for a wound infection to develop.

The routine use of antibiotics is discouraged.[7] Proper irrigation and careful wound preparation and repair are the best tools to prevent infection. Oral antibiotics should be prescribed for patients with human or animal bites, lacerations that involve the joints, and patients whose wounds are being considered for delayed primary closure.

References

1. Singer AJ, Hollander JE, Quinn JV. Evaluation and management of traumatic lacerations. *N Engl J Med.* 1997;337:1142-1148.
2. Howell JM, Chisholm CD. Wound care. *Emerg Med Clin North Am.* 1997; 15:417-425.
3. Gergen PJ, McQuillan GM, Kiely M, et al. A population-based serologic survey of immunity to tetanus in the United States. *N Engl J Med.* 1995;332:761-766.
4. Diphtheria, tetanus, and pertussis: recommendations for vaccine use and other preventive measures. Recommendations of the Immunization Practices Advisory Committee (ACIP). *MMWR Morb Mortal Wkly Rep.* 1991;40(RR 10):1-28.
5. Hill R, Conron R, Greissinger P, et al. Ultrasound for the detection of foreign bodies in human tissue. *Ann Emerg Med.* 1997;29:353-356.
6. Voit G, Irvine G, Beals RK. Saline load test for penetration of periarticular laceration. *J Bone Joint Surg.* 1996;78:732-733.
7. Cummings P, DelBeccaro MA. Antibiotics to prevent infection of simple wounds: a meta-analysis of randomized studies. *Am J Emerg Med.* 1995;13:396-400.

CHAPTER 6

Splinting and Casting

Kevin G. Rodgers, MD

Most fractures, dislocations, and tendon injuries of the hand require splinting as part of the initial emergency management. Splinting also is considered definitive therapy for many soft tissue injuries, infections, sprains, and acute and chronic inflammatory conditions. A well-applied splint reduces pain, bleeding, swelling, and inflammation by immobilizing the involved tissues. For a patient with a fracture, immobilization also prevents further damage to muscles, nerves, and blood vessels caused by the sharp ends of fractured bones; conversion of a closed fracture to an open one; and constriction of vascular structures by misaligned bone ends.

Applying true casts has become an uncommon practice in emergency departments. Emergency physicians instead apply more comfortable, easily applied splints that have fewer associated complications. Splints allow for swelling while maintaining adequate immobilization, which results in fewer episodes of compartment syndrome and other pressure-related complications. Just as splints are easier to apply than casts, they also are easier to remove (temporarily or at the end of treatment) and reapply if necessary. The advantages of splints combined with the potential complications of casting led to this change in practice.

Unfortunately, learning to apply splints is commonly an on-the-job experience. Most emergency departments do not have a formally trained cast technician available to apply splints 24 hours a day. Thus, splints often are made incorrectly and applied in a suboptimal and potentially injurious manner, leading to significant complications and potential litigation. This chapter reviews splinting principles, the types of splints that are used in common hand injuries, the potential complications, and patient instructions regarding splint use.

General Principles of Splinting

- All clothing and jewelry should be removed from the area of suspected injury. The area should be inspected for evidence of soft tissue swelling, ecchymosis, open wounds, deformity, and visible bone or foreign bodies.
- A detailed neurovascular examination distal to the site of injury should be documented, including capillary refill and two-point discrimination.
- Before splint application (and fracture reduction), the most appropriate method for providing an adequate degree of analgesia should be considered.
- All wounds should be irrigated and débrided as indicated and covered with a dry sterile dressing before a splint is applied. The consulting orthopedist should be consulted regarding all open wounds and the administration of antimicrobials considered for all open fractures, open joints, and tendon injuries.
- The splint must adequately immobilize the joint above and the joint below the suspected fracture or the bone above and the bone below a suspected joint injury.
- All rigid splints should be padded to prevent localized areas of pressure that lead to discomfort and potential pressure blister and ulcer formation.
- During splint application, there must be adequate staff to minimize movement and support the injured site until the limb is completely splinted and the splint is dry.
- A severely deformed fracture should be aligned with the use of constant gentle manual traction as the splint is applied so realignment can be incorporated into and maintained with the splint.
- If there is significant resistance to bony alignment on the application of traction, the bone should be splinted in the position of deformity.
- Finally, when in doubt, splint.

Figure 6-1.

Indications for immobilization of the hand.

Fracture
Dislocation
Subluxation
Sprain
Strain
Tendon disruption
Tendon laceration
Laceration across a joint
Severe contusion/abrasion
Bite
Joint infection
Puncture wound
Deep space infection
Acute arthritis
Tenosynovitis
Tendonitis
Carpal tunnel syndrome
Radial nerve palsy

Indications for Immobilization

The indications for splinting are described in greater detail in other chapters, but briefly, the purpose of a splint is to partially or fully immobilize the digits or hand to allow for healing of an injury. Figure 6-1 lists many of the indications for immobilization of the hand.

Equipment

- Strips or rolls of plaster of Paris in varying sizes (2, 3, 4, and 6 inches)
- Cast padding (different widths)
- Stockinette to protect the skin (different widths)
- Commercially available prefabricated splints with padding
- Prefabricated rolls of fiberglass splints with polypropylene padding
- Elastic bandages
- Adhesive tape
- Plaster knife
- Bucket

Splint Application

In general, the patient's clothing should be protected with a gown or other waterproof barrier. The extremity should be inspected and any wounds treated as appropriate with irrigation, débridement, repair, and a dressing before the splint is applied. Saline-soaked sterile dressings should be applied to open fracture sites.

Plaster of Paris Splints

Stockinette

A piece of stockinette should be measured and cut 3 to 4 inches longer than the length of the cast and a hole cut for the thumb at the appropriate level (Figure 6-2A). The stockinette is rolled up and placed on the arm above the most proximal level of the cast and then unrolled down the arm to the hand. Later, the stockinette can be folded back over the ends of the splint to create a smooth, nonirritating edge at the proximal and distal ends of the splint. Excessive stretching or wrinkling should be avoided because it could place undue pressure on bony prominences or produce friction blisters. In general, 3-inch stockinette is used for the upper extremity.

Padding

The extremity should be wrapped circumferentially with two or three layers of padding such as Webril (Webril undercast padding, The Kendall Company, Mansfield, Mass) or a similar product, with the previous rotation overlapped by 25% at each turn around the extremity (Figure 6-2B). This protects the skin and bony prominences and allows for swelling. Padding should extend beyond the edges of the splint so it can be folded back with the stockinette to form a smooth, padded edge. Extra padding should be added around joints and bony prominences or if excessive swelling is anticipated; felt can be used as an alternative. Webril also is placed between the digits to prevent maceration.

To avoid wrinkling, padding can be stretched or small tears can be made in the padding as each turn is made to adjust the angle and direction of the padding. At angles, the joint should be placed into the position it will be in within the splint; strips of padding are used to cover

Figure 6-2.

Plaster of Paris splint.

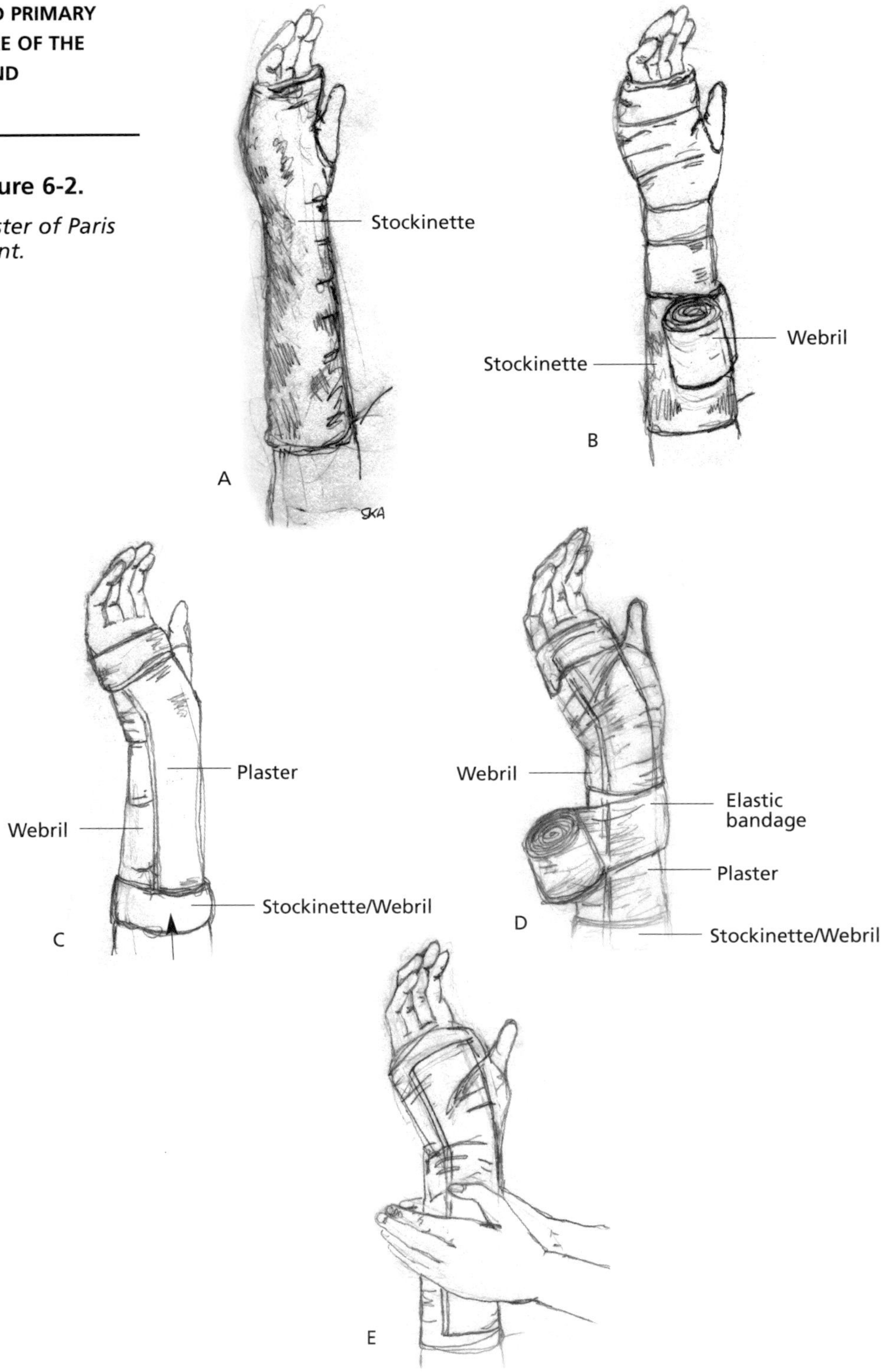

the areas that cannot be wrapped easily. Two-inch padding works well on the hand, and 3- or 4-inch padding works well on the remainder of the upper extremity. Circumferential padding by itself can cause ischemic injury in the presence of excessive swelling. This can be prevented by making a longitudinal cut in the padding along the entire length of the splint opposite the location of the splint.

Plaster Splints

The ideal width and length of the splint depend on the injured body part to be splinted. The splint should be cut slightly longer than the total length that will be needed; the splint is measured against the actual body part to obtain a length (some shrinkage will occur when the splints are wet). The splint width typically should be slightly wider than the diameter of the extremity. The thickness is based on the amount of strength that is required but should not exceed 12 layers because this is associated with an increased risk of burns. Also, the more layers that are used, the heavier and more uncomfortable the splint will be. For the upper extremity, typically eight layers are optimal in terms of strength, comfort, and potential for causing burns.

The splints are wet by submersion in fresh water until bubbles cease to form. Splints have different set times (fast setting is 5 to 8 minutes; extra fast setting is 2 to 4 minutes). The choice of fast-setting versus slow-setting plaster is dependent on the expertise of the person who applies the splint and how quickly the splint should set up: slow-setting plaster if manipulation or molding is required, and fast-setting plaster if rapid immobilization is needed for a fracture that has just been reduced. In general, slow-setting plaster is best for use in the emergency department because more time is allowed to apply and mold the splint and less heat is produced as it sets up. Setup time also can be affected by the temperature of the water; warm water hardens the plaster faster than does cold water.

The plaster splint is removed from the water and squeezed to remove the excess moisture. The splint is smoothed onto a flat surface to remove wrinkles and excess water and to help bond together the layers of plaster. At this point, the plaster splint can be wrapped in cast padding, gauze bandage, or stockinette; this prevents the elastic bandage from sticking to the plaster splint. The now-laminated splint is applied over the padding to the hand, wrist, or arm (Figure 6-2C). Although the splint usually sticks to the cast padding underneath, an extra hand may be needed to hold the splint in place while it is molded.

The next step is quite important and often overlooked. The splint must be molded to the contour of the extremity; the patient should be warned that the process of molding the splint may cause some discomfort. Any angles that are required for appropriate alignment and immobilization should be molded. Only the palm of the hand is to be used to mold and smooth the plaster because finger indentations may create pressure points. All manipulation of the plaster must be completed before it attains a creamy, thick consistency.

The excess stockinette and padding should be folded back over the edge of the splint to form a smooth, comfortable edge. Elastic bandages are applied in a distal-to-proximal manner to hold the splint in place (Figure 6-2D). The splint is supported with the palm of the hand while it cures (Figure 6-2E); the splint must not be wrapped or placed in any position that will decrease ventilation around the splint because this increases the amount of heat to which the skin is exposed.

Before discharge, the patient should be observed for the development of signs or symptoms of ischemic compromise or pressure discomfort. If either occurs, first, the elastic bandages should be loosened. If the ischemic symptoms persist, the cast padding and stockinette should be cut longitudinally along the entire length on the surface opposite the splint material. Once the symptoms resolve, tape can be used to loosely approximate the edges of the padding/stockinette, and the splint can be reapplied. For pressure discomfort, an extra one or two layers of padding can be added to the area. If the discomfort persists after reapplication of the splint, this is most likely due to an indentation in the splint, and a new splint should be made. Any complaint of increased discomfort or pain after splint application is abnormal and should be rectified before discharge. In addition, the splint should be checked to ensure it is maintaining adequate immobilization of the injury site.

Prefabricated Splints

Plaster

These commercially available prefabricated splints contain multiple sheets of plaster within a protective layer of foam rubber padding on one side and cloth on the other (for example, OCL splint products, M-PACT Worldwide Management Corp, Eudora, Kan). Advantages include rapid application, fewer steps, and less mess than regular plaster. Disadvantages include expense and some potential problems with the one-size-fits-all approach.

Because these splints are already padded, they can be applied directly to the skin (foam side to the skin) or over stockinette. The precut splint is wet by submersion in fresh water until bubbles cease to form. Prefabricated splints have varying set times just like regular plaster splints. Slow-setting splints are best for use in the emergency department because more time is allowed to apply and mold the splint and less heat is produced as it sets up. Setup time also can be affected by the temperature of the water; again, warm water hardens the plaster faster than does cold water.

The splint is removed from the water and squeezed to remove the excess moisture. The splint is smoothed onto a flat surface to remove wrinkles and excess water and to help bond together the layers of plaster. At this point, the prefabricated splint can be applied to the hand, wrist, or arm. An extra hand may be needed to hold the splint in place while it is molded. The splint is molded as previously described, with only the palm of the hand used to avoid pressure points. Elastic bandages are applied in a distal-to-proximal manner to hold the splint in place. The splint is supported with the palm of the hand while it cures. The splint must not be wrapped or placed in any position that will decrease ventilation around the splint because this increases the amount of heat to which the skin is exposed.

Fiberglass

Prefabricated rolls of fiberglass splints with polypropylene padding also are available (for example, Ortho-Glass, Smith & Nephew, Casting Division, Charlotte, NC). Similar to the prefabricated plaster splints, fiberglass splints can be applied rapidly with fewer steps and less mess. They also are stronger and lighter and can be washed and reapplied, and the padding keeps moisture away from the skin. Disadvantages include cost and the more rapid set time, which makes molding more difficult compared with plaster. The application is the same as for prefabricated plaster splints.

Common Types of Splints

Bulky Hand Dressing

The bulky hand dressing can be used to immobilize the hand in certain bony and soft tissue traumatic injuries. It also is a useful adjunct in the treatment of inflammatory and infectious conditions of the hand,

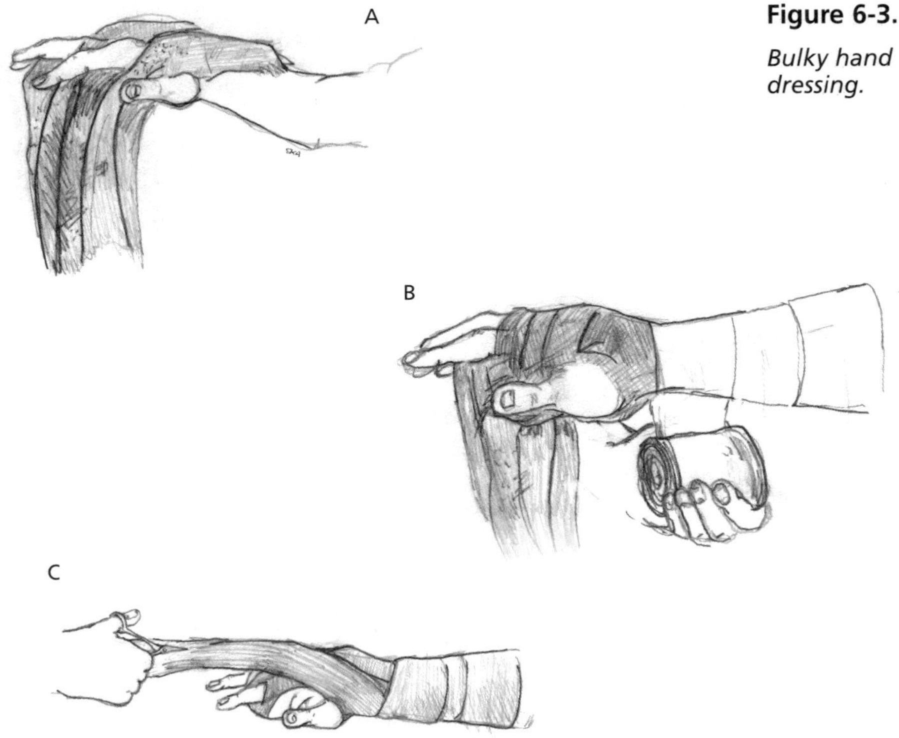

Figure 6-3.

Bulky hand dressing.

providing stabilization and a position that allows for maximal drainage. The equipment needed is readily available in the emergency department: gauze mesh pads, Kerlix rolls (The Kendall Company, Mansfield, Mass), and 3-inch elastic (Ace) bandages.

Application of the dressing begins with the placement of the unraveled gauze mesh between each of the fingers running longitudinally along the dorsal and volar surfaces of the hand (Figure 6-3A). Sufficient gauze fluffs are placed such that the fingers are comfortably separated.

Next, a small ball of gauze fluffs should be placed in the palmar space to simulate the position of function (20 to 30 degrees of wrist extension, 50 to 70 degrees of MCP flexion, and 5 to 10 degrees of PIP/DIP flexion). To achieve wrist extension, a Kerlix roll is gently wrapped circumferentially around the hand, then around the wrist (Figure 6-3B), and finally around the fingers. More Kerlix then is repeatedly applied back and forth from the volar wrist, around the hand and fingers, and back to the dorsal wrist, forming a bulky nonconstricting glove (Figure 6-3C).

The fingertips should protrude for documentation of neurovascular status. The Kerlix may be secured with tape running longitudinally between the fingers from the palmar side to the dorsal wrist, helping to maintain slight wrist extension. Another option is a minimally stretched Ace bandage with holes cut out for the fingers.

Foam-Backed Aluminum Splints

Foam-backed aluminum splints are used to immobilize bony and soft tissue phalangeal injuries. They can be cut to the appropriate length, applied on either the dorsal or volar surfaces, and secured to the digit between the joints with cloth tape (Figure 6-4). Sharp edges should be contoured and padded.

Short splints can be applied to the dorsal surface of the DIP joint (mallet finger; Figure 6-5) or the PIP joint (volar dislocation), splinting the joint in full extension. Wraparound or U-splints can be formed and applied to protect and immobilize the injured distal phalanx. Nondisplaced proximal and middle phalangeal fractures and stable PIP and DIP dislocations also can be immobilized with a volar or dorsal splint with the IP joints flexed at 5 to 30 degrees depending on the injury. If the splint includes the MCP joint, it should end just distal to the wrist joint and be secured with tape that runs circumferentially around the hand both proximal and distal to the thumb.

Figure 6-4.

Foam-backed aluminum splints.

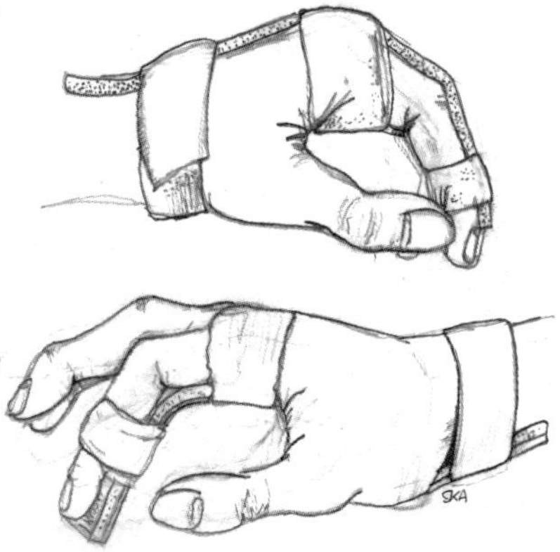

Preformed Mallet Finger Splints

Preformed mallet finger splints are available commercially and are easily applied to digits that have sustained disruption of the distal extensor tendon insertion (Figure 6-6). Once the splint is slipped into place, tape is applied to maintain the position.

Dynamic (Buddy-Taping) Splints

Dynamic splinting (buddy-taping) is a type of immobilization commonly used to treat collateral ligament sprains, stable IP dislocations, and nondisplaced proximal and middle phalangeal fractures. The injured finger is splinted to the adjacent normal finger; this provides support for the injured finger while allowing for full range of motion of the MCP joints and partial range of motion of the IP joints. A pad is placed between the two fingers, which then are taped together between the involved joints (Figure 6-7). Failure to place a pad between the taped fingers may result in a slow-healing pressure blister or ulcer.

Radial Gutter Splint

Radial gutter splints are indicated for the immobilization of second or third metacarpal fractures, unstable fractures of the proximal or middle phalanges of the index or middle finger, and MCP subluxations.

The only equipment needed is splinting material (either a 4-inch prefabricated splint or eight layers of 4-inch splints and stockinette), Webril, and Ace bandages. Several folds of Webril are placed between the index and middle fingers to prevent maceration. A length of splinting material (prefabricated splint or eight layers of plaster splints) is measured and cut to extend from the elbow to the fingertips. A large hole is cut in the splint to accommodate the thumb. If plaster splints are used, the arm should be prepared with stockinette and Webril as previously described, with the included fingers, hand, wrist, and forearm covered. The splint material is prepared and applied to the radial side of the forearm (Figure 6-8). If stockinette and Webril are used, the excess can be folded back to form a smooth, comfortable edge. This is secured with a snug but not tight Ace bandage. The fingertips must be free for neurovascular examination, and the thumb hole must be nonconstricting. The splint is molded to provide 20 degrees of wrist extension, 50 to 90

Figure 6-5.

Aluminum splint for mallet finger.

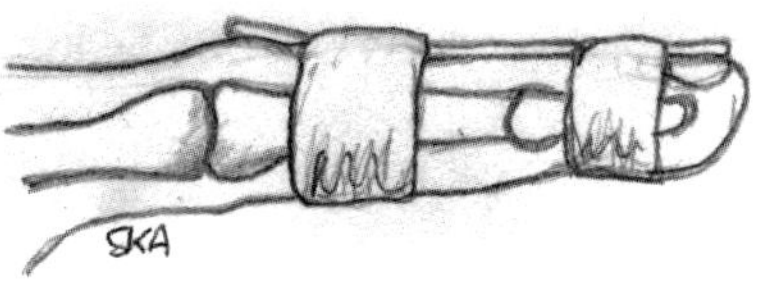

Figure 6-6.

Preformed mallet finger splint.

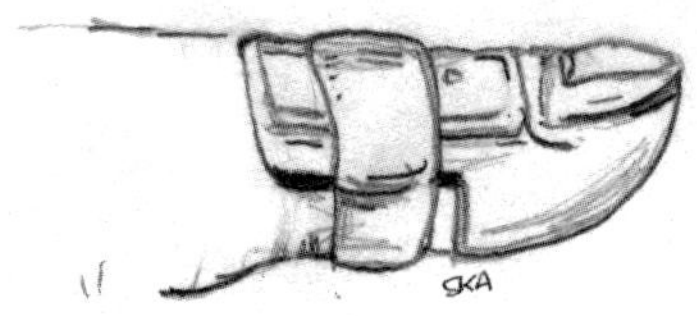

degrees of MCP flexion (depending on the injury), and 5 to 15 degrees of IP flexion.

Ulnar Gutter Splint

Ulnar gutter splints are indicated for the immobilization of fourth or fifth metacarpal fractures, unstable fractures of the proximal or middle phalanges of the ring or little finger, and MCP subluxations.

The only equipment needed is splinting material (either a 4-inch prefabricated splint or eight layers of 4-inch splints and stockinette), Webril, and Ace bandages. Several folds of Webril are placed between the ring and little fingers to prevent maceration. A length of splinting material (prefabricated splint or eight layers of plaster splints) is measured and cut to extend from the elbow to the fingertips. If plaster splints are used, the arm should be prepared with stockinette and Webril as previously described, with the involved fingers, hand, wrist, and forearm covered. The splint material is prepared and applied to the ulnar side of the forearm (Figure 6-9). If stockinette and Webril are used, the excess should be folded back to form a smooth, comfortable edge. This is secured with a snug but not tight Ace bandage. The fingertips must be free for neurovascular examination. The splint is molded to provide 20 degrees of wrist extension, 50 to 90 degrees of MCP flexion (depending on the injury), and 5 to 15 degrees of IP flexion.

Thumb Spica Splint

A thumb spica splint is used to immobilize fractures and dislocations that involve the first metacarpal or the proximal phalanx of the thumb and the MCP or CMC joint of the thumb, including scaphoid injuries. It also can be used as an adjunct in treating de Quervain disease (tenosynovitis).

The only equipment needed is splinting material (either a 4-inch prefabricated splint or eight layers of 4-inch splints and stockinette), Webril, and Ace bandages. Several folds of Webril are placed around the thumb, with care taken to pad the first web space well. A length of splinting material (prefabricated splint or eight layers of plaster splints) is measured and cut to extend from the thumbnail to the proximal forearm. If plaster splints are used, the arm should be prepared with stockinette (a hole is cut for the thumb) and Webril as previously described, with the thumb, hand, wrist, and forearm covered. The wrist is positioned in 15 to 20 degrees of extension and the thumb in the position of function (like holding a wine glass). The other digits are left free. The splint material is prepared and applied to the radial side of the forearm, wrist, and thumb, extending to the base of the

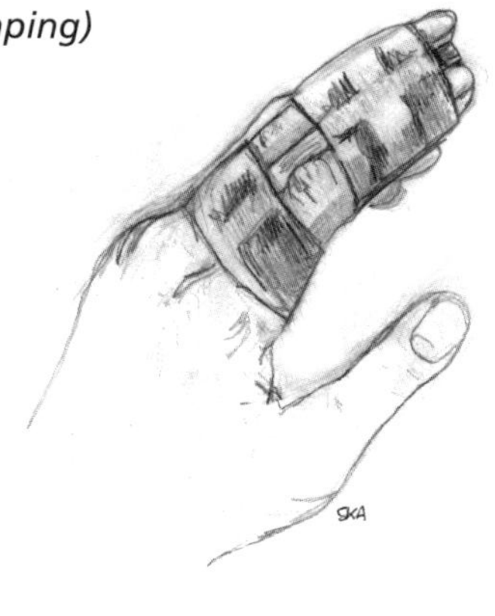

Figure 6-7.

Dynamic (buddy-taping) splint.

thumbnail (Figure 6-10). A 1- to 2-cm perpendicular cut is made on each side of the splint 1 cm distal to the first MCP joint. These cuts prevent the plaster from buckling when the plaster is wrapped around the thumb so it meets and overlaps on the medial side of the thumb. If stockinette and Webril are used, the excess should be folded back to form a smooth, comfortable edge. This is secured with a snug but not tight Ace bandage. The thumb tip must be free for neurovascular examination. The splint is molded to provide 15 to 20 degrees of wrist extension and the thumb in the wine glass position. Once the splint is molded, the patient might be asked to hold a can or bottle to maintain the position of function until the splint is dry.

Short Arm Volar Splint

Short arm volar splints are used to immobilize a variety of soft tissue injuries of the hand and wrist, carpal fractures, and fractures of the second through fifth metacarpal heads. A variation of this splint is the "cockup" splint, which places the wrist in hyperextension. It should never be used to treat acute soft tissue or bony injuries but may be used to treat a variety of chronic problems, including radial nerve palsy with wrist drop, tendonitis, and carpal tunnel syndrome.

The only equipment needed is splinting material (either a 3- or 4-inch prefabricated splint or eight layers of 3- or 4-inch splints and stockinette), Webril, and Ace bandages. A length of splinting material (prefabricated splint or eight layers of plaster splints) is measured and cut to extend from the proximal palmar crease (volar metacarpal heads) to the proximal forearm. If plaster splints are used, the arm should be prepared with stockinette (a hole is cut for the thumb) and Webril as previously described, with the hand, wrist, and forearm covered. The wrist is positioned in 15 to 20 degrees of extension. The digits are left free. The splint material is prepared and applied to the volar side of the forearm, wrist, and hand (Figure 6-11). If stockinette and Webril are used, the excess should be folded back to form a smooth, comfortable edge. The splint is secured with a snug but not tight Ace bandage. The splint is molded so it provides 15 to 20 degrees of wrist extension and

Figure 6-8.

Radial gutter splint.

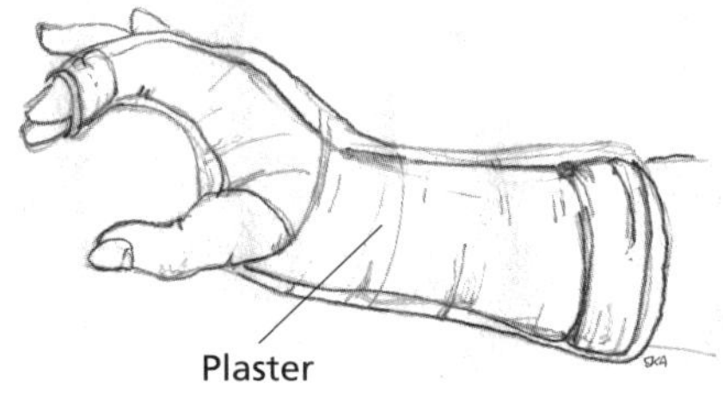

Figure 6-9.

Ulnar gutter splint.

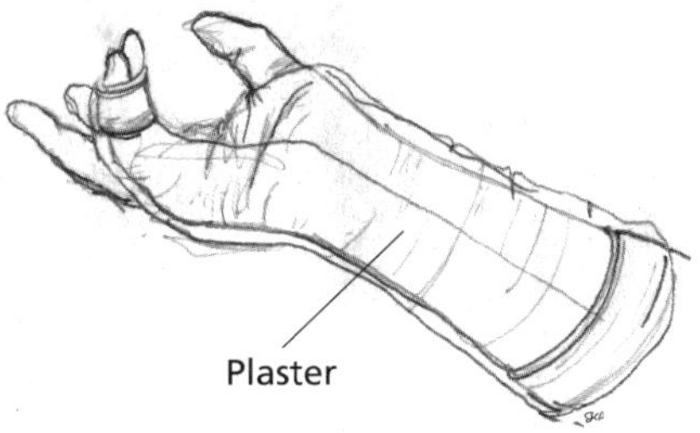

Table 6-1.

Metacarpal fractures.

Fracture	Type of Splint
Second-fifth metacarpal head fracture	Bulky hand dressing in the position of function: wrist extended 20 degrees, MCP joints flexed at 50-90 degrees, and PIP/DIP joints flexed at 5-15 degrees (with or without temporary immobilization depending on the need for open reduction and internal fixation)*
Fourth or fifth metacarpal neck fracture (after reduction of rotational deformity and/or significant angulation)	Ulnar gutter splint (or AP splints) to the fingertips with the MCP joints flexed 70-90 degrees, the IP joints extended, and the wrist extended to 20 degrees (similar to holding a tennis ball)*
Second or third metacarpal neck fracture (angulated)	Short arm volar splint or radial gutter splint from the elbow to the proximal phalanx with the wrist in 20 degrees of extension and the MCP joints in 50-90 degrees of flexion (temporary immobilization until anatomic reduction can be accomplished by an orthopedist)
Second-fifth metacarpal neck fracture (nonangulated)	Short arm volar splint or radial/ulnar gutter splint as described above*
Second-fifth metacarpal shaft fracture (transverse, spiral, oblique)	Gutter splint from the elbow to the fingertips with the joints in the position of function*
Second-fifth metacarpal shaft fracture (comminuted)	Bulky hand dressing in the position of function pending surgical repair
Second-fifth metacarpal base fracture	Bulky hand dressing in the position of function*
Thumb metacarpal fracture (extra-articular transverse, oblique, comminuted)	Short arm volar splint with digits in the position of function or thumb spica splint*
Thumb metacarpal fracture (intra-articular Bennett or Rolando)	Thumb spica splint pending surgical repair

*Obtain orthopedic followup care within 48 to 72 hours.

conforms to the contours of the wrist and palm. The edges along the forearm should be molded upward to form a gutter. For more serious injuries that require more stable immobilization, a dorsal splint may be added, creating a bivalve effect.

Splints for Specific Injuries

There are many different types of injuries to the wrist and hand; Tables 6-1, 6-2, and 6-3 match specific injuries with types of splints to be used, important positioning information, and expected time for followup care for specific injuries. Many splints are applied strictly as a temporary immobilization device pending definitive orthopedic intervention.

Complications

Although splints are applied to avoid vascular compromise and compartment syndrome, these complications can still occur. Webril can stretch and tear, but several layers of snugly applied Webril can compromise circulation just as efficiently as a circumferential cast. This also is true of Ace bandages. It is important to remember that a compartment syndrome can occur without excessive external compression from splinting material. Soft tissue edema and bleeding within the compartment may lead to elevated compartment pressures, resulting in compromised perfusion of muscles and nerves. Regardless of the cause, if tissues remain ischemic for a sufficient period of time, irreversible necrosis, permanent neurologic damage, and muscle contracture will occur.

Figure 6-10.
Thumb spica splint.

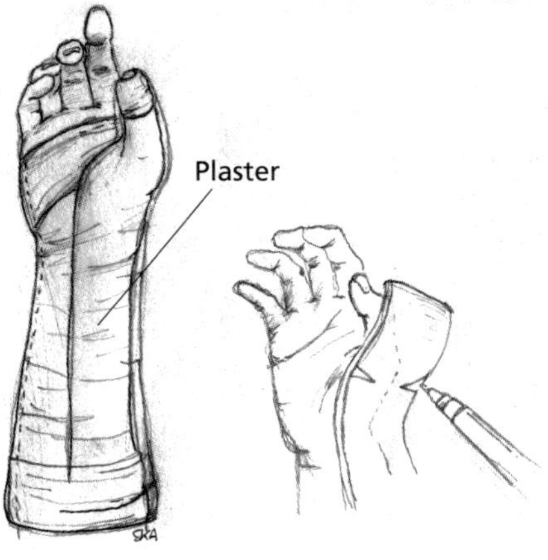

Figure 6-11.
Short arm volar splint.

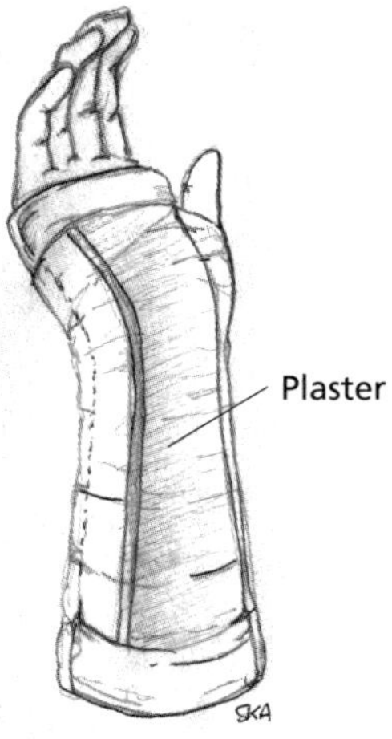

Table 6-2.

Phalangeal fractures and dislocations.

Fracture or Dislocation	Type of Splint
Distal phalanx fracture (tuft, transverse, longitudinal)	Removable wraparound AP foam-backed aluminum or preformed plastic splint that immobilizes the distal phalanx and the DIP joint for 2-4 weeks
Distal phalanx fracture (dorsal intra-articular mallet finger)	Preformed plastic mallet splint or foam-backed aluminum extension splint applied to the dorsal surface of the finger, which includes the distal and middle phalanges, for 6-8 weeks and protective splinting for 2-4 weeks (fractures that involve greater than 33% of the articular surface may require surgical fixation)
Distal phalanx fracture (volar intra-articular)	Volar foam-backed aluminum splint that immobilizes the DIP joint in 5-10 degrees of flexion for 6-8 weeks*
Middle phalanx fracture (nondisplaced)	Dynamic (buddy-taping) splint or radial/ulnar gutter splint with followup in 1 week
Middle phalanx fracture (nondisplaced comminuted, displaced, spiral, angulated)	Ulnar or radial gutter splint that incorporates the wrist and extends to the distal phalanx pending surgical repair
Middle phalanx fracture (intra-articular nondisplaced)	Dynamic splint or volar foam-backed aluminum splint that immobilizes the involved joint (DIP, PIP) in 5-10 degrees of flexion*
Middle phalanx fracture (intra-articular displaced or intra-articular comminuted basilar fracture)	Volar foam-backed aluminum splint that immobilizes the entire finger into the palm or a radial or ulnar gutter splint pending surgical repair
Proximal phalanx fracture (nondisplaced stable fracture)	Dorsal foam-backed aluminum splint extending from the metacarpal to the middle phalanx with the MCP joint flexed at 60 degrees and the PIP joint flexed at 30 degrees*
Proximal phalanx fracture (displaced or unstable)	Radial or ulnar gutter splint that incorporates the wrist pending surgical repair
Proximal phalanx fracture (nondisplaced stable intra-articular)	Dynamic (buddy-taping) splint with early range of motion exercises

Fracture or Dislocation	Type of Splint
Thumb sesamoid fracture	Volar foam-backed aluminum splint from the metacarpal to the distal phalanx with the IP joint flexed at 10-15 degrees and the MCP joint flexed at 30 degrees for 2-3 weeks
DIP dislocation	Volar foam-backed aluminum splint that immobilizes the DIP joint in 5-10 degrees of flexion for 2-3 weeks*
PIP dislocation (lateral or dorsal, stable after reduction)	Volar foam-backed aluminum splint that immobilizes the PIP joint in 30 degrees of flexion for 2-3 weeks and then dynamic (buddy-taping) splint for 1-2 weeks (joints unstable to active range of motion often require surgical repair)
PIP dislocation (volar: unable to extend the PIP on examination, associated with the development of boutonnière deformity)	Dorsal foam-backed aluminum splint that immobilizes the PIP joint in extension for 4-6 weeks (some prefer open reduction and internal fixation)
MCP subluxation (true dislocation requires open reduction)	Radial or ulnar gutter splint that immobilizes the MCP joint in 50-70 degrees of flexion for 7-10 days versus dynamic splinting with immediate range of motion exercises
Thumb IP dislocation	Volar foam-backed aluminum splint that immobilizes the IP joint in 5-10 degrees of flexion for 3 weeks
Thumb MCP dislocation (dorsal)	Volar foam-backed aluminum splint that immobilizes the PIP joint in 30 degrees of flexion for 4-6 weeks
Thumb MCP dislocation (lateral: gamekeeper thumb)	Thumb spica splint (often requires surgical repair)*
Thumb CMC dislocation (rare without Bennett or Rolando fracture)	Thumb spica splint (often requires K-wire fixation)*

*Obtain orthopedic followup care within 48 to 72 hours.

Patients and caregivers should be repeatedly educated on the signs and symptoms of compartment syndrome before discharge. Classic signs and symptoms include increased pain, numbness, tingling, pallor/cyanosis, decreased capillary refill, and weakness. Because many of these are late findings that appear after irreversible damage has occurred, it must be stressed that ***pain is the earliest sign and the hallmark sign of compartment syndrome.*** In contrast to fracture pain, compartment syndrome pain is deep, continuous, poorly localized, and difficult to control and commonly occurs away from the fracture site. Passive extension of the fingers typically exacerbates the pain.

The possibility of an evolving compartment syndrome is a true emergency. Any patient who experiences any increased pain should immediately release the elastic bandages that secure the splint. If the symptoms do not completely resolve in a short period of time, the patient should go to the emergency department immediately for evaluation.

Other complications include soreness over pressure points or binding areas that have been padded inadequately. This is easily rectified with additional Webril. Wounds, ulcers, or blisters that result from attempts to scratch or from objects trapped between the splint and the skin necessitate removal of the splint for examination and treatment.

Patient Instructions

Patients should be provided verbal and written instructions on splint care and potential complications such as compartment syndrome. The importance of elevating the extremity above the heart to decrease throbbing pain and to reduce swelling must be stressed (slings typically are detrimental in this regard). Elevation on several pillows at night is useful. Ice may be applied during the first 48 hours for 30 minutes at a time, but precautions should be taken to keep the splint dry (ice can be used in a sealable plastic bag). Depending on the type of injury, ice may be applied with the splint removed.

The patient must not apply stress to the splint for the first 24 hours, which is the time it takes to completely cure the splint. If the injury permits, the splint can be removed for showering or wound care and then reapplied. For nonremovable splints, care should be taken during bathing to keep the splint dry (the splint can be wrapped in a plastic trash bag). For splints that are applied over a wound, a window may be cut in the splint material over the wound to provide access for wound observation and care. When a wound window is used, the splint may require some reinforcement or additional layers. Cracked or

Table 6-3.

Other soft tissue injuries and conditions.

Soft Tissue Injury or Condition	Type of Splint
Tendon laceration, burns, hand infection	Bulky hand dressing*
de Quervain disease (tenosynovitis)	Thumb spica splint
Carpal tunnel syndrome, tendonitis, radial nerve palsy with wrist drop	Cockup splint

*Obtain orthopedic followup care within 48 to 72 hours.

broken splints serve no function and should be replaced or removed. Patients should be cautioned against attempts to scratch the skin inside the splint with any object. These attempts often result in wounds, which become infected, or objects break off, creating unwanted pressure points and possibly blisters or ulcers. Specific instructions should be given regarding the length of immobilization and when and with whom followup care should be obtained.

Additional Reading

Hart RG, Rittenberry TJ, Uehara DT. *Handbook of Orthopedic Emergencies.* Philadelphia, Pa: Lippincott-Raven; 1999.

Martin DS, Collins LD. *Management of Acute Hand Injuries.* St Louis, Mo: Mosby–Year Book; 1997.

Olson DA, Goga-Eppenstein P, Hill JP, et al. *Casting Protocols for the Upper and Lower Extremities: Rehabilitation Institute of Chicago Procedure Manual.* Gaithersburg, Md: Aspen Publishing; 1999.

Roberts JR, Hedges JR. *Clinical Procedures in Emergency Medicine.* 3rd ed. Philadelphia, Pa: WB Saunders; 1998.

Simon RR, Koenigsknecht SJ. *Emergency Orthopedics: The Extremities.* 3rd ed. Stamford, Conn: Appleton & Lange; 1996.

Steinberg CG, Akins CM, Barin DT. *Orthopedics in Primary Care.* 3rd ed. Philadelphia, Pa: Lippincott Williams & Wilkins; 1999.

Wilton J. *Hand Splinting.* Philadelphia, Pa: WB Saunders; 1997.

Wu KK. *Techniques in Surgical Casting and Splinting.* Philadelphia, Pa: Lea & Febiger; 1987.

CHAPTER 7

Principles of Hand Surgery

Wesley P. Eilbert, MD, FACEP

With the development of modern anesthesia in the 20th century, surgical intervention for hand injuries has become commonplace. Restoration of function is the primary goal of hand surgery. Surgical procedures of the hand can be divided into three categories: emergent, urgent, and elective. There is no indisputable agreement on these time frames and indications, but the following are general guidelines.

Conditions that require **emergent** surgical intervention are those that may lead to serious infection, neurologic damage, amputation, or impaired function if surgery is delayed. These conditions include open fractures, open joints, replantations, infections of the flexor tendon sheath, septic joints, compartment syndromes, injection injuries, and wounds from large penetrating foreign bodies that cannot be safely removed in the emergency department. **Urgent** procedures are those that should be performed within 2 weeks of the initial injury and include the repair of unstable fractures and dislocations, tendon repairs, and nerve repairs. **Elective** hand operations are those that may be performed without specific time constraints. Such situations include ganglion cyst excisions, old tendon lacerations or avulsions (chronic mallet finger), and longstanding fracture malunions.

Fractures

Treatment

The definitive treatment of any hand fracture should be delayed until the general condition of the patient has been stabilized. The goal of treatment of any fracture in the hand is to have the bone heal in a position such that its function is preserved with minimal soft tissue damage. Several treatment modalities are available to optimize fracture healing.

Splinting or Casting

This time-honored method is typically used for simple, closed, isolated, stable fractures. Fractures that will later require internal fixation may also be initially immobilized in this manner.

Pin or Wire Fixation

These methods usually are combined with splinting or casting. They are frequently used for the fixation of fragments in metaphyseal and epiphyseal fractures of the phalanges and metacarpals, fractures of the distal radius, and scaphoid fractures.

Screws

Screws can be used to attach plates to bone, bone to bone, and ligaments and tendons to bone. In the hand, screws are used primarily to compress bone fragments and to improve the mechanical stability of internal fixation.

Plates

Plates are used to provide stability to healing fractures after open reduction. They are commonly used in the hand to stabilize midshaft metacarpal fractures.

External Fixation

This method allows the fixation of bones when other forms of immobilization are impractical. Open fractures with extensive soft tissue injury, comminution, bone loss, or contamination frequently are treated in this manner.

Open Fractures

An open fracture is one in which a break in the integument and underlying soft tissue leads directly into the fracture and its hematoma. Various classification systems can be used to describe the severity of open fractures. In general, the greater the amount of contamination, bone exposure, and soft tissue damage, the greater the likelihood of resultant osteomyelitis. It often is difficult to determine whether a small wound in close proximity communicates with the fracture. Some advocate probing the wound with a sterile blunt instrument, although this is not generally recommended and should be undertaken with great caution. If any uncertainty exists, it is advisable to assume that the injury is an open fracture.

The management of open fractures should proceed without delay. Ultimately, prevention of osteomyelitis is the goal. Gross debris should be removed, and wound cultures should be obtained. The wound should be irrigated with saline and then covered with saline-soaked sterile gauze. Fractures should not be reduced before definitive débridement and irrigation. Tetanus prophylaxis should be administered as appropriate, and intravenous antibiotics should be administered as soon as possible. Most agree that a first-generation cephalosporin with the possible addition of an aminoglycoside provides adequate antimicrobial coverage. For fractures caused by "fight bite" injuries, ampicillin/sulbactam, ticarcillin/clavulanate, or clindamycin combined with ciprofloxacin may be used. Definitive management of open fractures involves débridement of the wound, copious irrigation, and the removal of any foreign bodies. Rarely, a minor open fracture can be treated in the emergency department, but the operating room is the appropriate site of treatment for the vast majority of open fractures.

Closed Fractures

Most closed fractures in the hand can be treated with closed reduction and immobilization. However, some closed fractures require either open reduction and internal fixation or closed manipulation with percutaneous pinning for optimal outcome. These procedures usually are performed on an urgent basis after initial immobilization in the emergency department.

Indications for Fixation

- The fracture is part of a major tendon or ligament avulsion.
- A displaced fracture involves a significant portion of an articular surface.
- Multiple fractures are present, and the hand cannot be held in a position of function without internal fixation.
- The interposition of tendons or other soft tissues prevents the realignment of a displaced fracture by closed methods.
- The fracture is displaced and has epiphyseal injuries known to have a propensity for growth arrest (Salter-Harris types III and IV).
- The fracture has a compartment syndrome that requires fasciotomy.

Contraindications to Surgical Reduction and Stabilization

- Osteoporotic bone is too fragile for stabilization by internal or external fixation.
- Significant damage of overlying skin caused by scarring, burns, dermatitis, or active infection exists, and internal fixation would result in the loss of soft tissue coverage or an exacerbation of infection.
- There is active infection or osteomyelitis.
- Fracture comminution is so severe that successful reconstruction is unlikely.
- The patient has an unstable medical condition in which the risks of surgery and anesthesia outweigh the possible benefits.

Tendon Injuries

Tendon injuries of the hand may be caused by lacerations, blunt trauma, or overloading of the musculotendon-bone system. Complete tendon transections require surgical repair for definitive treatment. The treatment of partial tendon transections is controversial. Partial flexor tendon lacerations require surgical repair, whereas extensor tendon lacerations are not as definitive. As a general rule, if a tendon is more than 50% transected, it should be repaired.

The timing of tendon repair is determined by the circumstances surrounding the initial injury. Primary repair, performed in the first 12 to 24 hours, is preferred. Delayed repair up to 2 to 3 weeks after injury is recommended for contaminated wounds and for those that involve skin loss, missing tissue, or an unstable bony skeleton.

Flexor Tendons

All flexor tendon transections should be repaired by a hand surgeon. If a delayed repair is planned, any overlying skin injury should be cleansed, irrigated, and closed loosely with nonabsorbable sutures. Then, to prevent further contraction of the tendon before it is repaired, the hand should be splinted posteriorly with the wrist flexed 30 degrees, the MCP joints flexed approximately 70 degrees, and the IP joint flexed at 10 to 15 degrees.

Extensor Tendons

Most extensor tendon transections should be repaired by a hand surgeon. Simple, clean lacerations of extensor tendons in zones I and VI can be repaired primarily in the emergency department under the following circumstances:

- The skin and tendon wounds are sharp and not heavily contaminated.
- The injury is less than 8 hours old.
- The two ends of the tendon are easily visualized.
- The individual performing the repair has experience with the procedure and has the appropriate instruments available.

If the involved extremity is repaired in the emergency department, it should be splinted as described later. If a delayed repair is planned, any associated skin injury should be treated as described for flexor tendon injuries.

Appropriate splinting of extensor tendon transections after primary repair or before delayed repair is important. The splinting technique is determined by the zone of injury, as follows:

- **Zone I and II injuries** should be treated with a dorsal splint, with the DIP joint maintained in slight hyperextension. The PIP and MCP joints need not be immobilized.
- **Zone III and IV injuries** should be splinted with the PIP joint in extension.
- **Zone V to VIII injuries** should be splinted with an adjacent finger. The wrist is splinted at 35 degrees of extension, and the MCP joint is splinted at 15 degrees of flexion with the IP joints slightly flexed.

Ligament Injuries and Dislocations

Ligament injuries in the hand can be classified simply as partial or complete tears.

Partial ligament tears can be treated initially with buddy-taping in mild cases or with immobilization in more severe cases.

Complete ligament tears can be treated with prolonged immobilization or surgical repair. These patients should be referred to a hand surgeon for definitive care.

Most joint dislocations in the hand can be reduced primarily in the emergency department. Reduction should be attempted as soon as possible. The urgency to reduce dislocated joints stems from two main considerations. First, in general, the longer the joint remains dislocated, the more difficult it is to reduce. Second, any neurovascular deficit involved with a dislocation may advance from temporary to permanent if treatment is delayed. Active range of motion of the joint should be tested after reduction. As a general rule, the presence of near-normal active range of motion implies that functional recovery will occur with conservative rather than with surgical treatment. Conservative treatment after reduction typically involves a period of buddy-taping or immobilization followed by active range of motion exercises.

Open reduction of acute dislocations is indicated in the following circumstances:

- The patient has an open dislocation, which requires extensive irrigation to reduce the risk of joint infection.
- Proper reduction cannot be achieved with closed techniques. This often occurs due to interposed soft tissue or osteochondral fragments.
- A stable reduction cannot be maintained. Associated fractures of the articular surfaces often are unstable and require open reduction and internal fixation to ensure stability of the reduction.
- Examination before closed reduction reveals no neurologic deficit, but a deficit is present after reduction.
- A circulatory deficit distal to the dislocation is found and persists after closed reduction. Further assessment of the vasculature is indicated, and vascular repair, if needed, should proceed on an emergent basis.

Infections

Because the hand has several closed spaces and compartments that allow for rapid "walling off" of infection, it is a part of the body that is frequently infected. As a general rule, most hand infections can be treated with nonsurgical therapy (antibiotics, immobilization, elevation) if it is administered within the first 24 to 48 hours of infection. Beyond this time, many hand infections require some form of incision and drainage, irrigation, or débridement. Another general surgical principle that holds true for hand infections is: "If there's pus, drain it."

Abscesses in the hand can be drained in the emergency department if they are superficial and do not extend into the deeper compartments of the hand. Paronychias, felons, and carbuncles on the dorsal surface of the hand fall into this category. Web space abscesses may be drained in the emergency department if the treating physician is experienced with the appropriate drainage technique. Deep space infections such as midpalmar and thenar space infections, ulnar and radial bursal infections, and infections in the dorsal subaponeurotic space should be referred to a hand surgeon for drainage on an emergent basis. Empiric antibiotics, usually a β-lactamase inhibitor such as ampicillin/sulbactam, should be administered while awaiting the drainage procedure.

Flexor tenosynovitis is a surgical emergency that requires prompt recognition and treatment. Treatment in the emergency department should include immobilization, elevation, and parenteral antibiotic therapy with a β-lactamase inhibitor. Emergent consultation with a hand surgeon should be obtained. Although some infections identified early in their course can be treated conservatively, many require open drainage and irrigation in the operating room.

Septic arthritis in the hand is frequently caused by direct inoculation from penetrating trauma or spread from a contiguous infection such as a felon. The treatment of septic arthritis requires hospitalization for the administration of intravenous antibiotics and drainage of the joint on an emergent basis. Most hand joints require open drainage in the operating room, although some may be managed with repeated aspiration and closed joint irrigation.

Necrotizing fasciitis and **gangrenous infections** of the hand are relatively rare, life-threatening surgical emergencies. Both require emergent débridement in the operating room and appropriate intravenous antibiotics.

Amputations

With the development of modern microvascular surgical techniques in the 1960s, the replantation of digits and limbs after traumatic amputation has become commonplace. With few exceptions, all amputated parts should be considered for replantation. Ultimately, the decision to attempt replantation should be made by a hand surgeon.

To prepare any severed part that may be replanted, the gross debris should be removed, and then the part should be cleansed gently with normal saline irrigation. It should then be wrapped in sterile gauze moistened with saline and placed in a plastic bag, and the bag should be placed on ice. Radiographs should be obtained of both the amputated part and the stump. Antibiotics that cover *Staphylococcus aureus* should be administered as prophylaxis.

Ischemia time is an important factor when replantation is being considered. Most digits can be successfully replanted after up to 8 hours of warm ischemia and up to 24 hours if cooled. Amputations that contain significant amounts of muscle, such as those of the forearm, are less tolerant of ischemia and must be replanted within 6 to 8 hours.

Patient characteristics such as hand dominance, occupation, and likely compliance with rehabilitation also must be considered. Elderly patients, patients with self-inflicted amputations, patients with chronic illnesses such as peripheral vascular disease or diabetes mellitus, and patients with other life-threatening injuries are poor candidates for replantation. Most replantations in children do well.

Characteristics of the amputation itself that favor replantation are as follows:

- Single digit amputations between the PIP and DIP joints (distal to the FDS insertion)
- Multiple digit amputations
- All thumb amputations
- Clean wrist and forearm amputations

Characteristics that do ***not*** favor replantation are as follows:

- Single digit amputations proximal to the FDS insertion

- Multilevel amputations
- Severe crush injuries

Soft Tissue Injuries Associated With Hand Trauma

Clenched Fist Injuries

Clenched fist, or fight bite, lacerations on the dorsal surface of the MCP joints are caused by one person striking another person in the teeth with a closed fist. These injuries are associated with a high incidence of infectious complications, including septic arthritis, tenosynovitis, osteomyelitis, and surgical amputation. Patients who present immediately after injury require a thorough examination with appropriate anesthesia to determine the extent of injury. It is important to realize that penetration of the deeper tissues occurs in a direct line while the fist is in a clenched position. If the skin wound is examined in the open hand position, it will lie significantly proximal to the underlying soft tissue and bony injury. For this reason, the hand must be evaluated in the clenched fist position to avoid missing communication with deeper wounds. Any patient with injury to the extensor tendon or joint capsule and those with an associated fracture should be evaluated emergently by a hand surgeon. Most of these injuries require further evaluation, débridement, and irrigation in the operating room. All patients should receive antibiotic prophylaxis with a β-lactamase inhibitor such as ampicillin/sulbactam. Any patient with evidence of infection more than 24 hours after sustaining a fight bite injury should be evaluated by a hand surgeon for emergent débridement and irrigation.

Peripheral Nerve Injuries

Classification

Neuropraxia is a mild blunt injury that produces nerve dysfunction without gross anatomic disruption. Full functional recovery usually occurs within days.

Axonotmesis is a more severe injury with interruption of the axons but preservation of the endoneural tube. Functional recovery of the nerve typically occurs within 1 year.

Neurotmesis is a complete severance of the nerve or damage to the point where spontaneous regeneration is impossible. Surgical repair is indicated.

Surgical Indications

Indications for surgical exploration of a peripheral nerve deficit are as follows:

- A sharp injury has obviously severed a nerve. The nerve may be repaired at the time of exploration or up to 2 weeks later. Repair is often delayed for grossly contaminated wounds.
- An avulsion or blast injury has rendered the condition of the nerve unknown. Exploration is required to identify the extent of nerve injury. Severed nerve ends can be identified and tagged to aid in future repair.

- There is a nerve deficit after a closed fracture, dislocation, or blunt injury, and no clinical or electrical evidence of regeneration has appeared after approximately 3 weeks.
- A nerve deficit was not present before closed reduction or casting of a fracture and becomes apparent later.
- A nerve deficit occurs after penetrating trauma such as a low-velocity gunshot wound, and evidence of regeneration does not appear after approximately 3 weeks.

Lacerations of digital nerves distal to the DIP flexion crease usually are left unrepaired because cross-innervation from the digital nerve on the other side of the finger usually provides adequate sensation.

Timing

The optimal timing of nerve repairs remains controversial. Most agree that early repair is preferable in clean wounds with adequate soft tissue coverage. Repairs performed more than 2 weeks after the injury have diminishing rates of success as a result of muscle atrophy and fibrosis of nerve stumps. All digits that have lost function as a result of a nerve injury should be splinted in a position of function to prevent further inadvertent injury.

Arterial Injuries

Penetrating trauma accounts for the majority of acute vascular injuries in the hand. Most closed fractures and dislocations of the wrist and hand do not result in significant vascular injury. Due to extensive collateral circulation, most isolated radial or ulnar artery injuries in the wrist and hand do not result in significant ischemia distal to the lesion. Likewise, most single digital artery lacerations do not require repair.

Critical arterial injuries result in distal tissue necrosis if they are not emergently repaired. Patients with these injuries present with the classic signs of arterial insufficiency: pallor, poikilothermy, paresthesias, pain, and pulselessness. A hand-held Doppler device is a convenient tool that can aid in the assessment of digital arterial flow. Typically, critical arterial injuries in the hand result from disruption of both the radial and ulnar arteries at the wrist, the palmar arch in the palm, or both digital arteries in a single digit.

Noncritical arterial injuries do not result in necrosis or amputation and can be repaired at the discretion of a hand surgeon. Relative indications for **arterial reconstruction** include the following:

- Evidence of suboptimal collateral circulation
- Previous injury to the collateral artery
- Associated major nerve injury
- Facilitation of healing of injuries distal to the disrupted artery

Compartment Syndromes

Diagnosis and Assessment

A compartment syndrome is a condition characterized by increased pressure within a closed fascial space that causes decreased perfusion of the enclosed tissues or tissues distal to the area, with potentially irreversible damage. In the hand, ten myofascial compartments can be defined, including the four dorsal interosseous, three palmar interosseous, one hypothenar, one thenar, and one adductor compartment. In addition, the fingers are compartmentalized by fascia at the flexor creases, and the carpal tunnel is a significant compartment at the level of the wrist. Compartment syndromes of the hand can easily be unrecognized and require a high degree of suspicion to secure a timely diagnosis.

The most common causes of compartment syndromes in the hand include the following:

- Fracture
- Crush injury
- Arterial injury or thrombosis that causes postischemic swelling
- Burns
- External compression caused by ill-fitting cast or bandage
- Snake envenomation

Clinical Features

The clinical features of compartment syndromes can be remembered by using the **six P's mnemonic device**, as follows:

- **Pain** out of proportion to the injury. Alert patients almost always complain of a severe and constant pain over the involved compartment.
- **Pain with passive stretching** of the involved muscle groups. However, this can be a nonspecific finding.
- **Paresis** or weakness of the involved muscles. This may be due to unrelated nerve damage or guarding secondary to pain.
- **Paresthesias** in the distribution of the nerve in the involved compartment. This is a relatively late finding. At the level of the wrist, both the median and ulnar nerves are a concern in the carpal tunnel.
- **Pulses intact.** Unlike arterial injuries, which can present with similar symptoms, distal pulses and capillary refill are preserved.
- **Pressure.** Swelling and palpable turgor over the compartment may be the first signs of a compartment syndrome. Direct measurement of intracompartment pressure offers the most objective means of diagnosis. Several devices and methods are available to measure compartment pressures.

Treatment

The only effective treatment for a compartment syndrome is surgical fasciotomy to relieve the pressure. In the wrist, an open carpal tunnel release decompresses the carpal tunnel. The intracompartment pressure threshold for fasciotomy is controversial. Some recommend that fasciotomy be performed when intracompartment pressure rises to within 20 to 40 mm Hg of the diastolic pressure.[1] Others believe that any intracompartment pressure greater than 30 mm Hg with positive clinical findings warrants treatment.[2]

High-Pressure Injection Injuries

Grease guns, spray guns, and diesel injectors account for most high-pressure injection injuries to the hand. Patients who present soon after injury often have pain out of proportion to a rather innocuous-appearing injection wound.

Radiographs of the hand should be obtained to help determine the extent of subcutaneous spread from the injection site. Parenteral antibiotics that cover the common skin flora should be administered. Immediate consultation with a hand surgeon should be obtained; most cases require emergent surgical decompression and débridement.

Burns

Burns of the hand can be caused by several mechanisms, including flame, electricity, flash, contact, chemicals, and steam. A determination of the depth of the burn at initial presentation guides management. The following sections describe the indications for surgical intervention.

Escharotomy

Circumferential full-thickness burns of the wrist, hand, or digits are at risk for distal ischemia secondary to edema. Edema may progress for up to 36 hours after a burn. The loss of pulses distal to the burn is an indication to perform an escharotomy. Quantitative monitoring of tissue pressures may be performed with a wick catheter or a similar device. If the pressure in the subcutaneous tissue under the burn exceeds 30 mm Hg on two separate readings, escharotomy is indicated.

Grafting

With the exception of injuries that cover less than 1% of the total body surface area, all full-thickness burns require skin grafting to heal. Skin grafting is typically performed on an urgent basis by a hand surgeon or plastic surgeon.

Electrical Burns

Electrical burns that conduct through the body deserve special mention. Although the entrance and exit wounds of these injuries may be unimpressive, there typically is extensive damage to the underlying muscles, nerves, and vessels. Early decompression with fasciotomy and débridement are almost always required.

References

1. Green DP, Hotchkiss RN, Pederson WC, eds. *Green's Operative Hand Surgery.* 4th ed. New York, NY: Churchill Livingstone; 1999.
2. Ortiz JA, Berger RA. Compartment syndrome of the hand and wrist. *Hand Clin.* 1998;14:3.

Additional Reading

Canale ST, ed. *Campbell's Operative Orthopedics.* 9th ed. St Louis, Mo: Mosby; 1998.

Chapman MW, Madison M, eds. *Operative Orthopedics.* 2nd ed. Philadelphia, Pa: JB Lippincott; 1993.

Hart RG, Rittenberry TJ, Uehara DT, eds. *Handbook of Orthopaedic Emergencies.* Philadelphia, Pa: Lippincott-Raven; 1998.

Uehara DT, ed. The hand in emergency medicine. *Emerg Med Clin North Am.* 1993;11:3.

CHAPTER 8

Long-Term Care and Rehabilitation

Wesley P. Eilbert, MD, FACEP

Treatment Modalities

Casts and Splints

Casts and splints are used to immobilize and to protect the injured part during the healing process. Potential complications include the following.

A **tight cast** typically is caused by swelling under a full-circumference cast. Pain is the first and most reliable symptom, and there should be no hesitation to bivalve a cast when a patient presents with this complaint. If relief is obtained with bivalving, the cast can be replaced and held in position with an elastic bandage. A new cast should be applied in 1 to 3 days.

Cast sores may be caused by indentations in the cast or splint or by a lack of adequate padding. Patients typically present with localized pain. Prompt removal of the cast or splint and inspection of the involved area are indicated.

Itching under the cast or splint occurs frequently and usually can be controlled with oral antipruritic agents or the application of warm air under the cast or splint with a blow dryer. The patient should be instructed not to attempt to relieve the itching by inserting a coat hanger or similar device under the cast or splint.

Prolonged immobilization can cause the loss of muscle strength, endurance, and ligamentous joint contracture. These problems can be avoided with the initiation of strength-enhancing and range of motion exercises as soon after the injury as possible.

External Fixation Devices

A main goal of outpatient care with these devices is to prevent pin track infections. Daily care of the pin sites includes cleansing with a mild soap and saline. Exposed portions of the pins should be wrapped with bulky gauze. Significant drainage from pin sites, alone or with mild cellulitis, can be treated with an oral first-generation cephalosporin and aggressive pin site hygiene. Cellulitis that involves more than mild erythema around the pin site should be treated with parenteral antibiotics. Any loose pins should be removed. Radiographic evidence, clinically significant pin loosening, or osteomyelitis should be treated with pin removal and a 10- to 14-day course of parenteral antibiotics.

Percutaneous Pins

Percutaneous pins used for fracture stabilization have a pin-track infection rate of 7% to 8%. Factors associated with pin-track infections are motion at the pin–bone interface, pin placement within the cortical bone, necrosis of the bone or soft tissue around the pin, and soft tissue tension at the site at which the pin exits the skin. Contributing factors are wound severity, amount of contamination, and delay in presentation, as well as systemic disease and noncompliance. Pin-track infections usually can be treated adequately with oral antibiotics that cover common skin flora. When outpatient therapy is unsuccessful, hospitalization for parenteral antibiotic administration, possible removal of the pin, and débridement of the pin track are warranted.

Internal Fixation

Deep infection after internal fixation of hand fractures is rare. Treatment involves hospitalization for parenteral antibiotics, possible implant removal and débridement of infected bone and soft tissue, and fracture stabilization, usually via external fixation.

Applications of Cold and Heat

The use of **ice or cold packs** is a time-honored treatment for acute musculoskeletal injuries. Cold decreases pain by impairing neuronal function and decreasing inflammation. A cold device should be applied for 10 to 20 minutes at 2-hour intervals. Maximum benefits are obtained with therapy within the first 24 to 48 hours after injury.

Forms of **heat therapy** can be classified as superficial (hot packs, heating pads, whirlpool baths) and deep (ultrasound). Heat can be used for analgesia and muscle relaxation and to facilitate reduction of chronic inflammation. Heat also increases blood flow and soft tissue extensibility. Heat should be used later (after the first 24 to 36 hours) in the course of treatment of musculoskeletal hand injuries.

Electrical Stimulation

Several different uses of electrical stimulation may be applied in the **rehabilitation** of hand injuries. Electrical stimulation has been used to facilitate muscle contraction after tendon repair, to improve range of motion and muscle strength after immobilization, and to aid in the resolution of chronic edema after cast removal.

Transcutaneous electrical nerve stimulation (TENS) is a form of electroanalgesia that involves the application of low-voltage electrical pulses through the skin to the nervous system. The TENS device may be used to control acute and chronic pain in the hand.

Therapeutic Exercise and Massage

Exercise is essential in the rehabilitation process after hand injuries.

Proper exercise strengthens injured bone and soft tissues, increases mobility, and prevents the detrimental effects of prolonged immobilization. Exercises that are used in the rehabilitation of specific injuries are discussed later.

Massage is an age-old therapeutic adjunct that is frequently used in the treatment of injuries such as burned hands, in chronically stiff hands, and in reflex sympathetic dystrophy.

Acute Pain Management

Many patients with acute musculoskeletal injuries of the hand obtain adequate pain relief with **RICE (rest, ice, compression, elevation) therapy**. An ice pack can be applied for 20 to 30 minutes every 1 to 2 hours while the patient is awake for the first day and then three or four times a day on the second day.

Most soft tissue injuries of the hand can be managed with **NSAIDs**. These medications have the added benefit of decreasing the inflammation associated with the injury, although side effects (gastric irritation, renal impairment) can limit their use.

Narcotic analgesics (acetaminophen/codeine, acetaminophen/hydrocodone, and others) can be used to treat more painful conditions such as fractures and burns. Caution should be used when prescribing these agents because they can be habit forming with prolonged use.

Reflex Sympathetic Dystrophy

Reflex sympathetic dystrophy is a syndrome of chronic pain, neurovascular disturbance, and dystrophic changes in the skin and bones that can occur after an injury. Other terms for this entity include causalgia, posttraumatic dystrophy, and shoulder-hand syndrome. Hand injuries are the most common cause of reflex sympathetic dystrophy, and those that involve significant soft tissue, nerve, or vascular injury may be at a higher risk. The exact pathogenesis of this condition is unknown, but it results in a dysfunction of the sympathetic nervous system in the hand and often the entire upper extremity.

Clinical Features

Reflex sympathetic dystrophy is frequently misdiagnosed in its early stages as symptoms of disuse caused by immobilization. The syndrome typically progresses through three stages.

Stage I lasts a few weeks to 6 months and is characterized by pain, often described as burning, that is out of proportion to the severity of the injury. Vasomotor instability can result in either pallor and cyanosis or redness and warmth. Pitting edema is often present. Decreased range of motion begins as a result of pain avoidance.

Stage II can develop as soon as 3 months after the onset of symptoms and typically lasts an additional 3 to 6 months. At this stage, the affected hand often develops a hard, brawny edema, with glossy skin and diminished growth of hair and nails. Pain and decreased range of motion are prominent features, and atrophy of muscle and subcutaneous tissue develops. Radiographic examination shows osteoporotic changes.

Stage III begins 9 to 12 months after the onset of symptoms and can last up to several years. This stage is marked by progressive and irreversible atrophic changes in muscle and soft tissue with marked loss of range of motion and extensive osteoporosis.

Treatment

Initiation of treatment before the onset of the trophic changes seen in stages II and III is of paramount importance to obtain functional recovery. Blocking of the associated sympathetic ganglion with a local anesthetic agent is both diagnostic and therapeutic and may be repeated multiple times. Several other pharmacologic interventions have been advocated, including corticosteroids, NSAIDs, tricyclic antidepressants, sympatholytic agents, β-blockers, and calcium channel blockers. A surgical sympathectomy may provide relief in recalcitrant cases when local anesthetic blockades have been effective but temporary. The cornerstone of the treatment of reflex sympathetic dystrophy is the establishment of a progressive exercise program for the affected hand; the treatments mentioned here serve only to provide sufficient analgesia to allow the initiation of such a program.

Fractures

Healing Stages

To better understand long-term fracture treatment, it is necessary to know the stages of healing.

The **inflammation stage** begins at the time of injury and lasts 3 to 4 days. During this stage, fracture hematoma formation occurs, and inflammatory cells predominate at the fracture site. Clinically, this stage ends when pain and swelling begin to subside.

The **soft callus stage** begins immediately after the inflammation stage and lasts approximately 1 month. This stage is marked by union of the fracture ends by fibrous and cartilaginous tissue. Clinically, this stage ends when the fracture is no longer grossly mobile.

The **hard callus stage** begins 3 to 4 weeks after the fracture and lasts 2 to 3 months. During this stage, the fibrocartilaginous union that was formed initially is replaced by a fibro-osseous union. At the end of this stage, the fracture is clinically and radiographically healed.

During the **remodeling stage**, the newly formed fibrous bone is reshaped and reorganized so that it more closely resembles the original bone. This process takes months to years to complete. Children have a much greater capacity to remodel bone than do adults. For this reason, angular deformities after initial reduction are not as great of a concern in children.

Long-Term Management

All fractures require observation throughout the healing period to ensure proper union. Repeat radiographic evaluations are performed during the course of treatment to ensure the maintenance of proper reduction.

Length of Immobilization

In general, splints and casts should remain in place until clinical union has occurred. Clinical union is demonstrated by lack of pain or movement at the fracture site. The length of time required for clinical union varies with the type of fracture, the age of the patient, and the specific bone involved. Guidelines for the length of immobilization required for some of the common hand fractures treated without fixation are as follows:

- **Distal phalanx**—3 to 4 weeks or until the finger is no longer sensitive to impact. If there is a dorsal avulsion fracture (mallet finger), 6 to 8 weeks of immobilization is typically required.
- **Middle and proximal phalangeal shaft**—3 to 4 weeks of buddy-taping for nondisplaced fractures. Four weeks of splinting usually is necessary for displaced fractures after closed reduction.
- **Metacarpal**—3 to 4 weeks for neck fractures, and at least 4 weeks, often longer, for shaft fractures.
- **Scaphoid**—10 to 12 weeks for nondisplaced distal and middle third fractures. Nondisplaced fractures of the proximal third require 12 to 20 weeks of immobilization.
- **Triquetrum**—2 to 4 weeks for dorsal avulsion fractures, and 4 to 6 weeks for transverse fractures through the body.
- **Distal radius (Colles fracture)**—4 to 6 weeks for nondisplaced fractures, and up to 8 weeks for displaced fractures that require closed reduction.

External Fixation Devices

Like other forms of immobilization, external fixation devices should remain in place until clinical union has occurred.

Internal Fixation Devices

Kirschner wires, or K-wires, which are commonly used for internal fixation in the hand, are typically left in place for 4 weeks with simple fractures. Other forms of internal fixation may be removed on an elective basis after sufficient healing of the fracture has occurred, unless the implant begins to cause complications such as fibrosis or pain.

Complications

Delayed Union

Delayed union occurs when an adequate amount of time has passed since the initial fracture and there is no clinical or radiographic evidence of the expected osseous union. Individual patient characteristics (age, systemic illness, nutritional status) affect healing rates. Several factors may predispose a fracture to delayed union, such as comminution, inadequate reduction, extensive soft tissue disruption, and inadequate immobilization or internal fixation. If conservative measures fail to stimulate fracture healing, surgical interventions such as stable fixation for compression of the fracture fragments or bone grafting may be necessary.

Nonunion

Nonunion is said to have occurred when all healing processes have ceased and bone continuity has not been restored. Causes of nonunion include infection, poor vascular supply, and other disruptive factors. Open hand fractures and fractures of the scaphoid are at a particular risk for this complication. **Pseudoarthrosis** is a rare form of nonunion in which dense scar tissue forms a false joint at the fracture site. The management of fracture nonunion involves the aggressive treatment of any associated infection and, frequently, surgical intervention such as internal fixation or bone grafting.

Malunion

Malunion is the healing of a fracture with deformity. Although many mild malunions require no treatment, intervention is indicated if the deformity interferes with hand or digit function or is cosmetically unacceptable to the patient. Three main types of malunion that occur in the hand are angulation, rotation, and exostoses.

Angulation is a relatively common complication of metacarpal and phalangeal fractures. The more proximal in the digit, the less acceptable is angulation, given the effect of projection of the angulation. For example, 2 to 3 degrees of angulation is of minimal cosmetic importance in a distal phalangeal fracture. However, the same degree of angulation in a proximal phalangeal fracture causes significant deformity, given the projection of the angulation over the length of the digit. A wedge osteotomy can be performed to correct these deformities.

Rotation occurs after metacarpal and phalangeal fractures, alone or in conjunction with angular deformities. A derotational osteotomy can be performed as a corrective procedure.

Exostoses are bony projections from the fracture site that form where the bone ends overlap. These may occur in conjunction with angular or rotational deformities. Exostoses may cause tendon attrition or irritation of other local structures. Treatment is simple excision of the bony prominence or corrective osteotomy if an angular or a rotational deformity also is present.

Avascular Necrosis

Avascular necrosis secondary to disruption of the blood supply to the bone is a concern with scaphoid fractures. Fractures of the proximal third of the scaphoid, oblique fractures, and fractures with significant displacement are at the greatest risk for this complication. Bone grafting may be indicated.

Tendon Adhesions and Joint Contractures

Without adequate fracture stabilization and early joint and tendon motion, all tissues in the zone of injury near a fracture tend toward healing as a single unit with confluent scarring. Fractures of the proximal phalanx and IP joint and those that require open reduction and internal fixation are at a particular risk for these complications. Therefore, proper joint positioning during immobilization and early range of motion exercises of adjacent joints are vital in the rehabilitation of hand fractures. In severe cases, tenolysis or contracture release may be necessary to restore proper function.

Infection

The incidence of infection after an open hand fracture is between 2% and 11%. Infection is more likely to occur in open fractures associated with extensive soft tissue injury or contamination and in comminuted fractures. Treatment involves débridement of the infected bone and soft tissue, parenteral antibiotics, and stabilization of the fracture, usually with external fixation. After the infection has cleared, bone grafting may be necessary if a segmental defect exists. Amputation ultimately may be necessary if the infection cannot otherwise be eradicated.

Rehabilitation

The recovery of range of motion and function is the primary goal of rehabilitation after hand fracture. The stages of rehabilitation typically proceed in the following order: recovery of motion and flexibility, recovery of strength and power, recovery of endurance, and return to routine activities. Recovery of motion is the most important component of the rehabilitation process.

Fracture stability must be ensured before beginning rehabilitative exercises. In general, patients with stable fractures or fractures treated with internal fixation may begin some motion 3 to 5 days after the injury or stabilizing procedure. Unstable fractures treated with closed reduction and immobilization may be mobilized once the fracture has healed sufficiently to provide some degree of stability. Dynamic splints and buddy-taping may be used to increase the functional use of the injured part while still providing some stabilization. A discussion of the specific treatment regimens for the various types of hand fractures is beyond the scope of this chapter, but a basic underlying principle is to advance therapy as limited by pain.

Tendon Injuries

Partial Tendon Transections

Partial tendon transections that do not require surgical repair typically are immobilized for 1 week and then reassessed. If the repeat examination reveals no abnormalities, immobilization is no longer necessary. If swelling, tenderness, or tendon function abnormality is noted, however, splinting should be continued for an additional 2 weeks.

Complete Tendon Transections

Flexor Tendon

After surgical repair, the wrist and involved digit usually are splinted in flexion, with active extension begun after 2 to 3 days. Active flexion exercises may begin after 3 to 4 weeks.

Extensor Tendon

Closed tendon injuries in zones I and II that are treated nonsurgically require 6 to 10 weeks of immobilization with the DIP joint in mild hyperextension. Surgically repaired extensor tendons typically require 3 to 4 weeks of postoperative splinting with the wrist and digit in extension.

Complications

Tendon adhesions and joint contractures may occur primarily as a result of immobilization. Delayed tendon rupture may result from overzealous therapy techniques or patient noncompliance.

Ligament Injuries

Ligament Tears

Partial ligament tears require 2 to 5 weeks of buddy-taping in mild cases. In more severe cases, 2 to 3 weeks of immobilization followed by a period of dynamic splinting or buddy-taping usually is necessary.

Complete ligament tears that require surgical repair (most often, injuries to the ulnar collateral ligament of the thumb) are immobilized for 4 to 6 weeks after surgery, followed by active range of motion and dynamic splinting.

Joint Dislocations

Interphalangeal and MCP dislocations that are treated with closed reduction typically are immobilized for 2 to 4 weeks, followed by active exercises. Those that require surgical intervention often are internally immobilized with a K-wire for 2 to 4 weeks after surgery, followed by limited range of motion.

Carpal dislocations (most often, lunate or perilunate dislocations) require 6 to 8 weeks of immobilization in a short arm cast after reduction.

Complications

Persistent swelling and stiffness are common after joint injuries, so range of motion exercises of the involved joint should begin as soon as feasible in the postinjury period. In severe cases, **arthrolysis** can be performed to free adhesions around the joint. **Arthrodesis** may be necessary to fuse a joint if there is chronic pain or instability after injury.

Replantations

Postoperative Care

Postoperative care of replantations involves the avoidance of stimuli known to cause vasospasm (caffeine, smoking, exposure to cold) for at least 3 weeks. The replanted part should remain in its initial dressing for 3 weeks because dressing changes also can evoke a vasospastic response. The part should be immobilized for 1 to 3 weeks, at which point some passive range of motion exercises typically are begun.

Complications

Vascular occlusion (arterial or venous) is the most common cause of replantation failure. Most vascular occlusions occur in the first 48 hours after surgery, while the patient is still hospitalized; however, occlusions can occur as late as 12 days after surgery. **Arterial occlusions** typically present with a cool, pale replanted part; **venous occlusions** usually are bluish-purple with brisk capillary refill. If an arterial occlusion is suspected, the affected arm should be lowered below the level of the heart. If a venous occlusion is suspected, the extremity should be elevated. If these conservative measures fail to improve circulation to the replanted part, a stellate ganglion block can be performed, or the patient may ultimately require surgical exploration of the neurovascular repairs. Long-term complications of replantation include malunion, nonunion, joint stiffness, tendon adhesions and rupture, and dysesthesias.

Peripheral Nerve Injuries

Nonsurgical Treatment

Patients who are not candidates for surgical repair typically are fitted with an orthosis to protect the paralyzed portion of the hand and to maximize its function. The most important aspect of long-term therapy in these patients is the maintenance of full passive range of motion in the involved joints and the prevention of contractures. **Tendon transfer**, in which a functioning muscle–tendon unit from another part of the hand is transferred to provide some function to the paralyzed part, can be performed to improve hand function.

Postoperative Care

After nerve repair or grafting, postoperative care involves the removal of all tension on the repaired nerve. The hand should be splinted for 3 to 4 weeks to achieve this goal, at which point gentle range of motion exercises may begin. Sensory reeducation therapy usually is necessary after nerve repair in the hand.

Burns

The main goals of long-term therapy of hand burns are the maintenance of range of motion, prevention of deformity, and restoration of function.

Splints often are applied at the first sign of decreased mobility or skin tightness as scar formation begins. The hand is splinted in an "anti-deformity" position (not the position of function) to apply tension to the burned area and to prevent scar contracture. Dynamic splinting can be used as the range of motion of the burned part increases.

Skin grafting frequently is necessary in the treatment of full-thickness burns and to cover areas that require scar excision to release contractures. Grafted areas require 5 to 7 days of immobilization after surgery, and then gentle active exercises may begin. Patients should be instructed to protect newly grafted skin from sun and cold exposure.

Scar compression is the primary means to prevent buildup of a hypertrophic scar, and elastic bandages or, ultimately, custom-fitted scar compression gloves are used. Scar compression should be continued for 12 to 18 months, until scar maturation is complete.

With **frostbite**, mummified tissue should be allowed to autoamputate; skin grafting may be necessary. Muscle fibrosis, especially of the intrinsic muscles of the hand, may occur. Surgical contracture release may be necessary if conservative measures (splinting and range of motion exercises) fail. Vasospastic and cold intolerance problems are the most common long-term sequelae; chronic pain, numbness or stiffness, excessive sweating, and abnormal skin color and nail appearance also occur.

Additional Reading

Boscheinen-Morrin J, Davey V, Conolly WB, eds. *The Hand: Fundamentals of Therapy.* Oxford, UK: Butterworth–Heinemann; 1992.

Clark GL, Wilgis EF, Aiello B, et al, eds. *Hand Rehabilitation: A Practical Guide.* New York, NY: Churchill Livingstone; 1997.

Freeland AE. *Hand Fractures: Repair, Reconstruction and Rehabilitation.* Philadelphia, Pa: Churchill Livingstone; 2000.

Hart RG, Rittenberry TJ, Uehara DT, eds. *Handbook of Orthopaedic Emergencies.* Philadelphia, Pa: Lippincott–Raven; 1999.

Hunter JM, Schneider LH, Mackin EJ, et al, eds. *Rehabilitation of the Hand: Surgery and Therapy.* St Louis, Mo: CV Mosby; 1990.

Light TR, ed. *Hand Surgery Update 2.* Rosemont, Ill: American Academy of Orthopaedic Surgeons, American Society for Surgery of the Hand; 1999.

CHAPTER 9

Metacarpal Fractures

James H. Sullivan, MD, FACEP, and George D. Tsonis, MD

The hand is an instrument of intention and expression. It gains much of its versatility from the combination of fixed and mobile elements, as described by Littler,[1] allowing the musculotendinous system of intrinsic and extrinsic units to move the different segments. The fixed elements include the distal carpal row and the second and third metacarpals. The mobile elements include the thumb, fingers, and fourth and fifth metacarpals. The structure of the metacarpals and their contributions to the fixed and mobile elements of the hand provide for a palm that can vary its degree of concavity, allow for the free movement of the thumb into opposition, and serve as the platform from which the digits perform. With the aid of the proximal limb, the hand becomes an extension of the brain, enhancing interactions with the outside world. In this central role, the hand often is injured through misadventure, accidental and otherwise, with metacarpal fractures frequently encountered. Fractures of the second through fifth metacarpals account for up to 36% of hand fractures, with fractures of the fifth metacarpal accounting for 20% of all hand fractures.[2] Although metacarpal fractures often are treated as minor injuries, inappropriate treatment may result in stiffness, malunion, and cosmetic or functional impairment, the consequences of which may result in prolonged disability.

Anatomy

The metacarpals radiate distally from their articulations with the distal carpal row and are numbered 1 through 5 from the thumb to the little finger. Each metacarpal is divided anatomically into a head, neck, shaft, and base.

The **metacarpal head** is bulbous and convex, sloping from dorsal to volar, and it articulates with the concave surface of the proximal phalangeal base. The metacarpal head is grooved in the midline on the volar surface for passage of the flexor tendons. The heads of metacarpals 2 through 5 are tethered to each other on their volar aspects by the transverse metacarpal ligament. On each side of the base of the head are small tubercles for the attachment of the collateral ligaments of the MCP joint. The metacarpal head resembles a cam in shape and function, causing the radius of the arc of rotation to change during flexion and extension of the proximal phalanx (Figure 9-1). When the MCP joint is in extension, the collateral ligaments are relaxed, allowing abduction and adduction of the phalanx. As the MCP joint is flexed, the collateral ligaments are progressively stretched to their tightest functional limit at 90 degrees. This anatomic point explains the MCP joint stiffening that occurs if the collateral ligaments are allowed to shorten by splinting the MCP joint in extension.

Proximal to the tubercle is the **metacarpal neck**, which is formed of softer cancellous bone, is angulated 15 degrees, and structurally is the weakest area of the metacarpal. When axial loads are applied to the hand by activities such as punching, the load is transmitted to this area of the metacarpal in response to the collapse into flexion of the IP and MCP joints.

The **metacarpal shafts** are prismoid and curved so that they are convex on the dorsal surface and concave on the volar surface. The radial and ulnar surfaces serve as the sites of attachment of the volar and dorsal interosseous muscles. These muscles are flexors of the MCP joint and account for the apex dorsal angulation seen in neck and shaft fractures (Figure 9-2).

The **metacarpal base** also is formed of soft cancellous bone. The bases of metacarpals 2 through 5 are cuboidal and broader dorsally than volarly. Ligaments that arise from the dorsal and volar carpal surfaces, as well as the interosseous muscles, stabilize the metacarpal articulations with the distal row of carpal bones. The base of the first metacarpal presents a concave-convex surface for articulation with the saddle-shaped articular surface of the trapezium. This allows great freedom in the movement of the thumb metacarpal, including flexion/extension in the plane of the palm, abduction/adduction at right angles to the palm, and circumduction and opposition.

The carpal articulations of the second and third metacarpals are practically fixed, making them a constituent of Littler's fixed elements, whereas the articulations of the fourth and fifth metacarpals allow for 15 and 25 degrees of movement, respectively, and make them part of the mobile elements. The mobility of the fourth and fifth CMC

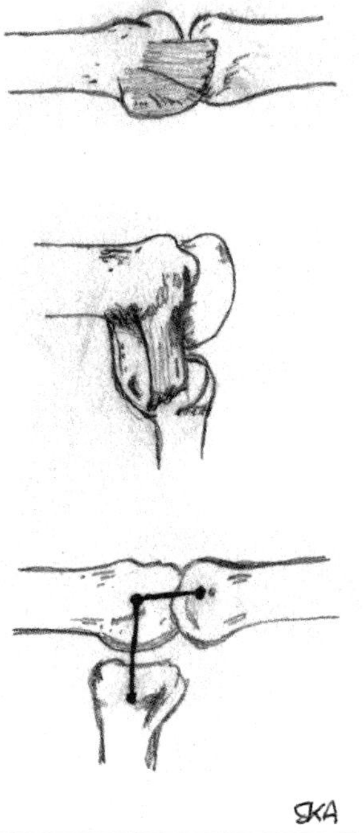

Figure 9-1.

The cam action of the metacarpal head results in steadily increasing collateral ligament tension as the proximal phalanx is flexed at the MCP joint. The integrity of the ligament is best tested in flexion.

joints allows these metacarpals to move away from the plane of the palm; this provides increased strength and security when objects are grasped firmly (Figure 9-3).

Mechanism of Injury

Fractures of the metacarpals are commonly classified according to location: head, neck, shaft, or base. Fractures may occur from direct blows, penetrating missiles, axial loads, and torsion applied to the phalanx and transmitted through the MCP joint collateral ligaments. These forces result in spiral, oblique, transverse, and comminuted patterns (Figure 9-4). Fractures may be single or multiple. Understanding the mechanism of injury helps to predict the type of fracture and the likely severity as well as the possible associated soft tissue injuries.

Physical Examination

Examination of the metacarpals should be directed to their functional elements, namely, as a platform for movement of the phalanges and as a base for grasping. Soft tissue injury and bony deformity should be sought. Palpation should be attempted, but edema and pain may make this problematic, so a low threshold for obtaining radiographs is advised. A subtle rotational component to the fracture can have a dramatic effect on the overlap of digits, thereby significantly affecting grasping functions as well as intricate movement of the fingers. To evaluate rotational deformity, the patient should flex the fingers into the palm. The nail plates are approximately coplanar. Another technique is to have the patient alternately flex the fingers into the palm. Axial lines, drawn through the digits, point toward the tubercle of the scaphoid. Although there may be significant intersubject and intrasubject variability, these techniques are helpful in the assessment of rotational deformity.

Treatment

The goal of treatment is to return the hand to pain-free range of motion with no loss of strength. Essential to the achievement of this goal is normal alignment and immobilization of the fracture fragments. This is not always possible due to the nature of the injuries encountered. Many metacarpal fractures can be treated with closed nonsurgical methods, and appropriate initial splinting plays a central role in the achievement of satisfactory results. Before splinting, soft tissue injuries should be treated and appropriate dressings applied. Soft padding is then applied over the anticipated area of the splint or immobilization device.

Figure 9-2.

Apex dorsal angulation occurs because of the volar force exerted by the interosseous muscles.

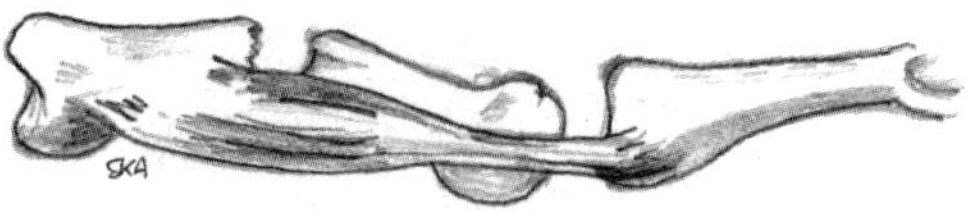

The splint can be made from plaster of Paris strips or commercially available splinting material. The preferred position of immobilization of the hand is the position of function: the wrist in 30 degrees of extension, MCP joints in 60 to 70 degrees of flexion, and the IP joints in 10 to 15 degrees of flexion. Muscles that originate in the forearm can deform metacarpal fracture sites, and splinting of the wrist in extension neutralizes these muscles. The flexion at the MCP and IP joints maintains the critical length of the collateral ligaments during immobilization and prevents undue contracture that would retard postimmobilization range of motion.

Splint types that are used include volar splints for metacarpal head fractures; some physicians add a dorsal splint to provide a more stable bivalve effect. The volar splint generally stops at the metacarpal heads, but some clinicians prefer to extend the splint to the fingertips and then fold it back and mold it to the palm. This allows the digits to move freely and to rest on the rounded end of the splint. The important point is to allow the thumb and fingers freedom of movement unless they are being immobilized because of injury. Radial and ulnar gutter splints are used for fractures of the neck, shaft, and base of the metacarpal. A thumb spica splint is used for fractures of the first metacarpal. When a metacarpal fracture is reducible but unstable, percutaneous K-wires may be used to stabilize it. For severe comminution or bone loss, open reduction and internal fixation with screws, wires, plates, or intramedullary devices is an option for the specialist. External fixation of metacarpal fractures generally is reserved for severe open fractures with associated soft tissue or bone loss.

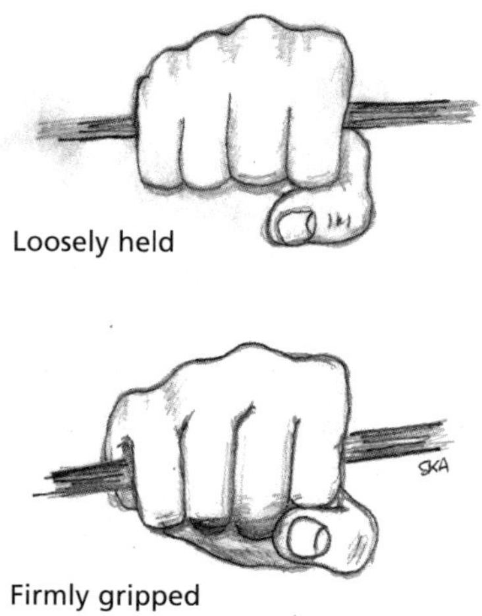

Figure 9-3.

On increasing the grip strength of the hand, flexion at the fourth and fifth MCP joints allows the grip to be more secure.

Second Through Fifth Metacarpal Fractures

Metacarpal Head

Mechanism of Injury

Direct or crushing force is the typical mechanism for these uncommon fractures, which usually are comminuted and intra-articular. The second metacarpal head is injured most frequently. Torque on the digit may cause the unusual collateral ligament avulsion fracture.

Evaluation

Standard radiographs generally delineate these fractures, although a Brewerton view may be needed if an avulsion fracture is suspected. Distraction views are sometimes ordered by the specialist, but due to pain, regional or general anesthesia is required. Care should be taken to assess the soft tissue injuries because extensor tendons are frequently injured.

Treatment

Because of the intra-articular predilection of this fracture, the standard treatment is open reduction and internal fixation with K-wires. Some fractures are so severely comminuted that restoration of the articular surface is not possible with open reduction. However, they may be improved with distraction and then are treated with external fixation or traction and immobilization. In cases in which distraction does not improve the fracture, a short period of immobilization and splinting followed by early mobilization is attempted so as to develop some sort of articulation while minimizing the loss of motion and pain. In the emergency department, attention should be paid to the associated soft tissue injuries and immobilization in the position of function. Because these fractures are intra-articular, patients should be referred to a specialist for early consultation. If these fractures are complicated with puncture wounds or lacerations, emergency consultation should be obtained for surgical débridement and irrigation. Prophylactic antibiotics should be administered if the wounds are potentially contaminated with oral flora.

Complications

Chronic residual pain, particularly on grasping, occurs frequently. Delayed rupture of extensor tendons due to crush injury also is possible and requires close followup care.

Metacarpal Neck

Mechanism of Injury

Metacarpal neck fractures usually are caused by an axial loading force applied to the metacarpal head and transmitted to the weaker neck region. The fourth and fifth metacarpals are injured more frequently than the second and third metacarpals because of the tendency to deliver a punch with a "roundhouse" motion, the impact of which is generally received by the head of the fifth or, less frequently, the fourth metacarpal. The fracture has apex dorsal angulation due to the concave volar surface and the deforming forces of the interosseous muscles. The more proximal the injury, the greater the deformity for any given angulation (Figure 9-5); conversely, the more distal the fracture, the greater the degree of angulation that is acceptable clinically. The volar surface usually is comminuted to some degree, and the pull of the interossei makes this fracture inherently unstable.

Evaluation

There is a definite gender predilection (92% male) for this injury and a tenden-

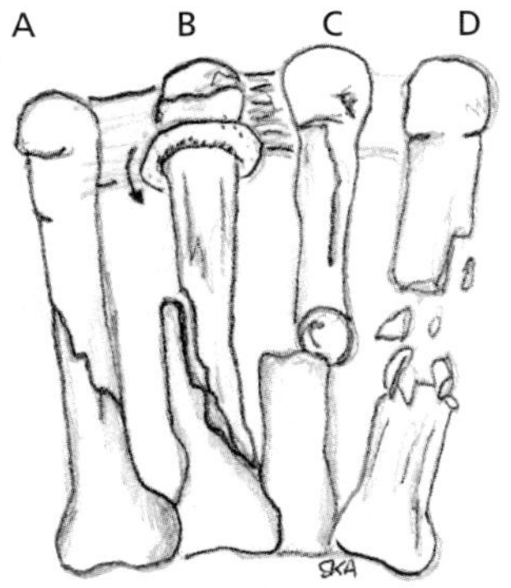

Figure 9-4.

Multiple fracture types, occurring singly or multiply.
A) *Oblique.*
B) *Spiral.*
C) *Transverse.*
D) *Comminuted.*

cy toward recidivism (as many as 27% have had a previous similar injury).[3] The history often reveals that the patient was pummeling an opponent or striking a solid surface such as a wall. Localized swelling, tenderness over the MCP joint, and, frequently, the metacarpal head palpated in the palm of the hand are found on physical examination. Because this is a clenched fist injury, particular attention should be paid to associated soft tissue injuries and the possibility of a foreign body or clenched fist bite.

Treatment

Treatment varies for fourth and fifth metacarpal neck fractures and for second and third metacarpal neck fractures. There are approximately 15 and 25 degrees of flexion/extension at the CMC joints available to the fourth and fifth metacarpals, respectively. This flexibility allows these metacarpals to move away from the plane of the palm on grasping, which allows greater toleration of angulation deformities. There is controversy regarding the treatment of fourth and fifth metacarpal neck fractures. Many advocate ulnar gutter splinting in the position of function or functional taping, citing more rapid mobilization and equal functional results.[4] Others propose reduction and immobilization for angulation of more than 30 degrees.[5] Normal neck angulation is 15 degrees; when the apparent angle of deformity is measured, this 15 degrees should be subtracted from the total measured angle. In the emergency department, if the physician chooses to reduce the fracture, the technique first described by Jahss in 1938 is used after adequate anesthesia is achieved with hematoma or nerve block. That technique is as follows:

- First, the metacarpal head is distracted to disimpact the fracture site.
- The MCP and PIP joints of the involved digit are fully flexed to 90 degrees.
- Pressure is directed dorsally through the shaft of the proximal phalanx to the metacarpal head.
- Simultaneously, the operator's other hand applies pressure on the dorsum of the metacarpal directed toward the volar surface.

The fracture then should be immobilized in an ulnar gutter splint in the position of function.

Neck fractures of the second and third metacarpals require anatomic reduction because these fixed elements of the hand have little motion and are unable to move out of the plane of the palm. Volar angulation of the second and third metacarpal heads of more than 15 degrees is likely to cause a painful grip and loss of strength. Even if nondisplaced, the tendency is for the fracture

Figure 9-5.

The more proximal the fracture, the more prominent the palmar displacement of the metacarpal head.

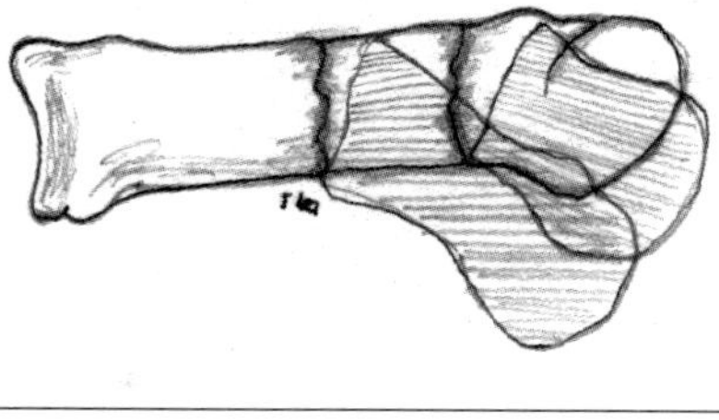

to angulate eventually. These fractures require close followup care to monitor fracture alignment. If reduction fails, percutaneous fixation is performed. In the emergency department, a radial gutter splint is used, with close followup care provided by a specialist.

Complications

Although most patients do not develop significant disability, loss of grip strength, intermittent pain, or deformity may occur. An uncommon but significant deformity that occurs with malunion of a severely angulated neck fracture is **clawing** (Figure 9-6). The severe angulation causes extreme MCP joint hyperextension, laxity of the extensor tendon, and resultant flexor dominance at the PIP joint. Regardless of the degree of deformity, if the patient can fully extend the digit without extensor lag at the PIP joint, the development of clawing is unlikely.

Metacarpal Shaft

Mechanism of Injury

Transverse metacarpal shaft fractures are the result of direct blows and often are accompanied by soft tissue injuries. Various factors that affect treatment include associated soft tissue injuries, number and configuration of fractures, and degree of displacement. Transverse shaft fractures angulate apex dorsal.

Oblique and spiral shaft fractures result from translational forces associated with twisting of the corresponding finger transmitted to the metacarpal shaft through the attachments of the collateral ligaments. These fractures tend to shorten and rotate, especially the second and fifth metacarpals, because they have support on only one side, by the transverse metacarpal ligament (Figure 9-7).

Comminuted shaft fractures generally are caused by crushing injuries or penetrating injuries inflicted by high-velocity projectiles. They frequently are associated with significant soft tissue injuries.

Evaluation

Because of the frequent association of soft tissue injuries with transverse and comminuted fractures, attention should be paid to the neurovascular and musculotendinous status of the hand. Oblique and spiral fractures may have associated injuries in the digit that was the origin of the translational force.

Figure 9-6.

With severe fracture angulation, hyperextension of the MCP joint is required to achieve neutral extension of the digit. The common extensor tendon is relaxed in hyperextension and is inadequate to resist flexor forces at the PIP, resulting in clawing.

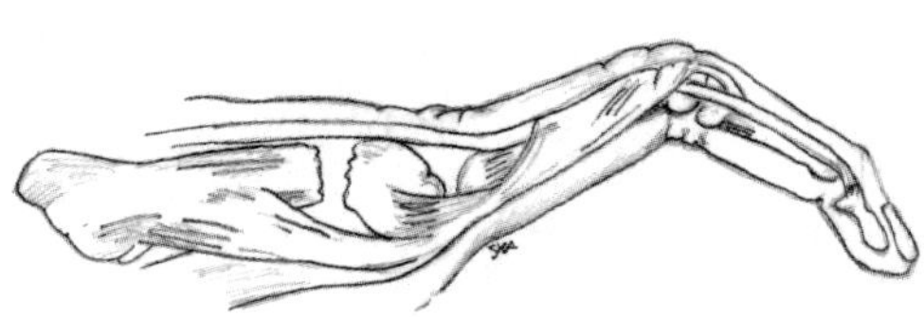

Treatment

Transverse fractures are subject to apex dorsal angulation for the same reasons as are metacarpal neck fractures (see Figure 9-2). Nondisplaced fractures of the second and third metacarpal shafts, as well as minimally displaced fractures of the fourth and fifth, are treated initially with immobilization using a dorsal and volar splint or the appropriate gutter splint. The splint should be in the position of function. Close followup care is recommended because these fractures tend to angulate despite immobilization. If a fracture requires reduction, many specialists still attempt closed reduction with splinting and reserve open reduction and internal fixation for failure to maintain reduction, noncompliant patients, open fractures, or multiple closed fractures.

Oblique and spiral nondisplaced fractures may be treated with splinting, but they have a tendency to shorten and rotate due to the pull of the intrinsic muscles. Many authors accept 5 mm of shortening; larger amounts of shortening lead to weakening of the intrinsic muscles and the transverse metacarpal arch. If acceptable reduction cannot be attained or maintained, either closed reduction and percutaneous fixation or open reduction and internal fixation may be performed. In the emergency department, care is directed toward splinting with a gutter splint or a dorsal and volar splint with early referral to a specialist.

Comminuted fractures, as a result of the loss of shaft integrity, shorten due to the pull of the intact interosseous muscles. Plaster splinting generally does not prevent this complication. In the emergency department, applying a bulky dressing is appropriate. Care must be taken to assess neurovascular and musculotendinous status because these fractures frequently are accompanied by significant soft tissue injuries. Edema is a common problem and is addressed with elevation. These fractures frequently require surgical repair and occasionally bone grafting. Immediate consultation with a specialist is recommended.

Figure 9-7.

Support of the metacarpals by the transverse metacarpal ligament.

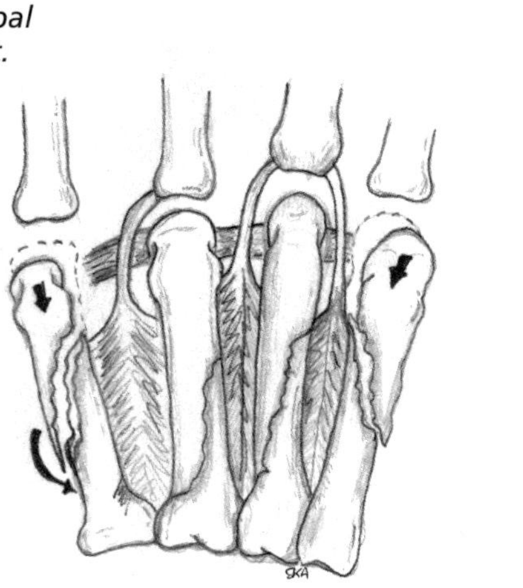

Because **multiple fractures** can be complicated by the loss of lateral support and a propensity for marked swelling and postinjury tendon adhesions, they frequently require open reduction and internal fixation to provide stability and a return to early motion.

Complications

Weakened grip, loss of mobility, rotational disability of digits, and chronic pain, as well as neurovascular and musculotendinous problems, may occur. Unusual complications include compartment syndromes, weakening of the dorsal metacarpal arch, and fracture nonunion.

Metacarpal Base

Mechanism of Injury

These fractures may be caused by falls on an outstretched hand, axial load injuries that drive the metacarpal shaft into the base, and direct blows to the metacarpal base.

Evaluation

The base of the metacarpal is stabilized by the intermetacarpal ligaments, intrinsic muscles, and fascia. Consequently, metacarpal base fractures usually are displaced minimally and typically are stable. These fractures may be difficult to visualize on the frontal projection radiograph of the hand because of the superimposition of the metacarpal bases on the distal row of carpal bones. Identification of these fractures may be aided by use of the Brewerton view or a CT scan. Careful assessment for intra-articular involvement should be performed, as well as assessment of rotational deformities. If the forces are severe, the examiner should be alert to the possibility of CMC joint dislocation as well. These patients present with severe edema and tenderness over the dorsum of the hand. A lateral radiograph of the hand reveals the fracture dislocation; fracture dislocation of the base of the metacarpal is rare and is unstable.

Special care is advised to not overlook the **baby Bennett fracture** of the base of the fifth metacarpal. This is analogous to a Bennett fracture, with distraction provided by the extensor carpi ulnaris. This intra-articular chip fracture requires anatomic realignment to avoid the occurrence of a significant amount of degenerative change in this important joint.

Treatment

In the emergency department, nondisplaced or minimally displaced fractures without intra-articular extension can be treated conservatively with a short arm splint that holds the MCP joints in flexion and the IP joints free with the wrist neutral. Early followup care is recommended. With displaced fractures, percutaneous K-wires may be used to maintain stability and to avoid CMC joint arthrosis. Rotational deformities must be sought because even a small amount of rotation at the metacarpal base is magnified many times at the flexed fingertip. The metacarpal base fracture with CMC joint dislocation generally is treated with closed reduction and percutaneous K-wire immobilization. Because this injury requires surgical intervention for stabilization, immediate consultation with a specialist is recommended.

Thumb Metacarpal Fractures

Anatomy

The mobility of the thumb, which acts to dissipate force, accounts for the low frequency of first metacarpal fractures. Because of the unique CMC joint anatomy, these fractures nearly always occur at the base. The CMC joint is a double saddle joint. The base of the first metacarpal is convex in the radioulnar plane (transverse) and concave in the dorsovolar plane (vertical). The trapezium is conversely convex in the vertical plane and concave in the transverse. The anterior oblique (volar) ligament and the first intermetacarpal ligament insert into the ulnar aspect of the first metacarpal base and stabilize the metacarpal by limiting abduction. These ligaments are so strong that fractures of the first metacarpal are much more common than pure dislocations. The abductor pollicis longus tendon inserts on the radial aspect of the metacarpal base and displaces the metacarpal proximally and dorsally during a fracture/dislocation (Bennett fracture).

Mechanism of Injury

Most fractures result from an axial loading force on the partially flexed metacarpal. This mechanism causes a levering force onto the base of the metacarpal and often occurs during a fistfight or a fall on the hand. Other less common mechanisms include direct blows, missiles, and torsion on the phalanx.

Evaluation

Lateral and oblique views and a true AP view of the thumb (Robert view) are needed for proper radiographic evaluation of the digit. The Robert view is performed with the hand in full pronation (the natural position of the hand when placed behind the back) and is needed with a slightly altered lateral view because the thumb is oriented in a different plane than the other digits. Thumb metacarpal fractures are classified into two groups: extra-articular (transverse, oblique, comminuted, and epiphyseal) and intra-articular (Bennett and Rolando fractures). Care must be taken to distinguish oblique fractures at the base without intra-articular extension from the Bennett fracture, which extends into the joint space, because treatment differs considerably. Evaluation in the emergency department should note associated soft tissue injuries and any rotational deformity. Urgent referral to a hand specialist should be arranged, with the hand immobilized in a thumb spica splint or a bulky dressing.

Treatment

Extra-Articular Fractures

Extra-articular fractures occur more frequently than intra-articular fractures and are more forgiving to treat. The injuries usually are located near the base and are transverse, oblique, comminuted, or epiphyseal. Most fractures are amenable to closed reduction and immobilization in a thumb spica cast for 4 weeks. Residual angulation up to 20 to 30 degrees is acceptable and leads to almost no limitation of motion, but rotational deformity is not as well tolerated. Some oblique fractures prove to be unstable, and these may require percutaneous pinning to maintain reduction. Fractures that are not located at the base are treated in a similar manner to those of the other metacarpals.[6]

Treatment in the emergency department consists of pain relief, immobilization in a thumb spica splint, and urgent referral to a hand specialist.

Intra-Articular Fractures

A **Bennett fracture** (Figure 9-8A) is an oblique fracture through the articular surface with dislocation of the metacarpal base. The volar fragment remains attached to the anterior oblique ligament, and the abductor pollicis longus tendon dislocates the metacarpal base proximally and dorsally. More than 20 different methods of treatment are described in the literature, ranging from early active motion without reduction to open reduction and internal fixation. Due to the deforming forces of the abductor pollicis longus tendon, the standard of care involves some sort of fixation. Most authors advocate attempts at closed reduction and percutaneous fixation with K-wires through the base of the metacarpal into the trapezium. If percutaneous efforts fail to maintain adequate reduction (no more than 2 to 3 mm of joint surface displacement), open reduction and internal fixation with AO screws is advised.[7] The thumb then is immobilized in a thumb spica cast for 4 to 6 weeks. Treatment in the emergency department includes pain relief, immobilization in a thumb spica splint, and referral to a hand specialist for definitive outpatient treatment.

A **Rolando fracture** (Figure 9-8B) is a comminuted intra-articular metacarpal base fracture. It is classically described as having either a T or Y configuration, but common use includes any multifragmented intra-articular metacarpal base fracture. These fractures occur less fre-

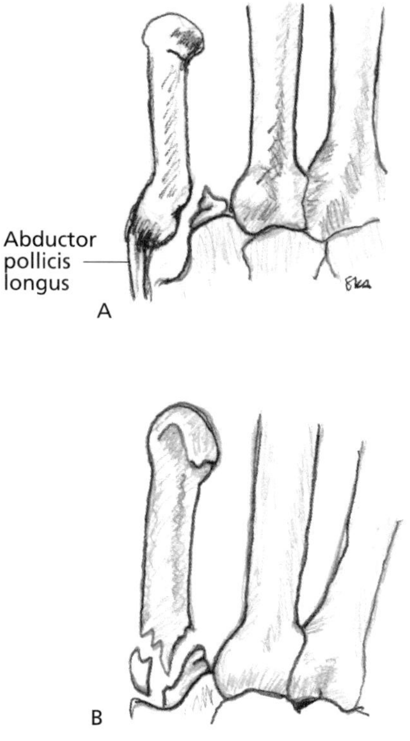

Figure 9-8.

A) *Bennett fracture. A volar articular fragment remains tethered to the anterior oblique ligament, whereas the metacarpal shaft is displaced by the traction of the abductor pollicis longus tendon.*
B) *Rolando fracture. Classically a T or Y intra-articular fracture but refers to any comminuted intra-articular first metacarpal fracture.*

quently than Bennett fractures. Treatment is determined by the number and size of the bone fragments; even with early intervention by a hand specialist, residual pain and some loss of mobility are common, and recovery to full function is difficult. With few and relatively larger bone fragments, open reduction and internal fixation may be attempted. For severely comminuted fractures, periods of external traction may be attempted if radiographs taken while traction is applied show some improvement in articular opposition. If no improvement with traction is seen on initial radiographs, a short period of molded immobilization to relieve pain is warranted.[7] Early active mobilization is advised to recreate some articular surface. Emergency department treatment includes pain relief, immobilization in a thumb spica splint, and urgent referral to a hand specialist for definitive treatment.

Complications

Complications can occur with both surgical and nonsurgical treatment of thumb metacarpal fractures. They include joint stiffness, residual pain, malunion, nonunion, motion compromise, and superficial and deep infections. Loss of motion can occur from adhesions and scarring of the muscle, but early mobilization of stable fractures increases the likelihood of recovery of full motion.[8] Complications are common with Rolando fractures, less common with Bennett fractures, and least likely with extra-articular first metacarpal fractures.

References

1. Littler JW. *Symposium on Reconstructive Hand Surgery.* Vol 9. St Louis, Mo: CV Mosby; 1974.
2. Greene TL. Metacarpal fractures. In: *Hand Surgery Update of the American Academy of Orthopaedic Surgeons.* Rosemont, Ill: American Academy of Orthopaedic Surgeons; 1996:11-15.
3. Williams JM, Greer SE. Boxer's fracture: an indicator of intentional and recurrent injury. *Am J Emerg Med.* 1999;17:357-360.
4. Braakman M. Is anatomical reduction of fractures of the fourth and fifth metacarpals useful? *Acta Orthopaed Belg.* 1997;63:106-109.
5. Ali A. The biomechanical effects of angulated boxer's fractures. *J Hand Surg.* 1999;24:835-844.
6. Mastey RD, Weiss AP, Akelman E. Primary care of hand and wrist athletic injuries. *Clin Sports Med.* 1997;16(4):705-724.
7. Lee SG, Jupiter JB. Phalangeal and metacarpal fractures of the hand. *Hand Clin.* 2000;16(3):323-332.
8. Hester PW, Blazar PE. Complications of hand and wrist surgery in the athlete. *Clin Sports Med.* 1999;18(4):811-829.

CHAPTER 10

Phalangeal Fractures

Todd H. Chaffin, MD, FACEP

The digits of the hand are complex anatomic structures that allow a wide range of sensory and motor skills in the performance of activities of daily living. It is for this reason that they are frequently injured and require physician evaluation. Emergency physicians must be skilled in obtaining a detailed history and performing a complete physical examination. Once these are accomplished, the physician should be able to either treat most digit injuries or determine which ones require referral to another specialist.

Injured digits exhibit remarkable healing and functional recovery[1] when treating physicians adhere to commonly accepted surgical techniques and proper immobilization procedures. The use of specialized wires, screws, and replantation techniques allows many injuries to heal with minimal morbidity. Even though these specialized surgical techniques typically are beyond the scope of emergency medicine practice, emergency physicians still can reduce morbidity by providing appropriate primary fracture management, wound care, prophylactic antibiotic therapy, and preservation of amputated parts.

Anatomy and Mechanics

Emergency physicians must have a reasonable understanding of hand anatomy so that they can initiate treatment and provide consulting physicians with suitable descriptions of fractures and associated soft tissue injuries.

History

The physician should elicit from the patient the time, location, and mechanism of injury; hand dominance; description of occupation; age; previous injuries; and preexisting conditions such as arthritis or impaired circulation. The patient's symptoms, such as numbness and loss of function, and the position of the digit at the time of injury also should be determined. The history also should include information on treatment provided before the patient's arrival in the emergency department, such as wound cleansing and digit manipulation, as well as environmental or chemical exposures, use of protective garments, and proper machine safety, if indicated. Information regarding activities or hobbies that are important to the patient is often overlooked in history-taking but is necessary for the patient's maximal functional outcome or prognosis.

Physical Examination

An optimal examination is performed under direct lighting with the extremity placed on an arm board and the affected digit anesthetized after neurovascular function has been assessed.

Inspection. The orientation of the digit relative to the position of function should be noted, along with any rotational deformity (Figure 10-1) or deviation. The presence of discoloration, soiling, swelling, ecchymosis, and soft tissue injuries is important.

Neurovascular assessment should include the Allen test, capillary refill, and two-point discrimination and light touch testing.

Tendon, ligament, and joint capsule injuries are evaluated using range of motion and stress testing and, if there is an open wound, direct inspection.

Wound exploration may be required to identify vital structure injury or the presence of gross contamination or foreign bodies.

Radiography

For most injuries, PA, lateral, and 45-degree externally rotated oblique views are necessary. The addition of stress, contralateral digit, and 45-degree internally rotated oblique views can be helpful when epiphyseal fractures, congenital anomalies, or certain fractures are in question.[2]

Diagnosis

A working diagnosis can be formulated after completion of the history, physical examination, radiography, and if necessary, wound exploration. Digit anesthesia may be required to assess tendon and joint function adequately. Pain relief can be achieved with a buffered, long-acting, non–epinephrine-containing anesthetic agent administered with a 27- to 30-gauge needle.

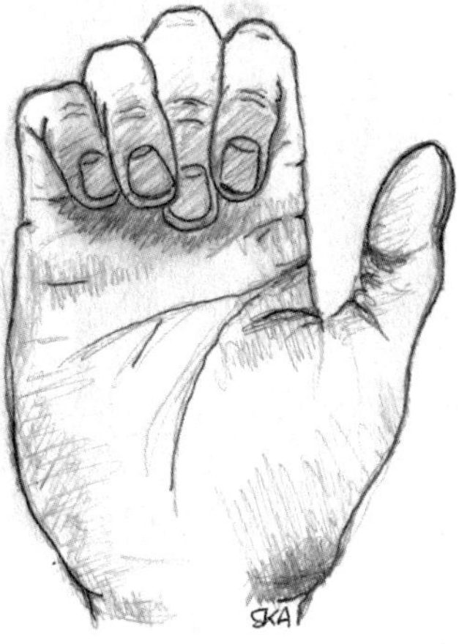

Figure 10-1.

Rotational deformity of the ring finger results in an abnormal position in flexion. Normally, the planes of the nails should be parallel, and the digits should point to the scaphoid tubercle.

Treatment Options

Indications for prompt specialty consultation include the following:

- Angulated or displaced fractures that do not maintain reduction
- Multiple fractures that require skeletal stabilization
- Displaced intra-articular fractures
- Spiral, rotated, or oblique fractures
- Neurovascular or tendon injuries or soft tissue loss of more than 1 cm^2
- Soft tissue loss that precludes adequate coverage or significant contamination
- Partial or complete amputations

Emergency Department Management

Pain management should be initiated promptly with elevation of the extremity and, when appropriate, intravenous narcotic administration and a digit/wrist nerve block.

Proper wound management includes foreign body removal (including rings), skin cleansing, and copious irrigation of open wounds. All wounds should be covered with antibiotic ointment, a nonadherent dressing, and a noncircumferential, loosely fitting gauze dressing. Postwound antibiotic administration and tetanus vaccination should be provided in the correct clinical setting.

The principles of immobilization are as follows[3]:

- A long finger splint suffices for most phalangeal fractures, except when deforming tendon forces are present. In this situation, immobilization of the wrist may also be required.
- A radial gutter splint with a hole for the thumb may be used for fractures of the index and middle fingers, and an ulnar gutter splint may be used for fractures that involve the ring and little fingers. If the patient is a child or if patient reliability is in question, a gauntlet cast can be used to immobilize the fracture and its adjacent digits.
- Isolated phalanx fractures can be splinted with a malleable, foam-backed metal splint for a reliable patient, and the adjacent, uninjured digit can be included (buddy-splinting) for extra stability and protection.
- Thumb fractures are best stabilized with a thumb spica splint or a radial gutter splint.

Proximal Phalanx Fractures

Proximal phalanx fractures (Figure 10-2) frequently result from a direct blow to the shaft or from hyperextension or torque forces. The proximal phalanx is responsible for positioning of the distal phalanx and has the greatest range of motion; for this reason, displaced and unstable fractures are poorly tolerated.

The following fractures require orthopedic referral[4]:

Nondisplaced stable fractures may be braced with a dorsal long finger splint that extends from the metacarpal through the middle phalanx, with the MCP joint at 60 degrees of flexion and the PIP joint at 30 degrees of flexion. With a reliable patient, dynamic splinting and early range of motion by buddy-taping to the adjacent uninjured digit are permissible.

Unstable or displaced fractures. Oblique, spiral, and angulated fractures (Figure 10-3A) may be splinted with a radial or an ulnar gutter splint, incorporating the wrist to eliminate deforming tendon forces. Reduction with longitudinal traction may be attempted.

Intra-articular MCP or PIP joint fractures (Figure 10-3B-D) are splinted similarly; however, some prefer buddy-taping to allow early range of motion if the intra-articular fracture is stable and has no step-off.

For **displaced fractures** (condylar or marginal), referral is mandatory because these fractures usually require internal fixation. They may be temporarily splinted with radial or ulnar gutter splints.

Sesamoid fractures of the thumb MCP joint (and, less commonly, of the index and little fingers) are uncommon and may be associated with proximal thumb fractures. They occur most often during sports activities when the joint receives a direct blow or is hyperextended. Radiographic detection may be missed unless the injury is sought specifically. Treatment consists of 2 to 3 weeks of immobilization in a dorsal or volar splint from the metacarpal to distal phalanx with the IP joint kept in 10 to 15 degrees of flexion.[5]

Middle Phalanx Fractures

Middle phalanx fractures (Figure 10-4) can occur from a direct blow or axial loading or hyperdeviation forces. Such fractures frequently involve the neck, proximal waist, or intra-articular structures. These

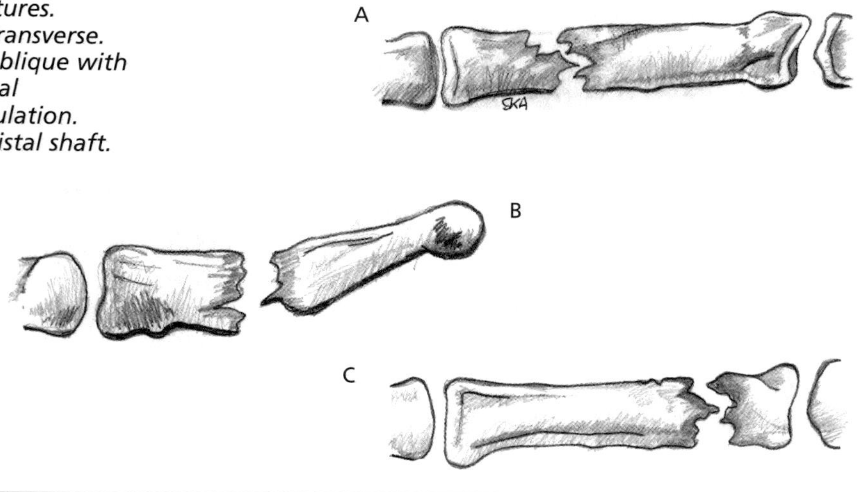

Figure 10-2.
Proximal phalanx fractures.
A) *Transverse.*
B) *Oblique with dorsal angulation.*
C) *Distal shaft.*

injuries are divided into nondisplaced stable (usually transverse) and displaced unstable (spiral, oblique, angulated, intra-articular) fractures. Displaced or unstable fractures result from deforming tendon forces that traverse the fracture site.

Nondisplaced stable fractures are treated with dynamic splinting by buddy-taping to an adjacent uninjured digit. This provides stability as well as joint motion, which limits complications of joint stiffness. To ensure proper alignment, these fractures require close followup care and repeat radiographs in 10 to 14 days. Comminuted fractures may appear stable but can be unstable and are best splinted with a gutter splint to incorporate the wrist as well as the injured digit. These fractures also should be followed closely, with repeat radiographs performed in 10 to 14 days.

Angulated, displaced, and spiral fractures are considered unstable and should be immobilized with a radial or an ulnar gutter splint and referred for surgical stabilization.

Intra-articular basilar and condylar fractures (Figure 10-5) involve cartilaginous or ligamentous structures and are at risk for suboptimal

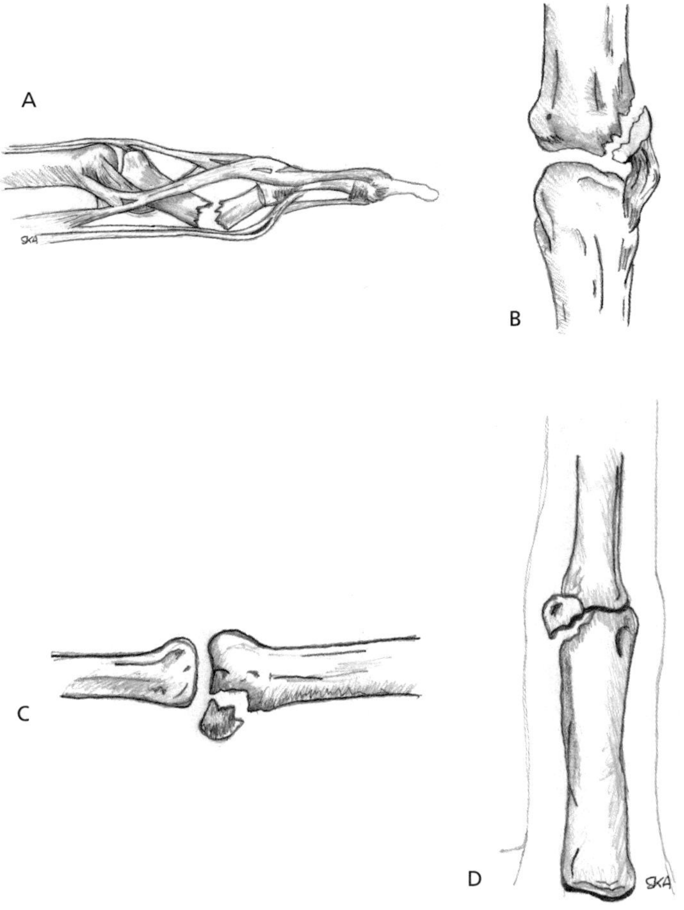

Figure 10-3.

Proximal phalanx fractures. **A)** *Volar angulated midshaft fracture resulting from opposing extensor and flexor tendon forces.* **B)** *Marginal.* **C)** *Volar.* **D)** *Displaced condylar.*

outcomes unless treated appropriately. If the fracture is displaced (step-off of 1 mm or more), surgical treatment may be indicated. In a nondisplaced fracture, a long finger splint in the position of function suffices, followed by early mobilization. Some recommend dynamic splinting, except for base fractures. These fractures should be immobilized in a long finger splint and referred because they are prone to healing with complications and may require specialized splinting techniques. Displaced fractures are splinted in radial or ulnar gutter splints and referred for possible surgical stabilization.

Displaced volar intra-articular base fractures of the middle phalanx typically result from a dorsal PIP joint dislocation and, depending on ligament damage, may result in joint instability. A large fracture fragment carries most of the collateral ligament with it, resulting in an unstable PIP joint. Some recommend internal fixation for fractures that involve more than 25% of the articular surface; others treat conservatively with splinting. Emergency department treatment consists of immobilization in an aluminum splint or a gutter splint and prompt orthopedic referral (see Chapter 11 for a complete discussion).

Displaced dorsal intra-articular avulsion fractures of the middle phalanx result in avulsion of the central tendon from its insertion on the proximal middle phalangeal base. If undiagnosed, the PIP joint falls into flexion and the lateral bands slip volar to the equator of the PIP joint. In this position, they act as flexors of the PIP joint and extensors

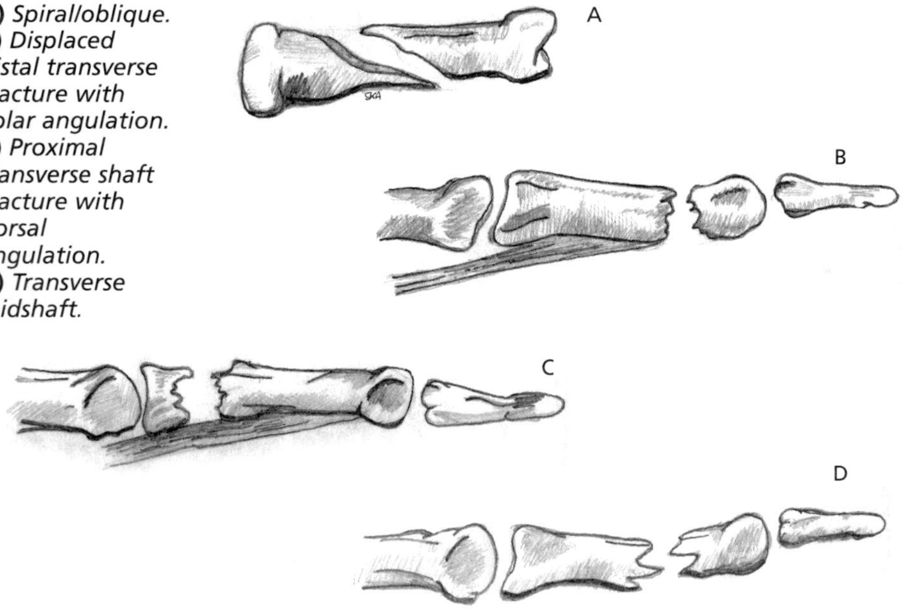

Figure 10-4.
Middle phalanx fractures.
A) *Spiral/oblique.*
B) *Displaced distal transverse fracture with volar angulation.*
C) *Proximal transverse shaft fracture with dorsal angulation.*
D) *Transverse midshaft.*

of the DIP joint, resulting in a boutonnière deformity. Acute injuries are treated with internal fixation. Emergency department treatment of dorsal middle phalangeal fractures consists of immobilization with the wrist in 30 degrees of extension and the MCP and PIP joints in full extension, followed by prompt orthopedic referral (see Chapter 11).

Distal Phalanx Fractures

These fractures result from a direct blow to the extended tip or dorsal surface and can be divided into the following categories: comminuted (usually the tuft), transverse, longitudinal, and intra-articular (Figure 10-6).

Comminuted (tuft) fractures frequently involve the nail bed. The fracture itself is stable because fibrous septae and the nail act as a splint. Treatment consists of 2 to 4 weeks of protection with a cage or molded aluminum splint that encloses the distal phalanx yet allows DIP motion. The presence of a subungual hematoma implies a nail bed injury that may require surgical repair. Most agree that, if the nail plate has been avulsed from its bed or from beneath the eponychial fold, the nail plate should be removed and the nail bed repaired with fine absorbable suture. Some believe that a subungual hematoma that involves 25% to 50% or more of the nail bed requires nail removal and nail bed repair. Others recommend simple evacuation through nail trephination with a

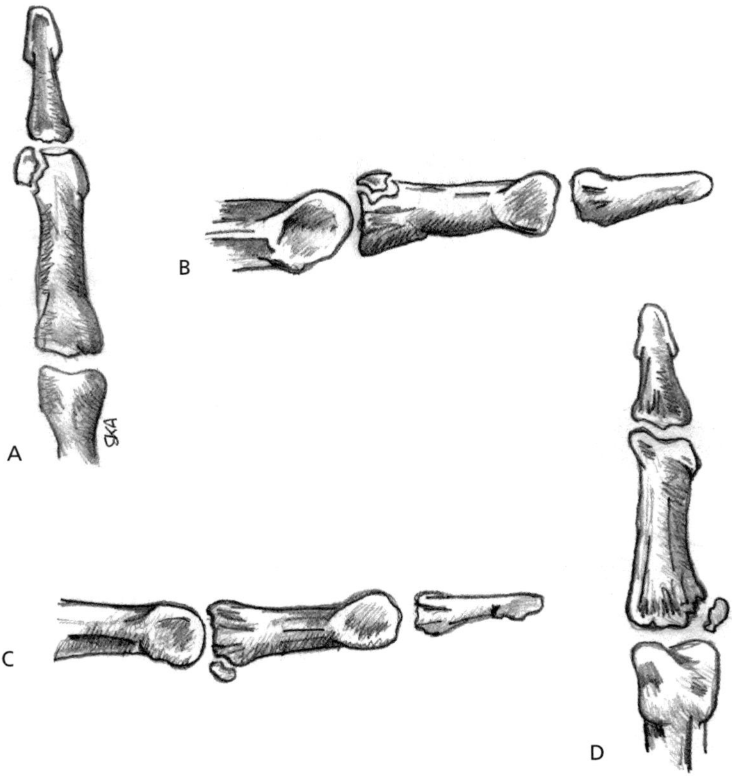

Figure 10-5.

Intra-articular middle phalanx fractures.
A) *Displaced condylar.*
B) *Dorsal avulsion fracture.*
C) *Volar avulsion fracture.*
D) *Marginal avulsion fracture.*

nail drill or heated cautery tip.[6,7] The weight of evidence is shifting to this more conservative approach in injuries in which the nail and nail margin are intact. Simple trephination provides substantial pain relief and an acceptable long-term functional and cosmetic result. Although this procedure technically creates an open fracture, it is one of the few situations in which prophylactic antibiotic coverage is unwarranted. If the nail is removed, a stent should be placed beneath the eponychial fold for 10 days by using the original nail or nonadhering gauze. This prevents nail bed adhesions, assists in nail regrowth, and may limit new nail deformity.

Transverse fractures often are nondisplaced and require only protective splinting of the distal phalanx for 2 weeks or until the fracture is painless and stable (4 to 6 weeks). Displaced transverse fractures should be reduced, but this may be difficult due to interposed adipose tissue. If the fracture cannot be reduced by manipulation or remains unstable after reduction, the distal phalanx should be splinted and the patient referred to a surgeon for pinning. If repeat radiographs reveal that reduction is satisfactory, treatment should proceed as for a nondisplaced fracture. Often, when displaced fractures are treated conservatively, they heal by a fibrous union that eventually provides a stable, painless phalanx; however, this may take 6 months or longer.

Longitudinal fractures traverse the length of the phalanx and generally are nondisplaced. A splint should be placed from the middle to the distal phalanges, leaving the PIP joint free. The splint remains for 3 to 4 weeks, followed by passive range of motion exercise until the digit is painless. Displaced fractures may be difficult to reduce and are best referred to a surgeon after similar splinting for possible pinning.

Intra-articular fractures are divided into dorsal injuries (mallet finger) and volar fractures. **Mallet finger** deformity (Figure 10-7) results from tendon or bone injuries that prevent full DIP extension and appear to have a DIP flexion deformity. Overstretching or tendon rupture without a fracture may produce a mallet finger deformity. The exact diagnosis is confirmed with radiography.

With regard to treatment, many divide these fractures into those that involve less than or more than 33% of the articular surface; fractures that involve more than 33% of the articular surface are treated surgically with K-wire fixation. This practice is questioned by

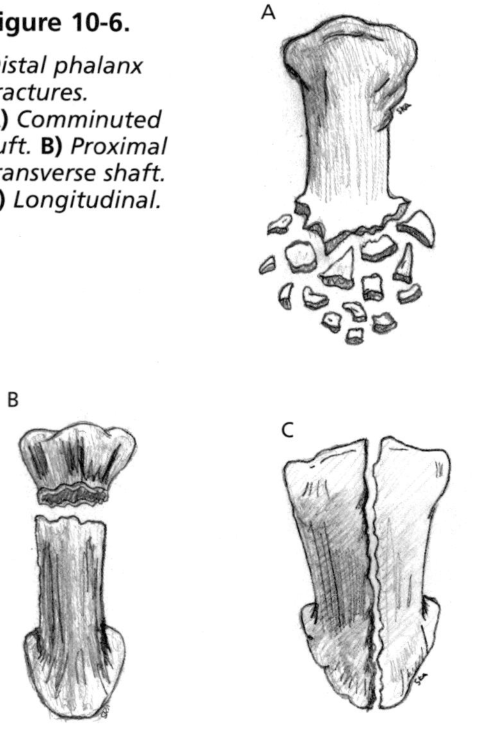

Figure 10-6.

Distal phalanx fractures. **A)** *Comminuted tuft.* **B)** *Proximal transverse shaft.* **C)** *Longitudinal.*

some,[8] who have had considerable success treating mallet finger injuries conservatively with dorsal splinting, even when the distal phalanx is subluxed volarly, reserving surgery for those injuries that fail conservative treatment. Regardless of the type of injury, mallet finger deformity should be splinted in slight hyperextension with a middle-to-distal phalangeal splint with the PIP joint free (Figure 10-8). Several commercial splints are available, but a simple aluminum or paper clip splint may be fashioned and applied. With conservative treatment, the splint must be left on for 6 to 8 weeks, followed by nocturnal protective splinting for 2 to 4 weeks. The patient must be advised not to test the DIP joint prematurely because this can disrupt any bone healing that has occurred and may lead to a failed union. All such fractures require close followup care. If a failed union does occur, surgical treatment is indicated.

Volar fractures usually are of the avulsion type (Figure 10-9). As long as there is some DIP joint flexion, these fractures may be treated for 6 to 8 weeks with dorsal or volar splinting, with only the DIP joint immobilized and kept in partial flexion (5 to 10 degrees).

Profundus tendon rupture from volar injuries and displaced avulsion fractures may be missed unless the function of the profundus tendon is tested properly. Digital radiographs may show minimal bone involvement; on occasion, the avulsed fragment retracts proximally giving the appearance of an avulsion fracture of the proximal or middle phalanx. These injuries require a splint that incorporates the wrist with the finger maintained in flexion, along with referral for prompt surgical repair.

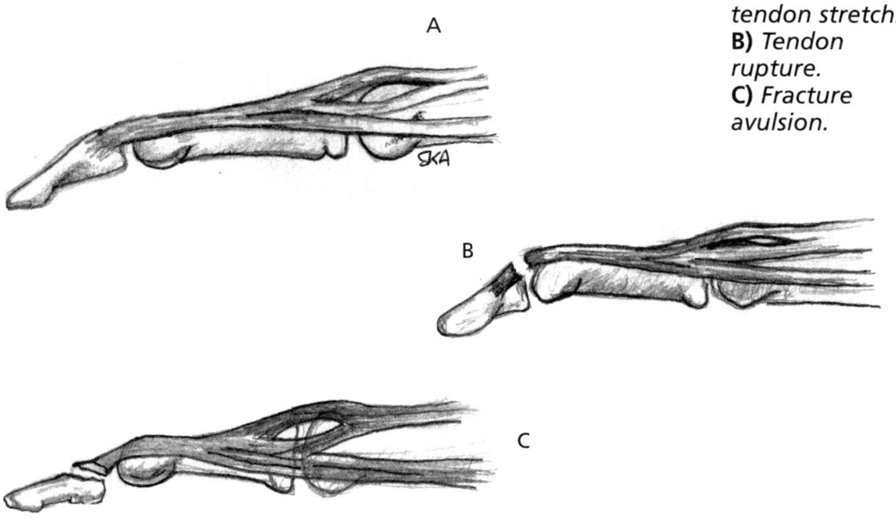

Figure 10-7.

Mallet finger deformity resulting from: **A)** *Extensor tendon stretch.* **B)** *Tendon rupture.* **C)** *Fracture avulsion.*

Complications

The complications associated with phalangeal fractures are the same as those for other fractures. However, the following complications should be noted:

- Callus formation can impede tendon or joint motion.
- Compartment syndrome can occur with circumferential dressings, crush injuries, or casts. Direct inspection of the digit is indicated if signs of impaired circulation are present.
- Infections are uncommon when standard wound care practices, including irrigation and exploration, are followed.
- Malunion can occur in fractures that are angulated, displaced, rotated, or shortened.
- Nonunion can result from interposed soft tissue between fracture ends or uncorrected displaced fractures. Distal phalangeal fractures often show delayed union; however, a stable fibrous union is normal.
- Periarticular injuries can result in arthritis, joint deformity, or stiffness.

Special Situations

Amputations

Amputations can be managed initially in the emergency department. Distal phalanx injuries heal satisfactorily, with or without grafting or with primary wound closure. Even when some bone is exposed, these injuries can be treated with antibiotic ointment and a nonadherent dressing and given adequate time to heal by secondary intention.[9] This may take several months. If primary closure is performed, some rongeuring may be required to provide adequate skin closure. Splinting for protection is required, as is specialty consultation. Indications for replantation are best

Figure 10-8.

Proper splinting technique for mallet finger deformity.

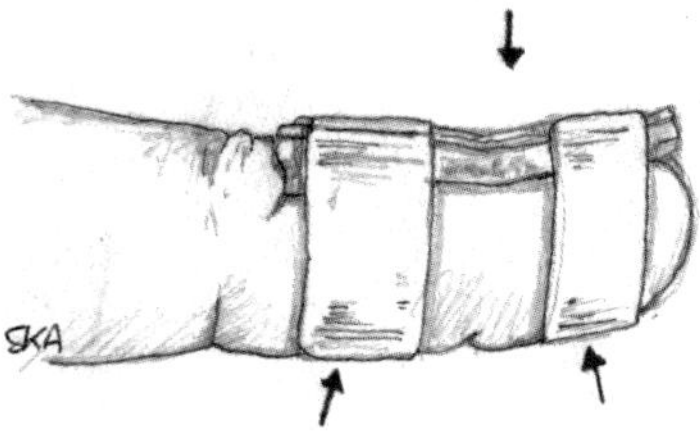

Figure 10-9.

Volar fracture with retraction of the avulsed fragment by the profundus tendon.

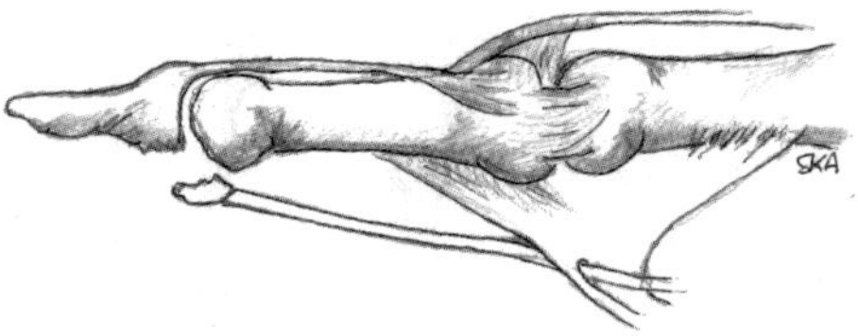

discussed with a consultant if the time since the injury is less than 12 hours. Indications for replantation include the following:

- Pediatric patients
- Amputations distal to the superficialis tendon insertion on the middle phalanx
- Multiple digits
- Thumb
- Patients without significant psychiatric or preexisting medical conditions

Elderly Patients

Fractures in elderly persons occur when osteopenic bone is subjected to trauma from a fall. Every effort should be made to avoid unnecessary immobilization of adjacent joints or digits and to mobilize injuries as soon as possible. Prolonged rehabilitation, reduced function, and chronic stiffness are common in this age group.

Pediatric Patients

Because children have enhanced healing potential, pediatric injuries often can be treated conservatively, as long as there is no displacement or rotation. However, followup care provided by a specialist is recommended. Depending on the child's age, immobilization from the elbow or wrist should be a consideration in this relatively noncompliant age group.[10]

Salter-Harris fractures are common and should be kept in mind before diagnosing a sprain, which may be less common than an actual fracture. The physician should look closely for periepiphyseal cortical disruption or buckling, which indicates the presence of a fracture.

Transverse, nonangulated, and nondisplaced fractures usually are stable and can be treated with gutter splinting or buddy-taping. A followup radiograph in 1 week is indicated to check for misalignment.

Greenstick fractures, without angulation, are treated with gutter splinting or buddy-taping, with followup radiographs in 10 days.

Disposition

To provide appropriate referrals, decrease morbidity, and limit medical-legal concerns, emergency physicians must have a detailed understanding of fracture management. One thing that is often neglected is the need to engage the patient in a discussion regarding his or her injury, potential complications, and outcome expectations. This proactive discussion should be documented in the medical record and include the following:

- Analgesics provided to cover the expected duration of pain. For most injuries, a digit block with a long-acting anesthetic agent provides several hours of complete pain relief, followed by hydrocodone for several days.
- The patient must be instructed to elevate the extremity above heart level for the first 24 hours.
- The patient also must be informed of potential complications, such as cosmetic appearance, deformity, infection, and digit stiffness,

and rehabilitation needs. If the fingernail growth plate has been disrupted, the patient must be advised of possible nail deformity.

- Office appointments with the referral physician for repeat radiographs and injury and splint rechecks, wound checks (within 48 hours), and suture removal (at 8 to 10 days) should be made before the patient is discharged.
- If indicated, postwound antibiotic coverage for 3 days may be started in the emergency department.
- The patient should be given instructions for standard wound care and cast or splint precautions, along with instructions to seek medical care immediately if unexpected symptoms or questions develop.
- Some patients need instructions regarding work restrictions for work-related injuries. Many companies provide modified work or light duty, of which the physician may be unaware. For this reason, it is better to provide a restriction that allows the patient to use the uninjured extremity or allows for light duty with the injured extremity. If modified or restricted work is unavailable, it is the employer's responsibility to decide whether the patient should be given time off work (see Chapter 22).
- Smoking and alcohol use should be discontinued due to the adverse effects on circulation and healing.

Rehabilitation and Long-Term Care

Most fractures heal satisfactorily with little morbidity. Rehabilitation may be required, especially if the digit injury has been immobilized. Referral to a skilled physical or occupational therapist often is required for such complications and is best prescribed by the physician who provides followup care.

References

1. Ip W, Ng K, Chow S. A prospective study of 924 digital fractures of the hand. *Injury.* 1996;27(4):279-285.
2. Street J. Radiographs of phalangeal fractures: importance of the internally rotated oblique projection for diagnosis. *Am J Radiol.* 1993;160:575.
3. Harrison BP, Hilliard MW. Emergency department evaluation and treatment of hand injuries. *Emerg Med Clin North Am.* 1999;17(4):793-822.
4. Schenck R. Classification of fractures and dislocations of the proximal interphalangeal joint. *Hand Clinics.* 1994;10(2):179-185.
5. Dong P, Seeger L, Shapiro M, et al. Fractures of the sesamoid bones of the thumb. *Am J Sports Med.* 1995;23(3):336-339.
6. Meek S, White M. Subungual haematomas: is simple trephining enough? *J Accid Emerg Med.* 1998;15:269-271.
7. Rosner SE, Gellman H. Comparison of nail bed repair versus nail trephination for subungual hematomas in children. *J Hand Surgery.* 1999;24A(6):1166-1170.
8. Lubahn J, Hood J. Fractures of the distal interphalangeal joint. *Clin Orthop Rel Res.* 1996;327:12-20.
9. Mennen U, Wiese A. Fingertip injuries, management with semi-occlusive dressing. *J Hand Surg [Br].* 1993;18B(4):416-422.
10. Morrissy R, Weinstein S, eds. *Lovell and Winter's Pediatric Orthopaedics.* 4th ed. Philadelphia, Pa: Lippincott; 1996.

CHAPTER 11

Joint Injuries

Arthur F. Proust, MD, FACEP

Emergency department visits for the care of hand injuries are common. These injuries range from apparent benign sprains to complex fracture-dislocations and crush injuries. Optimal treatment should be initiated promptly because, more than any other anatomic area, the hand is exposed to more potential dangers and requires precise movement to meet daily demands. However, the severity of injury may not be readily apparent. Subtle injuries to the joints are often missed compared with injuries that produce gross deformities or radiographic abnormalities. Indeed, because the healing of joint structures is often imperfect and unpredictable, early recognition and treatment are crucial to the restoration of full function.

Initial Evaluation and Management

History

A precise history helps lead to an accurate diagnosis. The type and extent of injury often are determined by the direction and magnitude of force to the joint. For example, intra-articular fractures are the result of an axial load. A lateral force may produce a lateral dislocation or collateral ligament injury. Volar plate tears and dorsal dislocations are the result of a hyperextension mechanism. The severity of injury may be predicted by the onset of pain, swelling, and ecchymosis.

A history that includes certain sporting activities or occupations may predispose or provide clues to specific injuries. For example, ulnar collateral ligament injuries of the thumb MCP joint often are the result of radial stress applied from a ski pole; this injury once was known to occur in British gamekeepers.

Physical Examination

Visual inspection to detect deformity, swelling, and ecchymosis may pinpoint the site of injury. Examination of the injured hand may be deterred by pain produced by the dense sensory fibers. Acute swelling and pain may camouflage an existing deformity or a dislocation. Functional impairment is implied by an abnormal carriage of the hand.

Active range of motion is a test of joint stability. This is most readily assessed with digital anesthesia, which eliminates the influence of pain. Although significant ligament injury may be present, near-normal active range of motion implies that functional recovery will occur with conservative rather than surgical treatment.[1] Finally, the evaluation of sensory function and determination of the point of maximal tenderness should be completed before a digital block is used.

Passive range of motion and ligament stressing can determine the location and degree of ligament injury. Volar plate and collateral ligament integrity are assessed by anteroposterior and radial-ulnar stress, respectively. This is accomplished in both extension and moderate flexion to eliminate volar plate stabilization. It also must be done gently so as not to produce a complete tear.

Radiography

Indications for radiography include swelling and tenderness and a suspicious mechanism. Standard views include AP, oblique, and, most important for individual digits, a **true lateral**. Failure to obtain this radiographic view leads to many errors in the diagnosis of joint injuries. Lateral views of the hand are not adequate because superimposition of the three other digits conceals important details. Oblique views may reveal injuries such as condylar fractures, but lateral views can delineate the presence or extent of chip fractures at the bases of the phalanges, as well as subluxations or fracture-subluxations of the PIP joint. Ligament disruption also can be demonstrated with stress radiographs.

Management Principles

Most joint injuries of the hand are managed conservatively, that is, with buddy-taping or immobilization followed by active range of motion exercises. Indications for surgical repair include complex or irreducible dislocations, joint instability after reduction, and displaced or large intra-articular fractures. The benefit of the procedure must always outweigh the residual surgical effects of limitation of motion caused by postsurgical periarticular fibrosis.

Residual joint stiffness and diminished flexion are the usual long-term sequelae of joint injuries to the hand. With this in mind, immobilization should include 60 to 70 degrees of flexion of the MCP joints and 30 to 35 degrees of flexion of the IP joints. Uninvolved joints should have minimal, if any, immobilization. Therapy guided toward active range of motion is encouraged because prolonged swelling and stiffness often accompany even minor joint injuries.

Partial Ligament Injuries

With incomplete ligament tears or **sprains**, anatomic continuity is maintained. There is sufficient capsular support to resist displacement with stress.

Treatment

Depending on injury severity, an acutely injured ligament requires 2 to 3 weeks of buddy-taping or immobilization for optimal healing. The goals of treatment include time to allow soft tissue healing and proper exercises to restore maximal joint motion.

Interphalangeal joints are best splinted in 30 to 35 degrees of flexion. Metacarpophalangeal joints are splinted in 60 to 70 degrees of flexion, and the thumb MCP joint is splinted in 30 degrees of flexion. Aluminum splints or volar plaster can be used.

Active range of motion exercises are recommended after immobilization. A mobile splint, with the injured digit taped to an adjacent digit, for approximately 5 to 7 days may be necessary depending on persistent soft tissue reaction. Buddy-taping with active range of motion from the outset has been advocated as an alternative.

Complications

Persistent swelling and stiffness for 6 to 12 months after severe partial tears are the most common complications. Periarticular fibrosis may develop and produce some permanent swelling and joint movement restriction. Permanent limitation of range of motion can occur with neglect or with patients who fail to exercise properly.

Interphalangeal Joint Injuries

The PIP and DIP joints are structurally identical. The IP joints are **uniaxial hinge joints** that move in a sagittal plane. The PIP joint flexes to approximately 105 degrees from full extension, but the DIP joint flexes no more than 90 degrees. This difference is secondary to the FDP tendon, which inserts closer to the articulation of the DIP joint than the FDS tendon, which inserts distal to the volar plate.

Interphalangeal joint stability in response to lateral and oblique stresses is caused in part by a doubling of the proximal bicondylar transverse phalangeal vertical diameter. Also, the central tongue-and-groove mechanism resists shearing and rotary forces.

The sturdy, quadrangular **collateral ligaments** along with the fibrocartilaginous volar plate further augment IP joint stability and strength (Figure 11-1). The collateral ligaments are parallel

Figure 11-1.

Interphalangeal joint anatomy. Note the boxlike configuration of the collateral ligaments and the accessory ligaments that merge into the volar plate, which is anchored proximally by the check ligaments.

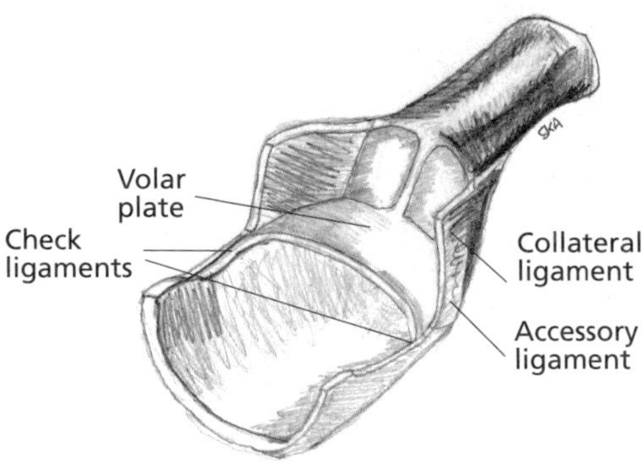

radial and ulnar fibers arising from the radial and ulnar aspects of the proximal condyles. They insert onto the volar base of the more distal phalanx and to the margins of the volar plate. Triangular, distinct, thin **accessory collateral ligaments** extend in a volar orientation and insert along the proximal volar plate to complete the lateral wall of the IP joint capsule. The fibrous **volar plate** forms the floor of the joint; it is 2 to 3 mm thick at its distal phalangeal insertion before tapering to a thin membranous sheet proximally. Thus, during maximal flexion, the volar plate can fold onto itself.

A pair of resilient **check ligaments** firmly attached to the proximal volar periosteum arise from the radial and ulnar aspects of the proximal volar plate. These ligaments are both supple enough to fold onto themselves during maximal IP flexion and strong enough to resist IP hyperextension.

The taut volar plate and the volar fibers of the collateral ligament stabilize the IP joint in extension. In flexion, the joint is stabilized by the capsular fibers stretched over the condylar flare. Hyperextension may be averted by the volar plate and the check and accessory ligaments.

Distal Interphalangeal Joint

The DIP joint is stabilized in all positions by adjacent flexor and extensor tendon insertions, strong collateral ligaments, and the short lever arm of the distal phalanx. Dislocations of the DIP joint are uncommon; however, when dislocations do occur, they are almost always dorsal, although they may present laterally in a jackknife manner. These dislocations often are open as a result of skin shear from the underlying firmly anchored osteocutaneous fibers. Radiographs are used to determine whether frequently associated mallet fracture-dislocations are present.

A **closed reduction** is almost always stable because both flexor and extensor tendons remain attached to the distal phalanx. After **digital nerve block**, reduction takes place with hyperextension and the application of longitudinal traction distracting the bayonet-opposed distal phalanx. This is followed by dorsal pressure to the base of the distal phalanx to achieve reduction. **Functional stability**, tested by active range of motion, reveals that enough ligament fibers remain to allow healing with minimal fibrosis. Two to 3 weeks of DIP joint immobilization in 30 degrees of flexion usually are sufficient.

Postreduction instability in response to active range of motion can occur with either open or closed DIP joint dislocations. This is indicative of complete and multiple ligament disruption that requires surgical repair.

Treatment for a patient with an **open DIP dislocation** should be directed toward surgical débridement of devitalized and contaminated tissue, copious wound irrigation, and gentle reduction. Prophylactic antibiotics are recommended. Immobilization is performed as described.

Open reduction is required for irreducible DIP dislocations. Three mechanisms have been reported:

- Dorsal dislocation with the volar plate interposed in the joint

- FDP tendon entrapment seen in DIP dislocations with collateral ligament rupture
- Osteochondral fragment or sesamoid bone interposition within the joint

Chronic (unreduced) DIP dislocations are those of 3 weeks' duration or longer. Closed reduction is ultimately unsuccessful, requiring open reduction through a dorsal exposure. Because of periarticular soft tissue contracture, surgical intervention may be technically challenging. The prognosis for joint mobility is poor.

Proximal Interphalangeal Joint

The PIP joint is the most frequently injured joint in the hand. The exact incidence is not known because reductions frequently are performed on the playing field and medical care is never solicited. The most common mechanism of injury is an axial load and hyperextension.

The PIP joint occupies a position of importance in the hand with function that is dependent on mobility; in no other area is the anatomy as complex and interrelated. Integrity is maintained by the junction of the volar plate at the base of the middle phalanx and the collateral ligament system (Figure 11-1). This boxlike configuration forms a strong three-dimensional hinge. For joint instability to occur, there must be disruption of at least two of the three supporting structures.[1]

Injuries to the PIP joint involve combinations of collateral ligament injuries, volar plate injuries, dislocations, and fracture-dislocations. The most important clinical consideration is to determine which injuries are stable and which are not.

Lateral Dislocations

A lateral dislocation occurs with radial or ulnar directed force to the extended joint. This ruptures one collateral ligament and a major portion of the volar plate insertion, causing the middle phalanx to pivot and assume an oblique orientation. Radial collateral ligament ruptures occur six times more frequently than ulnar collateral ligament ruptures.

The joint often reduces spontaneously; otherwise, longitudinal traction easily provides reduction. Despite disruption of the ligament box complex, with few exceptions the ligaments return to their normal position with realignment of the joint. Lateral stability is enhanced by the flexor tendon, its sheath, the lateral bands, and retinacular ligaments of the extensor mechanism. After reduction, however, ligament disruption may not be appreciated because active flexion and extension usually are not limited. Postreduction films are mandatory to confirm reduction; small avulsion fractures may occur.

Under digital anesthesia, suspected or confirmed lateral PIP dislocations should have each collateral ligament stressed in full extension. The degree of angulation provides an accurate assessment of ligament injury that directly relates to the duration of immobilization and prognosis. Two weeks of complete immobilization, followed by 1 week of partial immobilization (buddy-taping to an adjacent finger on the affected side) at 30 degrees of flexion, is indicated if the joint is stable. Joints that are stable to active range of motion but unstable to stress require 3 to 5 weeks of complete immobilization followed by an additional 3 weeks of guarded active motion with buddy-taping. Joints that are unstable to active range of motion require prompt orthopedic referral for possible surgical repair.

The patient should be advised that residual stiffness, pain, and swelling may last for a number of months after the injury. A protective splint should be advocated if the patient wants an early return to the activity that produced the injury.

Dorsal Dislocations

Dorsal dislocation is the most common type of dislocation of the PIP joint. The mechanism of injury is hyperextension of the joint with a concomitant longitudinal compression, as commonly occurs in ball-handling sports. The physician may not see the dislocation because it is likely to have been reduced by a trainer, a coach, or the patient. It is important for the examining physician to ascertain the orientation of digit displacement because dorsal and volar dislocations are treated differently.

Figure 11-2.

Scheme of dorsal IP joint dislocation. **A)** *Normal anatomy of the lateral capsule consisting of the accessory (a) and the collateral (c) ligaments.* **B)** *Stable dorsal dislocation. The distal phalanx is displaced dorsally as both the volar plate and one collateral ligament tear.* **C)** *Unstable dorsal dislocation. Note the bayonet displacement of the more distal phalanx with few, if any, intact ligament fibers. Postreduction stability is unlikely.*

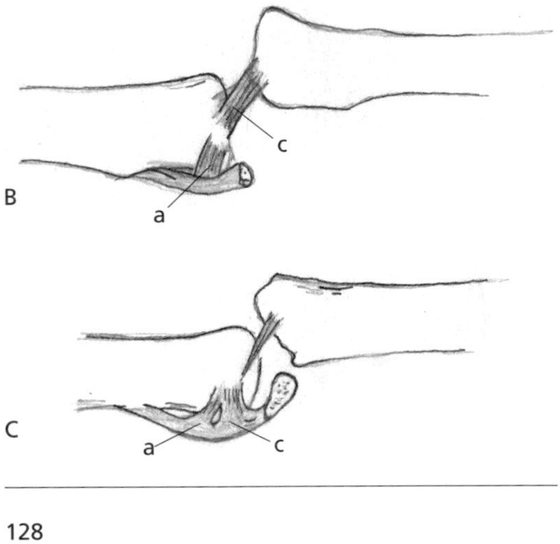

Rupture of the volar plate with a coexisting collateral ligament tear occurs with PIP joint dislocations (Figure 11-2). The middle phalanx assumes a bayonet-type dorsal displacement. The volar plate may be torn either at its membranous and fibrocartilaginous junction proximally or at its distal attachment on the base of the middle phalanx. A small avulsion fracture may occur with the latter, is rarely displaced, and is not an indication for open repair.

Closed reduction of the PIP joint is enhanced with digital anesthesia. It is accomplished with mild hyperextension and longitudinal traction applied to the middle phalanx, followed by dorsal pressure to the base of the middle phalanx. Closed reduction usually is easily accomplished and has a good prognosis. Stability assessment, immobilization, and complications are as noted with lateral dislocations.

Other Injuries

Fracture-dislocations. Dorsal fracture-dislocations can be the most disabling injuries to the PIP joint. The usual mechanism is from an axial load. The fracture occurs at the volar articular surface of the base of the middle phalanx.

Several classification systems have been proposed for categorizing dorsal fracture-dislocations.[2,3] Common to these categorizations is the point regarding stability. Fractures that involve 40% or more of the articular surface are unstable because a greater portion of the collateral ligament insertion is detached from the middle phalanx (Figure 11-2).[2,3] Because radiographs fail to demonstrate cartilaginous injury, the size of the fracture is not the only criterion for determining future joint function.

Because of the possible disabling nature of these injuries, orthopedic referral is mandatory. Treatment of the acute injury is controversial and without consensus; both closed and surgical techniques have been described.[2,3] However, most recommend surgical repair for injuries that are unstable in flexion with any degree of subluxation.

Open dislocations. The severity of open dislocations of the PIP joint usually is underestimated. Débridement, parenteral antibiotics, and surgical reduction are recommended.

Complex dislocations. Irreducible or complex dislocations of the PIP joint are uncommon. The volar plate or the flexor tendons are the structures that often impede reduction.

Volar Plate Tears

Disruption of the volar plate can arise without a dislocation of the PIP joint. The mechanism is a hyperextension force when a force is applied at the end of a digit. A horizontal volar skin laceration over the PIP joint should elevate the index of suspicion that this injury has taken place. Volar plate injuries cause a hyperextension deformity at the PIP joint on extension of the digit; pain and locking are observed with flexion. Hyperextension at the PIP joint requires assessment of the stability of the volar plate under digital anesthesia, even when a laceration is not present. Radiography may reveal a small bone fragment avulsed from the base of the middle phalanx. This must be differentiated from the more serious fracture-dislocation of the PIP joint. In extension, radiographs may show an abnormal hyperextension when compared with the normal side.

The PIP joint should be splinted in 30 degrees of flexion for 3 to 5 weeks. An alternative is to splint the PIP joint for 3 weeks followed by active flexion in an extension block splint at 15 degrees of flexion for 2 additional weeks. Most patients regain full range of motion with residual effects persisting for several months. Permanent swelling of the joint may be expected. Open injuries require orthopedic referral.

Volar Dislocations

Volar dislocations of the PIP joint are relatively rare and often missed. They may occur as either pure dislocations or fracture-dislocations. For this injury to occur, the **central slip** of the extensor mechanism is disrupted (Figure 11-3). The proximal phalangeal head ruptures through the retinacular fibers between the lateral band and central tendon. In addition, at least one collateral ligament is ruptured, the volar plate may be torn, or the lateral band may be caught in the joint resisting reduction. The potential for a boutonnière deformity (late complication) exists since the central slip is detached at its insertion.

If a patient presents following field reduction without the presence of a fracture to indicate a volar dislocation, the digit will mistakenly be immobilized in flexion as if a dorsal dislocation had occurred. This enhances the likelihood of the development of a boutonnière deformity. A key finding to note is that the patient is unable to extend the PIP joint against resistance.

Controversy exists in the literature regarding closed versus open reduction. Some advocate open reduction with repair of the central slip and transarticular pinning in extension for all volar PIP dislocations.[4] Others recommend conservative treatment (as with closed boutonnière injuries) of the PIP joint in extension for 4 to 6 weeks followed by dynamic PIP extension splinting during the day, static splinting at night, and active range of motion exercises. Open reduction is reserved for irreducible dislocations, incongruent joint surfaces after reduction, and an active extension lag of more than 30 degrees. Emergency treatment consists of ice, elevation, and splinting in extension with urgent referral to an orthopedist.

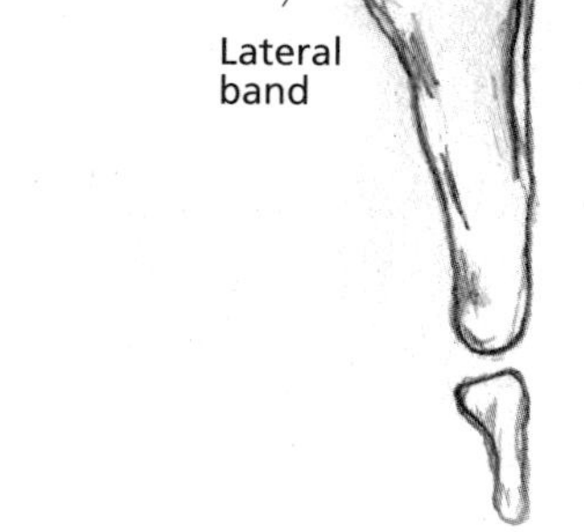

Figure 11-3.

Volar dislocation of the PIP joint. The proximal phalangeal head ruptures through the retinacular fibers between the lateral band and central tendon. The lateral band is interposed, blocking reduction.

Metacarpophalangeal Joint Injuries

The MCP joint is condyloid with the globular cam-shaped head of the metacarpal articulating with the concave base of the proximal phalanx. In contrast to the IP joints, full flexion and extension are permitted, along with significant abduction, adduction, and limited circumduction. The configuration of the metacarpal head (broader at its volar surface) allows the eccentric dorsally oriented collateral ligaments to remain taut in flexion and lax in extension (Figure 11-4). Therefore, limited lateral movement is allowed only in extension; the joint remains more stable in flexion.

The supporting structures for each joint consist of a capsule dorsally, a fibrocartilaginous volar plate, and a combination of ligaments, sagittal bands, and intrinsic tendons radially and ulnarly. The ability to resist hyperextension forces is limited because of the bony contour of the MCP joint, lack of check ligaments, and the thinner proximal volar plate. This is in contrast to the ability of the MCP joint to resist ulnar and radial stress. Strong collateral ligaments are present, along with a thicker distal volar plate that extends between adjacent metacarpals to form the deep **transverse metacarpal ligament**. Also, a buttressing effect occurs between adjacent rays, especially to the third and fourth MCP joints. Finally, flexors and extensors provide dynamic stability; lumbrical and interosseous muscles add to radial and ulnar stability.

The MCP joint is where primary digit flexion occurs; therefore, residual stiffness causes functional impairment. Early diagnosis, appropriate treatment, and rehabilitation are essential for optimal recovery.

Collateral Ligament

Isolated injuries to the collateral ligaments of the MCP joints are rare because of the protection afforded within the web space and adjacent rays. These injuries usually occur from hyperextension forces applied to the MCP joint while the digit is in extension.

Localized swelling and tenderness over the involved collateral ligament suggest the diagnosis. The most significant sign is pain in response to radial or ulnar stress with the MCP joint in extension with or without instability. Usually, no radiographic abnormality is present, although small avulsion fractures of the metacarpal head or intra-articular fractures of the base of the proximal phalanx may be present.

Conservative treatment with the MCP joint splinted in 60 to 70 degrees of flexion for 3 weeks is recommended if a significant avulsion fracture is not present. Surgical treatment is recommended if the fracture is displaced more than 2 to 3 mm or involves more than 20% of the articular surface and is displaced or rotated. Surgery also is reserved for unstable injuries and for chronic pain.

Dorsal Dislocations

Two types of dorsal MCP dislocations occur: simple and complex. Simple dislocations can be reduced by closed manipulation; complex dislocations are irreducible and require open reduction. Both types are caused by hyperextension forces that result in proximal volar plate tears.

Figure 11-4.

Scheme of the collateral ligament of the MCP joint depicting the dorsal eccentric origin of the collateral ligament attached to the cam-shaped metacarpal head. The collateral ligaments are lax in extension and taut in flexion.

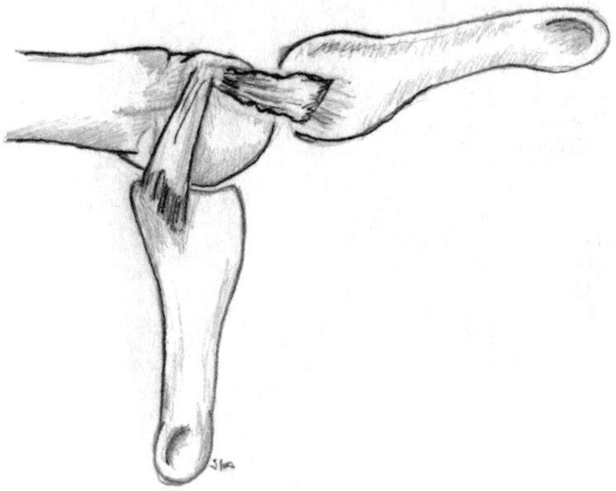

Simple

Simple dorsal dislocations of the MCP joint are more precisely subluxations because the articular surfaces are still in partial contact. The proximal phalanx is locked in 60 to 90 degrees of hyperextension on the dorsum of the metacarpal head. Clinically, a greater degree of hyperextension is present than in complex MCP dislocations. Radiographically, the joint space is narrow without the presence of an interposed sesamoid.

Closed reduction is achieved by first flexing the wrist to relax the flexor tendons and then applying pressure to the dorsum of the proximal phalanx in a distal and ulnar direction, sliding the joint into flexion. Traction/countertraction must be avoided because it may cause the volar plate to be interposed in the joint, converting a reducible to an irreducible dislocation.

Various authors advocate reduction achieved with a wrist block because pain can hinder reduction and lead to an inaccurate assumption that a complex dislocation is present.

A course of 7 to 10 days of immobilization of the MCP joint in 60 to 70 degrees of flexion is acceptable. Some prefer immediate active range of motion, with hyperextension prevented by buddy-taping. Recurrent simple MCP dislocations and chronic symptoms after simple MCP dislocations are rare. Orthopedic referral is recommended.

Complex

In complex MCP joint dislocations, the metacarpal head ruptures through the volar plate, which then occupies the joint space. The lumbrical on the radial aspect and the long flexor tendon on the ulnar aspect buttonhole the metacarpal head (Figure 11-5). The dislocation is irreducible because of the interposition of the volar plate within the MCP joint. In addition, longitudinal traction further entraps the metacarpal head in the ring formed by the lumbrical and the long flexor tendon.[5,6]

Complex MCP dislocations can be recognized by moderate hyperextension and a dorsal bayonet position. Pathognomonic findings are volar dimpling of the palmar skin at the proximal palmar crease and the radiographic presence of a sesamoid within the widened MCP joint space.

Complex MCP dislocations occur most commonly in the index finger, followed by the thumb and little finger. Rarely, MCP dislocations occur in the middle and ring fingers.

Figure 11-5.

Complex dislocation of the MCP joint depicting the interposition of the volar plate within the joint space.

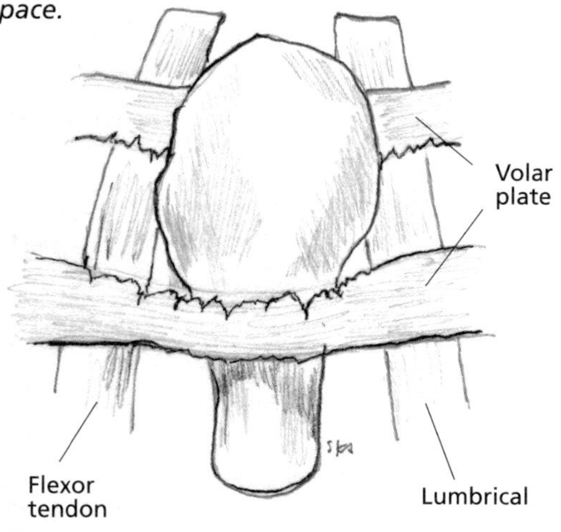

Reduction of complex MCP dislocations can be accomplished only with open techniques. After surgery, the joint is stable and requires no immobilization. Early active range of motion is advocated, with the affected digit protected with buddy-taping.

Carpometacarpal Joint Injuries

The CMC joints of the index, middle, and ring fingers are **arthrodial diarthroses** or **gliding joints**. The little finger is a **modified saddle joint**. The bases of the metacarpals articulate with each other and the distal carpal row in an interlocking complex to form the base of the transverse metacarpal arch of the hand.

The third metacarpocapitate joint functions as the stable central post of the hand, with essentially no movement possible. Limited anteroposterior gliding occurs at the base of the second metacarpotrapezoid joint. The saddle joint articulations between the bases of the fourth and fifth metacarpals are more mobile, having approximately 10 to 20 degrees of flexion and extension, respectively, and a few degrees of supination when opposing the thumb.

The joints are bolstered by tough dorsal and volar intermetacarpal and CMC ligaments. Wrist flexors and extensors provide additional support at the bases of the metacarpals.

Two important soft tissue structures are of significance when surgical intervention is required. The motor branch of the ulnar nerve is found volar to the fifth CMC joint as it courses around the hook of the hamate. The deep palmar arterial arch lies volar to the third CMC joint.

Dislocations

Dislocations of the CMC joints are uncommon and frequently missed. The mechanism of injury usually is the result of high-speed trauma as occurs with falls, crushing injuries, and motorcycle crashes. Closed-fist trauma also may result in CMC dislocations. Every combination of CMC dislocation has been described; isolated individual dislocations of the four joints may occur, with the fifth CMC joint dislocation presenting most frequently. Dorsal dislocations are more common than are volar dislocations. Avulsion fractures at the bases of the metacarpals or adjacent carpal bones often accompany these injuries.[3]

Clinical Diagnosis

Typically the patient presents with marked dorsal swelling that usually conceals the deformity at the metacarpal base. Maximal tenderness also is noted at the metacarpal bases. There may be no obvious deformity, and the severity of the injury may be unrecognized initially. Most of these dislocations are dorsal. With multiple dislocations, circulatory assessment is extremely important. Ulnar nerve integrity should be assessed with fifth metacarpohamate joint dislocations. Associated injuries to the median nerve and avulsions of the wrist extensor tendons also have been described.

Radiographic Diagnosis

Initial radiographic views of the hand should include the PA, oblique, and the extremely important lateral view to help delineate displacement of the metacarpal base. Other views, including multiple obliques, along with tomography and CT scans have been useful in demonstrating displacement and degree of intra-articular comminution.

An important consideration, similar to the Monteggia and Galeazzi fracture-dislocations of the forearm, is that the displaced fracture of one metacarpal can coexist with an adjacent CMC joint dislocation. This may arise because the metacarpals are tethered both proximally and distally. If one metacarpal is shortened or significantly angulated, dislocation at the base of the adjacent metacarpal must be ruled out.

Treatment

Emergency department treatment consists of ice, elevation, and analgesic agents. Orthopedic referral is mandatory because reduction is difficult to maintain due to joint instability. There is a particularly high incidence of lost reduction, especially for the second and third metacarpals, because of the contraction of the extensor carpi radialis longus and brevis tendons. Cast immobilization alone often is inadequate after reduction. Thus, percutaneous K-wire fixation is recommended for a minimum of 6 to 8 weeks.[3]

Thumb Joint Injuries

Interphalangeal Joint

The IP joint of the thumb is a hinge joint with a range of motion in a sagittal plane identical to that of the DIP joints of the fingers. Lateral stability is afforded by the collateral ligament and volar plate configuration (Figure 11-1). Clelland fibers also reinforce lateral stability.

Interphalangeal dislocations of the thumb usually are caused by hyperextension of the joint and dislocation of the distal phalanx dorsally. With a dorsal dislocation, the volar plate remains attached to the distal phalanx; a tear occurs at the proximal volar plate and the condylar origin of the collateral ligament. Shear stresses on the skin usually produce open dislocations.

Closed reduction usually is simple and easily achieved with either digital anesthesia or a median nerve block. Reduction is accomplished by accentuating the deformity, applying traction, and flexing the joint. After reduction, active range of motion testing determines stability and excludes the rare flexor pollicis longus tendon rupture. The joint usually remains stable because the volar plate remains attached to the distal phalanx. The IP joint should be immobilized in approximately 30 degrees of flexion for 3 weeks.[7]

Surgical management is required for irreducible IP dislocations. Open injuries should be treated surgically with irrigation and débridement.

Metacarpophalangeal Joint

The MCP joint of the thumb is a hybrid of a **ginglymus** and a condyloid joint. Flexion, extension, abduction, adduction, and limited rotation are possible. This joint has the most variable range of motion of all the joints in the hand; the maximal extension to maximal flexion varies from 5 to 100 degrees, with an average of 75 degrees.

The broad transverse diameter of the first metacarpal condyle is a major contributor to lateral joint stability. Also, joint stability is provided by the enhanced tensile strength of the volar plate and collateral ligaments. The **intrinsic flexor-adductor muscles** adjacent to the sesamoids help maintain the integrity of the proximal volar plate analogous to the paired check ligaments at the digital PIP joints. Fibers from the adductor pollicis muscle merge with the dorsal aponeurosis to form the adductor aponeurosis. Overlying the ulnar collateral ligament, the **adductor aponeurosis** provides active stabilization. Finally, dynamic stability is provided by the **thenar intrinsic muscles**, which stabilize the joint even with volar plate disruption.

Despite substantial stabilization, the oblique orientation of the thumb makes the MCP joint five times more vulnerable to radially directed stress. The force of strong opposition that is essential to provide a forceful pinch-grip requires firm resistance to hyperextension. Two basic types of ligament injury may occur: dorsal dislocation as a result of volar plate disruption and lateral or jackknife dislocation secondary to a unilateral collateral ligament tear.

Dorsal Dislocations

Dorsal dislocation of the thumb MCP joint is caused by either an extreme hyperextension injury or shearing stress that causes rupture of the volar supporting structures. Displacement is directly proportional to the degree of disruption. The volar plate usually avulses proximal to the sesamoid insertion but can rupture distally. Displacement varies from a subluxation of the phalanx to a complete dislocation. The characteristic bayonet orientation of the phalanx overriding dorsal and parallel to the metacarpal occurs with complete rupture of the volar plate and one of the collateral ligaments.

Closed reduction can be accomplished following a digital block. With the wrist and IP joint flexed to relax the flexor tendons, the thumb metacarpal is adducted and flexed into the palm and dorsal pressure is applied over the proximal phalanx. Reduction is achieved by pushing the base of the proximal phalanx over the metacarpal head. Traction/countertraction must be avoided because it may cause the volar plate to be interposed in the joint, converting a reducible dislocation to an irreducible one.

Stability is assessed by active range of motion along with stress of the MCP joint after reduction to assess ulnar and radial collateral ligament integrity. A course of 4 to 6 weeks of immobilization in flexion is recommended for stable joints, with orthopedic referral. Open repair is reserved for unstable joints, significant lateral instability (more than 40 degrees), and irreducible dislocations.

Collateral Ligament Injuries

Radial and ulnar collateral ligament injuries of the thumb MCP joint are common and present with subtle physical findings. The dislocation that ensues from rupture of a collateral ligament and volar plate is transient and, in many instances, unrecognized and, therefore, untreated. Ulnar collateral ligament ruptures have been characterized as occurring 10 times more frequently than radial collateral ligament ruptures. However, one recent report noted a much higher occurrence of radial collateral ligament injury.[8] The loss of ulnar collateral ligament support is quite disabling because it reduces the ability of the thumb to resist stress, which is necessary for a strong pinch. Complete disruption of either ligament is likely to result in both static and dynamic joint instability, leading to a sequence of painful deformity followed by articular degeneration.

Historically, ulnar collateral ligament injury was termed **gamekeeper thumb** because it was the result of repeated radial stress from breaking the necks of wild game. The term **ski pole thumb** or **skier thumb** currently reflects the most common mechanism of injury and is, in fact, one of the most common skiing injuries.

Figure 11-6.

Ulnar collateral ligament injury to the thumb MCP joint. **A)** *Depiction of the collateral ligament mechanism.* **B)** *Ulnar collateral ligament rupture at its insertion.* **C)** *Intact ligament, but distal attachment avulses a bone fragment.*

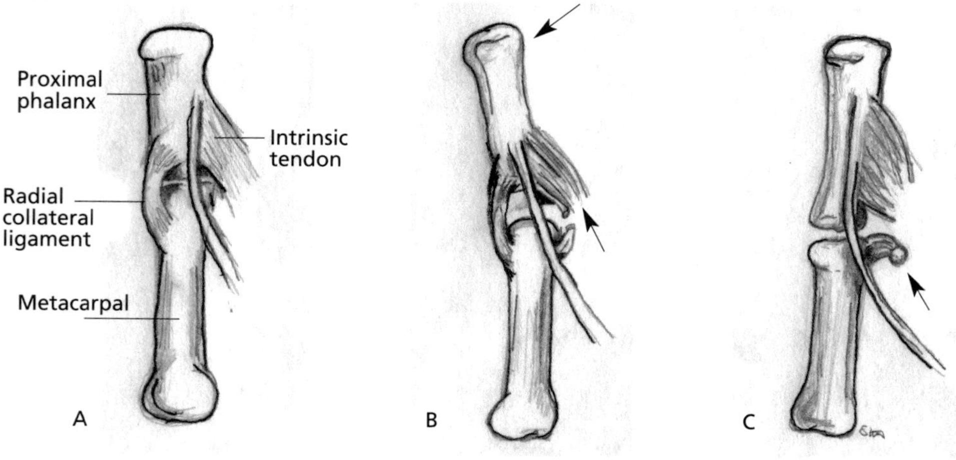

The diagnosis is pursued with physical examination and stress radiographs; most of these dislocations reduce spontaneously. The patient typically presents with a painful, swollen MCP joint of the thumb, with the point of maximal tenderness over the ulnar collateral ligament.

Radiographs may reveal an avulsion fracture at the base of the proximal phalanx where the ulnar collateral ligament inserts. More often, stress radiographs are necessary to reveal the injury because the rupture occurs within the ligament itself (Figure 11-6). After radial and median nerve wrist blocks, the collateral ligament is stressed with the MCP joint in 20 to 30 degrees of flexion to eliminate the stabilizing effect of the volar plate. The uninjured thumb should be tested for comparison because great variability exists in MCP joint range of motion.[7,9]

Greater than 30 degrees of lateral laxity coupled with 33% or greater subluxation of the proximal phalanx relative to the metacarpal head as measured on the stress radiographs indicates complete collateral ligament disruption. This is a surgical indication even if stability exists through active range of motion. Integrity of both collateral ligaments of the thumb is necessary for full function.[8]

The **Stener lesion** is another indication for surgical repair. Stener noted that the adductor aponeurosis becomes interposed between the two ends of the ruptured ulnar collateral ligament most frequently where the distal ligament attaches to the proximal phalanx. This results in inadequate healing, a lax residual ligament, and a poor outcome because the ligament ends will not approximate in two thirds of cases.[7] The incidence of the Stener lesion ranges from 14% to 83%.

The thumb is immobilized in a thumb spica cast for 3 to 4 weeks with the IP joint free for conservative treatment of incomplete collateral ligament tears and after surgical repair of complete tears. A removable splint to allow active range of motion is applied for an additional 5 weeks.

Carpometacarpal Joint

The CMC joint of the thumb is a biologic **universal joint** with the concave metacarpal base seated onto the saddle of the trapezium. This configuration allows for wide range of motion, including circumduction. However, the joint is stable enough to resist the combined force of the four fingers. The principal ligament support is the **anterior oblique CMC ligament**. Its stabilizing force is equivalent to the IP volar plate. Dorsal support is provided by the **posterior oblique CMC ligament**, which is reinforced by insertion of the abductor pollicis longus tendon.

Thumb CMC dislocations without fractures are uncommon. The mechanism is postulated to be secondary to a longitudinal force directed along the metacarpal shaft with the basal joint in slight flexion. The anterior oblique CMC ligament and opponens pollicis muscles are the deterrents to subluxation. Because of the tensile strength of these structures, the longitudinal force more commonly produces fracture-dislocations, such as the **Bennett fracture**.

Injuries of the volar ligament of the thumb CMC joint may be partial or complete. Complete rupture allows the entire thumb metacarpal to dislocate dorsally and radially; partial rupture permits varying degrees of displacement. Stress radiographs may aid in the diagnosis.

If the patient has acute posttraumatic pain in the CMC joint without clinical instability and radiographic evidence of subluxation, a partial volar ligament tear should be considered and treated accordingly. The joint should be immobilized with the metacarpal in abduction and extension for 4 weeks.[3] Orthopedic referral is recommended.

Closed reduction of the thumb CMC joint is simple but often is unstable, especially to active range of motion. Percutaneous K-wire fixation of the trapeziometacarpal joint is used to maintain reduction. A thumb spica cast is worn for 4 to 6 weeks; at the end of this time, the pins are removed, but the joint remains protected for an additional 8 to 10 weeks.[3]

Summary

Optimal treatment of joint injuries of the hand is essential to prevent long-term functional disability. Complex intra-articular geometry, strong yet flexible supporting ligamentous structures, and dynamic extensors and flexors provide joint stabilization. A thorough history to ascertain the mechanism of injury may be helpful in providing an index of suspicion for specific injuries. Important aspects of the physical examination include assessment for swelling, deformity, and neurovascular status. Active and gentle passive range of motion under anesthetic block is key to determine joint stability. Standard radiographic views include AP and oblique and, for individual digits, a true lateral. Except for ulnar collateral ligament rupture of the thumb MCP joint, stable joints are treated with conservative measures that include appropriate immobilization and referral to hand surgeons. Indications for surgical repair include complex dislocations, unstable joints, and dislocations associated with large or displaced intra-articular fractures.

References

1. Eaton RG. *Joint Injuries of the Hand.* Springfield, Ill: Charles C Thomas; 1972.
2. Glickel SF, Barron OA. Proximal interphalangeal joint fracture dislocations. *Hand Clin.* 2000;16:3.
3. Palmer RE. Joint injuries of the hand in athletes. *Clin Sports Med.* 1998;17:3.
4. Kahler DM, McCue FC. Metacarpophalangeal and proximal interphalangeal joint injuries of the hand, including the thumb. *Clin Sports Med.* 1992;11:57.
5. Wolov RB. Complex dislocations of the metacarpophalangeal joints. *Orthoped Rev.* 1988;17:770.
6. Viegas SF, Heare TC, Calhoun JH. Complex fracture-dislocation of a fifth metacarpophalangeal joint: case report and literature review. *J Trauma.* 1989;29:521.
7. Langford SA, Whitaker JH, Toby EB. Thumb injuries in the athlete. *Clin Sports Med.* 1998;17:3.
8. Melone Jr CP, Bedner S, Basuk RS. Thumb collateral ligament injuries. An anatomic basis for treatment. *Hand Clin.* 2000;16:3.
9. Kozin SH, Bishop AT. Gamekeeper's thumb. Early diagnosis and treatment. *Orthoped Rev.* 1994;23:797.

CHAPTER 12

Wrist Injuries

Robert Escarza, MD, and Harold W. Chin, MD, FACEP

Wrist injuries are common, and their evaluation in the emergency department is facilitated by a solid working knowledge of general and functional anatomy, injury mechanism, and radiologic nuances. An understanding of the limitations of the physical examination and radiography also is necessary. Clinical examination often is more reliable than radiographs in some conditions, although the reliability of the examination can be impaired by swelling and poorly localized pain. Even subtle injuries may lead to significant impairment if they are not properly diagnosed and treated. Therefore, an understanding of the complexities of the wrist and the mechanisms of injury helps clinicians avoid these pitfalls.

Anatomy

The wrist includes the distal radius, the ulna, and the carpal bones. The **distal radius** ends in a smooth articulation with the scaphoid and lunate; the **ulna** is separated from the carpals, lunate, and triquetrum by the **triangular fibrocartilage complex**. This complex also is the main stabilizer of the **distal radioulnar joint**.

The **carpal bones** are arranged in two functional rows (Figure 12-1). The proximal row (radial to ulnar) comprises the scaphoid, lunate, triquetrum, and pisiform. In a similar manner, the distal row is composed of the trapezium, trapezoid, capitate, and hamate. Three significant extrinsic ligaments support the carpal bones. Two are volar and support the lunate and capitate, respectively; the third is dorsal and less important in wrist stability. Intrinsic ligaments also help stabilize each carpal articulation.

Movement of the wrist is divided evenly between the proximal and distal carpal rows and the radiocarpal joint. The proximal carpal row is the mobile middle link in this system, making it inherently unstable, which accounts for its propensity for injury. The scaphoid, which bears the largest radial articulation and bridges the carpal rows, is the carpal bone that is most often stressed. This explains why the most common carpal injuries involve the scaphoid and scapholunate joint.

Physical Examination

Mechanism of injury is an often ignored but helpful aspect of the evaluation of a wrist injury. Most injuries are caused by a fall on an outstretched hand. Age can predispose patients to certain types of injury. For example, children often injure the radial epiphysis, sparing the still-cartilaginous carpals. Young adults tend to injure the scaphoid and stabilizing ligaments, and older adults more frequently fracture the radius.[1] Armed with a knowledge of topographic anatomy, the examining physician can pinpoint areas of tenderness, which helps determine potential injury. Then, appropriate radiographic studies can be obtained to confirm the diagnosis.

Dorsal Surface

The **anatomic snuffbox** is the most visible feature on the radial aspect of the wrist. The scaphoid is palpable within a triangle formed at its base by the bony radial styloid, the extensor pollicis brevis tendon radially, and the extensor pollicis longus tendon on its ulnar aspect. The extensor pollicis longus tendon crosses around a bony prominence on

Figure 12-1.

Key elements on a normal PA view of the wrist. **A)** *The carpal bones form three smooth arcs.* **B)** *Each carpal bone is separated by uniform 1- to 2-mm spaces.* **C)** *The scaphoid has an elongated shape.* **D)** *The distal radius has an ulnar inclination of 13 to 30 degrees.* **E)** *The radial styloid projects 8 to 18 mm. At least half of the lunate articulates with the distal radius.*

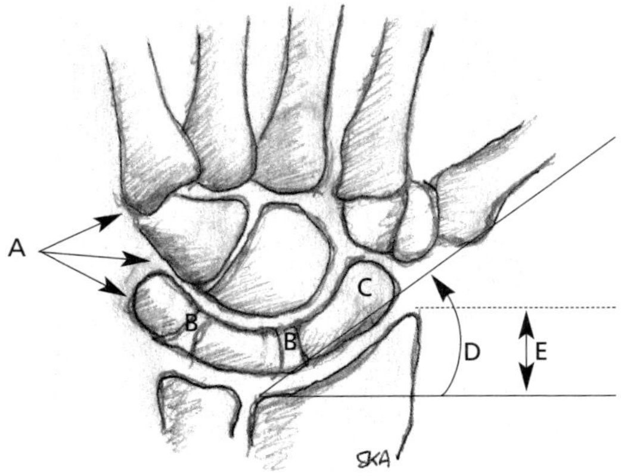

the distal radius, known as **Lister's tubercle**. The area immediately distal to this point marks the junction of the scapholunate joint. Just ulnar to Lister's tubercle, the lunate and capitate are palpable in the shallow indentation present in the middle of the wrist. The bony prominence on the ulnar aspect of the wrist is the **ulnar styloid**. The triquetrum is palpable immediately distal to this landmark.

Volar Surface

The proximal flexor crease of the wrist identifies the location of the proximal carpal row. The bony prominence at the base of the hypothenar eminence is the **pisiform**. The **hook of the hamate** is palpable approximately 1 to 2 cm distal at a 45-degree angle radial to the pisiform. The bony prominence at the base of the thenar eminence is the **scaphotrapezial ridge**.

Radiography

Clinical evaluation should dictate which radiographic views to order to support a diagnosis. Proper positioning must be ensured because inadequate positioning can create misleading artifacts. The standard PA, lateral, and oblique views are adequate in most cases. Nonstandard views and motion studies are useful for profiling specific carpal injuries.

Posteroanterior View

On a properly positioned PA view, the axis of the third metacarpal should parallel the axis of the radius. There should be no overlap between the radius and the ulna at its distal articulation. In addition to disruption of the bony cortex, the following items should be examined on the PA view (see Figure 12-1):

- The carpals form three smooth arcs. The proximal and distal articular surfaces of the scaphoid, lunate, and triquetrum form two arcs; the third is formed by the proximal surface of the capitate and hamate.
- The carpals are separated in a relatively uniform manner by a 1- to 2-mm joint space. Any disruption of this space suggests ligament injury, fracture, dislocation, or improper positioning.
- The scaphoid has an elongated shape in its normal palmarly flexed position. Fractures or ligament disruption may cause further palmar rotation, making the scaphoid appear shortened on the PA view. Injuries to the scaphoid also may obscure the **scaphoid fat stripe**, a linear or triangular collection of fat that is distal to the radial styloid and parallel to the radial border of the scaphoid.[2,3]
- **Radial inclination** of 13 to 30 degrees (average 22 degrees) and **radial styloid length** of 8 to 18 mm (average 13 mm). The average radial styloid length of 13 mm creates the average radial inclination of 22 degrees (see Figure 12-1). Distal radial fractures can change these measurements.
- At least half of the lunate makes contact with the distal radius. Injuries to either the radiocarpal support ligaments or the triangular fibrocartilage complex can cause an ulnar shift of the carpals

(ulnar translocation). These injuries also may produce shear stress and fracture the lunate.

Lateral View

The lateral radiograph is the most important view in the assessment of wrist injuries. On a properly positioned lateral radiograph, the hand should be in a neutral position, and the radius and ulna should overlap completely. The degree of fracture angulation, displacement, and carpal alignment are best seen in this view. Key elements of the examination are as follows (Figure 12-2):

- **Three C's sign**. The axes of the radius, lunate, and capitate should be in a straight line, and highlighted articular surfaces appear as three C's in a row. Torn ligaments and dislocations disrupt this normal articular pattern.
- The **capitolunate angle** is less than 10 to 20 degrees. The scaphoid is flexed toward the palm and forms a scapholunate angle of 30 to 60 degrees with the lunate. Deviation from these measurements results from ligament injuries, carpal instability, and improper positioning.
- The radius has a **volar tilt** of 1 to 23 degrees (average 14 degrees). Angulated radial fractures alter this measurement. A goal of fracture reduction is to restore this angle to prevent functional impairment.

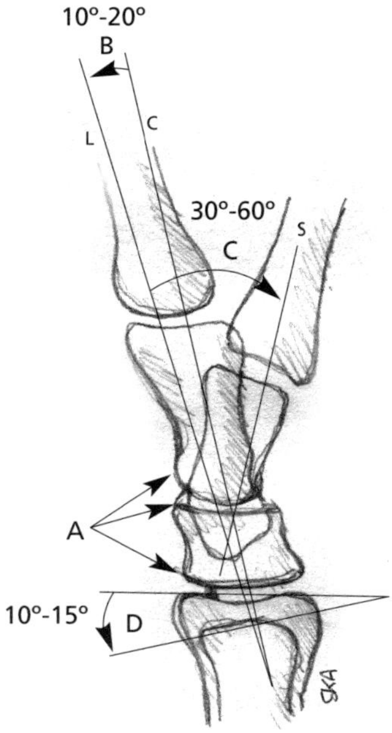

Figure 12-2.

Key elements on a normal lateral view. **A)** *The three C's sign.* **B)** *A capitolunate angle of less than 20 degrees.* **C)** *A scapholunate angle of 30 to 60 degrees.* **D)** *A radial volar tilt of 10 to 15 degrees.*

Oblique View

Oblique views are taken in partial pronation or supination to project the scaphotrapezial joint or pisiform, respectively, away from other carpals.

Scaphoid View

This is a PA view of the wrist in ulnar deviation. This position causes the scaphoid to elongate on the radiograph by changing it from its normal palmar-flexed position to a more upright position. This view helps reveal more subtle scaphoid fractures and should be ordered routinely when a scaphoid fracture is suspected clinically.

Power Grip Compression View

This is a stress view of the wrist in the PA projection with the hand held in a tightly clenched fist. This positioning pushes the capitate into the proximal carpal row and may force the carpals apart in the presence of a scapholunate ligament injury.

Carpal Tunnel View

A tangential view through the carpal tunnel is used to visualize the pisiform and the hook of the hamate.

Motion Studies

These are dynamic views of the wrist in flexion, extension, and radial and ulnar deviation. They demonstrate carpal movement at the radiocarpal and midcarpal joints and may reveal an occult ligament injury.

Fractures of the Carpal Bones

Fractures of the carpal bones can be subtle and escape early detection. Missed fractures can result in early degenerative arthritis and a chronically painful wrist. The various carpal fractures are discussed here in order of decreasing frequency.

Scaphoid Fracture

Fractures of the scaphoid account for 60% to 70% of carpal bone fractures and, among all wrist fractures, are second only to distal radius fractures.[4]

Anatomy

The scaphoid is an irregular, oblong bone that articulates with five other bones. Because articular fractures generally are more difficult to heal, this large articular surface area accounts for the propensity for potential morbidity in the face of injury. As discussed, the scaphoid forms a mobile link between the two carpal rows, exposing it more than all other carpals to injury. Blood is supplied from branches of the distal radial, palmar, and superficial palmar arteries that enter the distal portion of the bone, so proximal scaphoid fractures are at high risk for avascular necrosis following injury.

Mechanism

A fall on an outstretched hand with the wrist in extension or an axial load to the thumb causes this fracture.

Examination

No clinical maneuver is pathognomonic, but various maneuvers and findings can increase the overall suspicion for a scaphoid injury. Pain on the radial aspect of the wrist is common. There is well localized tenderness in the anatomic snuffbox, and palpation during ulnar deviation may be helpful in this examination. Pain in the snuffbox with resistance to pronation/supination or with axial loading of the thumb also is suggestive of injury.[5] Edema may obscure the snuffbox, so a comparison with the uninvolved wrist may be helpful.

Radiography

Standard and scaphoid views should be obtained to detect cortical disruption. Loss of the scaphoid fat stripe is suggestive of injury. Approximately two thirds of fractures involve the waist or midportion of the bone; 22% involve the proximal third, and the remaining 10% involve the distal third. One of 10 patients has accompanying injuries to the radius, ulna, neighboring carpals, or ligaments.[5,6]

Treatment

As many as 10% of initial radiographs may fail to demonstrate a fracture that is present.[4] Treatment therefore should be dictated by clinical suspicion. As many as 15% of suspected occult scaphoid injuries are confirmed in followup studies within 1 week.[4] Classic teaching calls for a long arm thumb spica splint as the treatment of choice; however, newer studies show questionable benefit from either extension of the splint above the elbow or inclusion of the thumb.[5] A short arm thumb spica splint is adequate treatment in the emergency department for scaphoid fractures, but consultation with an orthopedic specialist is prudent to determine the preferred splinting method. Wrist position also is controversial, but most advocate a neutral position rather than either pronation or supination.[5] Unstable fractures require orthopedic consultation; these include fractures that are displaced more than 1 mm; rotated, angulated, or shortened; or accompanied by a carpal instability due to ligament disruption.

Complications

Avascular necrosis (especially with proximal third fractures), delayed union, nonunion, and malunion are the greatest concerns.

Triquetrum Fracture

Anatomy

The triquetrum is encased by strong ligamentous attachments on its dorsal and volar aspects and by the triangular fibrocartilage complex on the ulnar aspect.

Mechanism

Typically the mechanism of injury is a direct blow to the dorsum of the wrist or a fall on an outstretched hand with hyperextension of the wrist. Dorsal chip and body fractures commonly occur. They also may be seen in combination with the arc fractures that occur with perilunate dislocations. Impingement fracture by the ulnar styloid or hamate also occurs; the mechanism of injury is a fall with the wrist in extension and ulnar deviation.

Examination

Evaluation reveals swelling and tenderness to palpation over the dorsum of the wrist just distal to the ulnar styloid.

Radiography

A chip or an avulsion fracture is most common and easily seen dorsally on either the lateral or oblique view. A small fragment of bone dorsal to the lunate should be sought. Fractures through the body usually are nondisplaced and seen on the PA view.

Treatment

Most triquetrum fractures have little long-term significance. Emergency treatment consists of a short arm splint. Later, a short arm cast is applied for 6 weeks. Fractures associated with perilunate dislocation require immediate orthopedic consultation and internal fixation.

Complications

Nonunion may occur, but it is rare. Avascular necrosis has not been reported.

Lunate Fracture

Anatomy

The lunate is well protected by its position in the lunate fossa, by the triangular fibrocartilage complex, and by strong ligamentous attachments to the triquetrum and scaphoid. Lunate fractures often are associated with injury to other carpals. Blood is supplied through the distal portion of the bone on its volar and dorsal surfaces.

Mechanism

A fall on an outstretched, dorsiflexed hand is the most common mechanism.

Examination

There is localized pain in the shallow indentation over the middorsum of the wrist, just distal and ulnar to Lister's tubercle. Flexion of the wrist, which brings the lunate closer to the palpating digit, may assist in the examination. Pain with axial compression of the middle finger also is suggestive of injury.

Radiography

A lunate fracture may be difficult to visualize on standard radiographs because of overlapping structures. Bone scans, CT, or MRI may be necessary if an injury is suspected clinically.

Treatment

Because occult injuries are common, treatment parallels that for a scaphoid fracture and is based mostly on clinical suspicion. A thumb spica splint is sufficient emergency treatment. Orthopedic followup care is mandatory for all suspected lunate fractures because of the complications of avascular necrosis and nonunion.

Complications

Avascular necrosis can occur due to the distal blood supply to the lunate. A special type of avascular necrosis known as **Kienböck disease** results from either an ignored or a missed acute fracture or repetitive lunate trauma that results in microfractures of the bone. Osteoarthritis, lunate collapse, chronic pain, and decreased grip strength may result.

Pisiform Fracture

Anatomy

A pisiform fracture is a sesamoid bone enveloped by the flexor carpi ulnaris tendon. Its dorsal surface articulates with the triquetrum, forming the **pisotriquetrum joint**. Along with the hook of the hamate, it forms the side walls of **Guyon's canal**, through which the ulnar nerve and artery course.

Mechanism

A fall on an outstretched hand with the hypothenar eminence as the point of impact is the most common injury mechanism. The three types of fractures that occur are avulsion, transverse, and comminuted.

Examination

There is no deformity and only mild swelling. Point tenderness is elicited over the proximal aspect of the hypothenar eminence.

Radiography

A pisiform fracture may be seen on a lateral or an oblique view but is best visualized using the carpal tunnel view.

Treatment

Pisiform fractures typically respond well to treatment. A compression dressing or short arm splint with the wrist in partial flexion and ulnar deviation is sufficient for emergency treatment. Later, a short arm cast applied for 4 to 6 weeks is recommended.

Complications

Nonunion, malunion, delayed union, and chronic pain occur occasionally. There is a remote possibility of ulnar nerve injury in Guyon's canal.

Hamate Fracture

This fracture usually involves the hook of the hamate. Body fractures are rare and typically are associated with severe injuries, such as fracture of the fourth or fifth metacarpal or CMC joint dislocations.

Anatomy

The hamate articulates with the fourth and fifth metacarpals distally, the lunate and triquetrum proximally, and the capitate radially. This triangular bone has a palmar bony process, the **hamulus**, or hook of the hamate. As mentioned previously, the hook of the hamate and the pisiform form the walls of Guyon's canal, which contains the ulnar nerve and artery.

Mechanism

The most common mechanism is a direct blow from the interrupted swing of a racquet, baseball bat, golf club, or tool, which compresses the hypothenar eminence and fractures the hook of the hamate. Axial force directed along the shaft of the fourth or fifth metacarpal may result in a fracture-dislocation at the articulation of the metacarpal and the distal hamate. Body fractures also occur with direct trauma.

Examination

There is point tenderness over the hamate. The hook of the hamate is located 1 to 2 cm distal and radial to the pisiform.

Radiography

This fracture may be seen on a PA view, but it is best visualized on a carpal tunnel view. It is missed frequently; CT or a bone scan may be required.

Treatment

Treatment with a compression dressing or short arm splint is sufficient for hamulus and nondisplaced body fractures. Displaced body fractures and those associated with fracture-dislocations of the metacarpals require immediate orthopedic consultation.

Complications

Nonunion and malunion of the hook of the hamate are common and require excision of the fragment. Ulnar nerve compression with associated intrinsic muscle weakness sometimes occurs.

Trapezium Fracture

Anatomy

The trapezium is a trapezoid-shaped bone that articulates with the first and second metacarpals, scaphoid, and trapezoid. Its articulation with the first metacarpal is saddle shaped and allows a great deal of motion.

Mechanism

Fractures of the trapezium include vertical, comminuted, and avulsion. The mechanism of injury may be direct trauma to the radiodorsal aspect of the hand or a fall on an outstretched hand with the wrist in hyperextension. Articular fractures may occur as a result of forces transmitted through an adducted thumb, driving the first metacarpal into the trapezium. There may be an associated fracture-dislocation of the first metacarpal or a fracture of the distal radius.

Examination

Passive thumb movement and axial compression of the thumb are painful. There is point tenderness at the base of the thenar eminence and at the apex of the anatomic snuffbox.

Radiography

The fracture is best seen on a pronated oblique view.

Treatment

Emergency treatment of a nondisplaced fracture consists of immobilization in a thumb spica splint and orthopedic referral. Definitive care consists of a thumb spica cast for 6 weeks. A displaced fracture requires anatomic reduction, so open reduction and internal fixation is performed.

Complications

Nonunion is a possible complication.

Capitate Fracture

Anatomy

The capitate is the largest carpal bone. It is located centrally and articulates with seven bones: the second, third, and fourth metacarpals distally, the scaphoid and lunate proximally, the hamate ulnarly, and the trapezoid radially. Anatomically, the capitate is divided into three parts: proximal head, neck, and distal body. Blood is supplied through the body, so neck fractures may result in avascular necrosis of the head. Isolated fractures are rare. Fractures usually occur in combination with scaphoid fractures, which is known as the **scaphocapitate syndrome**.

Mechanism

An isolated fracture or a fracture associated with metacarpal or other carpal bone fractures results from direct trauma to the dorsum of the wrist. Another possible injury is the scaphocapitate syndrome, which typically is caused by a fall on an outstretched hand with the wrist in dorsiflexion and radial deviation. In this injury, the scaphoid fractures first, followed by the capitate (usually at the neck), and then if the force is sufficient, the capitate is displaced posteriorly to create a perilunate dislocation with associated arc fractures.

Examination

Diffuse tenderness and swelling are noted over the dorsum of the wrist. Axial traction and compression along the shaft of the third metacarpal will cause pain.

Radiography

Posteroanterior, lateral, and scaphoid views should be obtained. The lateral view is best to reveal fractures, which occur most often in the neck. Fractures often are missed, being overshadowed by a more obvious scaphoid fracture or perilunate dislocation. The head of the capitate and the proximal scaphoid may rotate together, possibly as much as 180 degrees.

Treatment

The rare isolated, nondisplaced fracture is treated with a short arm splint. Displaced fractures and the scaphocapitate syndrome require open reduction and internal fixation.

Complications

Avascular necrosis, nonunion, malunion, and complications associated with scaphoid fractures and perilunate dislocations are possible.

Trapezoid Fracture

Anatomy

The trapezoid is a wedge-shaped bone that articulates with the second metacarpal distally, the trapezium radially, the capitate ulnarly, and the scaphoid proximally. Fractures are very rare, accounting for approximately 1% of all carpal bone fractures.

Mechanism

Fractures and dorsal dislocations usually are produced by an axial load along the second metacarpal. Direct trauma also may cause a fracture or dislocation of the trapezoid.

Examination

There is tenderness on the radial aspect of the wrist. Pain with axial compression of the index finger is highly suggestive.

Radiography

Trapezoid fractures are difficult to detect with plain radiography because they are rare and because the carpal bones and the second metacarpal base overlap. Oblique radiographs, CT, or a bone scan may be necessary to identify the injury.

Treatment

Emergency treatment consists of a thumb spica splint until orthopedic followup care is obtained. Displaced fractures require open reduction and internal fixation.

Complications

Nonunion is a possible complication.

Ligament Injuries

Most ligament injuries occur around the lunate in a predictable, sequential pattern caused by varying degrees of force. A fall on an outstretched hand in dorsiflexion is the most common mechanism. Injuries range from isolated ligament tears to lunate and perilunate dislocations.

Scapholunate Ligament Instability

This is the most common soft tissue wrist injury.

Anatomy

Each carpal row is held together as a unit by intrinsic ligaments. The **triquetrolunate** and **scapholunate intrinsic ligaments** of the proximal row are particularly important because they, along with the extrinsic ligaments, are the main wrist supports. These ligaments hold the lunate tightly between the scaphoid and triquetrum in a deli-

Figure 12-3.

Classic radiographic findings with scapholunate dissociation.
A) *Increase in the scapholunate space to 3 mm or more.*
B) *Cortical ring sign, with the scaphoid also appearing shortened due to rotation.*

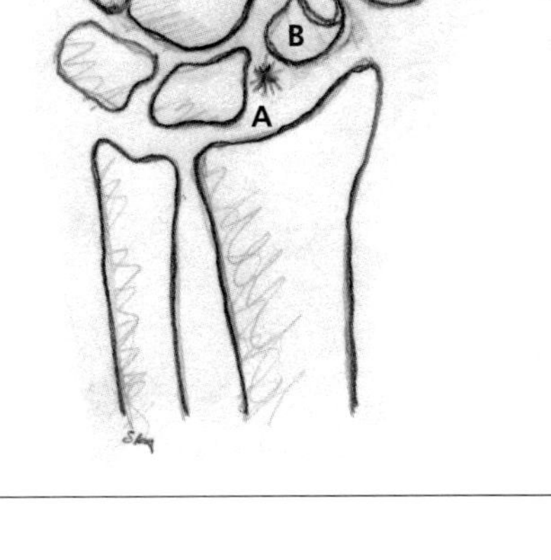

Figure 12-4.

A) *Normal wrist. Axes of the radius (R), lunate (L), and capitate (C) are colinear. The capitolunate (CL) angle is less than 20 degrees, and the scapholunate (SL) angle is between 30 and 60 degrees.*
B) *Dorsal intercalated segment instability. The lunate (L) tilts dorsal and slides palmar, thus increasing the capitolunate angle. The axes of the radius (R), lunate, and capitate (C) take on a zigzag pattern.*
C) *Volar intercalated segment instability. The lunate (L) tilts palmar and the capitolunate angle increases, but the scapholunate angle is maintained. The zigzag pattern is in the opposite direction.*

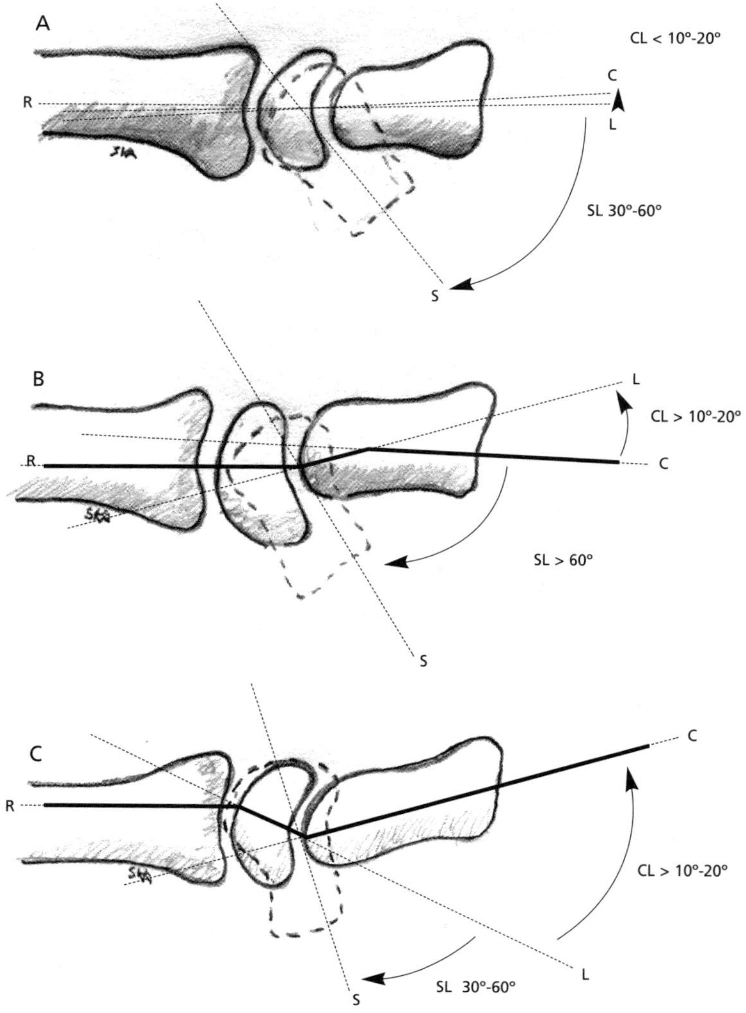

cate balance of flexion (scapholunate) and extension (triquetrolunate) forces.

Mechanism

A fall on an outstretched hand with slight ulnar deviation of the wrist is the typical mechanism of injury.

Examination

Pain and swelling are noted along the dorsoradial aspect of the wrist. The patient may complain of a clicking sensation with movement. Palpation just distal to Lister's tubercle elicits pain. **Ballottement**, or dorsally directed pressure, of the scaphoid also may produce pain at the scapholunate articulation.

Radiography

The injury may manifest in any one of three radiographic patterns (Figure 12-3):

- **Scapholunate dissociation**. On the PA view, an increase in the joint space of 3 mm or more may be present. This is called the **Terry Thomas sign**, named for a British comedian who had a large gap between his front teeth.[7] Partial tears may not be revealed without a power grip compression view, which pushes the capitate into the proximal row and forces the lunate and scaphoid apart if the ligament is torn. This reveals separation of the scapholunate joint space of greater than 3 mm.
- **Rotary subluxation of the scaphoid**. This is best seen on a lateral projection. The scaphoid tilts in a palmar direction, increasing the scapholunate angle to more than 60 degrees (normal 30 to 60 degrees). On the PA view, the scaphoid rotates toward the observer, making the bone appear shorter, with a dense cortical ring around its center. This is the **cortical ring sign**.
- **Dorsal intercalated segment instability**. On a lateral view, the scaphoid normally is in a flexed position, and this imparts a flexion torque on the lunate that is balanced by an extension torque from the triquetrum (Figure 12-4A). When the scapholunate ligament is disrupted, so is the flexion force on the lunate. The lunate subsequently rotates dorsally from this unopposed extension force. The pathology is best illustrated on the lateral view, in which the lunate has a dorsal tilt and the capitolunate and scapholunate angles are increased. The normal linear arrangement of the axes of the radius, lunate, and capitate takes on a skewed zigzag pattern (Figure 12-4B).

Treatment

The application of a radial gutter or short arm volar splint is adequate until close orthopedic followup care is obtained. This injury may be pinned percutaneously, but most acute injuries require open reduction and direct ligament repair.

Complications

Failure to diagnose this injury can result in early degenerative arthritis and chronic pain of the wrist.

Triquetrolunate Ligament Instability

This is the ulnar counterpart to the scapholunate injury, but it occurs much less frequently.

Anatomy

This intrinsic ligament joins the triquetrum and lunate and provides the previously mentioned extension torque on the lunate.

Mechanism

A fall on an outstretched hand with the wrist in extension and hypothenar impact is the most common mechanism of injury.

Examination

Local tenderness is present just distal to the ulnar styloid. In severe injuries, a painful click can be elicited by moving the triquetrum back and forth.

Radiography

With tears of the triquetrolunate, volar radiolunotriquetral, and dorsal radiotriquetral ligaments, a pattern of **volar intercalated segment instability** is present and is best seen on a lateral radiograph. Disruption of the triquetrolunate ligament causes the lunate to tilt in a volar direction in response to the unopposed flexion torque imparted by the scapholunate ligament. The capitolunate angle is increased, but the scapholunate angle remains unchanged. The linear arrangement of the axes is skewed into a zigzag pattern opposite that observed with scapholunate ligament tears (Figure 12-4C).

Treatment

The application of an ulnar gutter or a volar splint with close orthopedic followup care is necessary. Cast immobilization for 6 to 8 weeks followed by splint immobilization for 6 to 8 more weeks typically is satisfactory; however, some injuries require open reduction and internal fixation.

Complications

Failure to recognize this injury may result in early degenerative arthritis and chronic wrist pain.

Perilunate and Lunate Dislocations

With enough applied force, ligament disruptions continue around the lunate and culminate in these dislocation injuries.

Anatomy

In addition to the intrinsic ligaments that link the carpal bones, there are extrinsic ligamentous bands, two volar and one dorsal, that connect the carpal bones to the radius and ulna. One volar band connects the distal radius and ulna to the proximal carpal row, and the other volar band connects them to the distal carpal row. These ligaments act as slings to support the respective carpal bones. There is an inherently weak area between the two ligamentous bands known as the **space of Poirier**. This space is closed when the wrist is flexed but open when it is extended. It is through this space that the lunate displaces, which explains why forced extension is responsible for the injury.

Mechanism

A fall on an outstretched hand in dorsiflexion is the most common mechanism of injury. Perilunate instability is a progressive injury that starts with tears of the scapholunate ligament, followed by a disruption of ligaments of the capitate and triquetrum in succession. This can displace the capitate dorsal to the lunate, creating a perilunate dislocation, or the capitate can push the lunate off the radius into the palm as it rebounds, creating a lunate dislocation. Any number of other carpal fracture-dislocations also can result from this injury mechanism.

Examination

Diffuse swelling, pain, and tenderness to palpation are noted. Contrary to what might be expected, there often is no highly visible gross deformity of the wrist. Except for swelling, the wrist may appear misleadingly normal.

Radiography

With a perilunate dislocation, on the PA view, the capitolunate joint space is obliterated. The scaphoid may appear shortened or fractured, and other fractures may be present. The lateral view shows the capitate posterior to the lunate, while the lunate maintains articulation with the radius (Figure 12-5).

With a lunate dislocation, on the PA view, the lunate has a triangular shape, or **piece of pie sign**, which is pathognomonic for lunate dislocation. The lateral view shows the lunate pushed off the radius into the palm. This is the **spilled teacup sign** (Figure 12-6). Fractures to surrounding carpals also are possible.

Treatment

Some injuries can be treated with closed reduction and a long arm splint, but open reduction and internal fixation with ligament repair is the usual approach. Emergency treatment consists of ice, elevation, immobilization, pain medication, and immediate orthopedic consultation.

Complications

Carpal instability patterns and early degenerative arthritis, in addition to the complications associated with individual carpal fractures such as delayed union, nonunion, malunion, and avascular necrosis, are possible. Lunate dislocation may compress the median nerve in the carpal tunnel. Other possible injuries include ulnar neuropathy and vascular injuries.

Figure 12-5.

Perilunate dislocation. The PA view shows overlap of the lunate and capitate. The lateral view shows the lunate (L) maintaining articulation with the radius while the capitate (C) is displaced dorsal to the lunate.

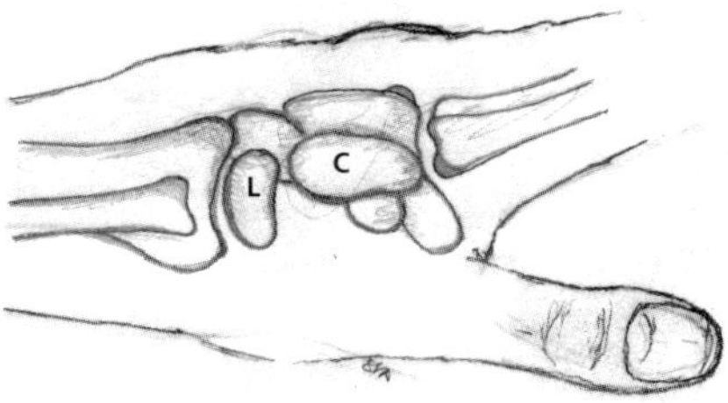

Fractures of the Distal Radius and Ulna

First described in 1814,[8] fractures of the distal radius and ulna are quite common and account for as many as 15% of all fractures. Peak occurrence is in elderly persons, and incidence rises in the winter when icy walkways increase the risk of falls.[1]

Colles Fracture

This is the most common wrist fracture; it is a fracture of the distal radial metaphysis with dorsal displacement and angulation (Figure 12-7).

Anatomy

The distal radial articular surface consists of two concavities that accommodate the scaphoid and lunate and a small notch that articulates with the ulna. The distal articular surface has an average alignment to the long axis of 22 degrees of inclination and an average volar tilt of 14 degrees (see Figure 12-1).

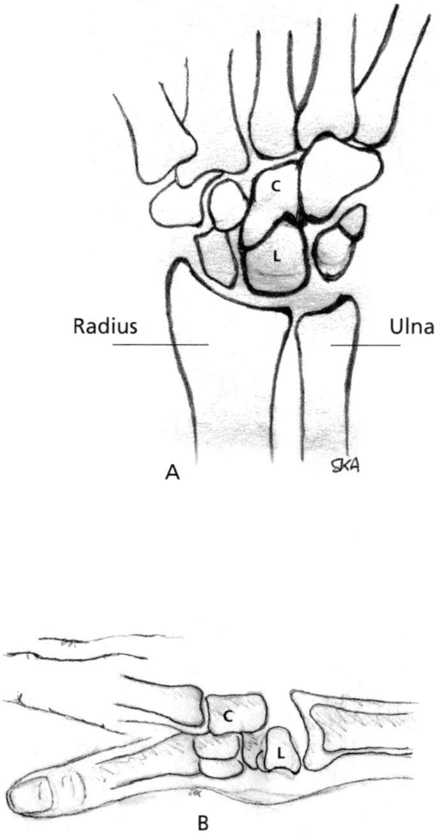

Figure 12-6.

Lunate dislocation. **A)** *The PA view reveals pathognomonic triangular shape of the lunate (piece of pie sign).* **B)** *The lateral view shows the lunate (L) tilting into the palm (spilled teacup sign) with the capitate (C) displaced dorsally.*

Mechanism

A fall on an outstretched hand with the wrist in dorsiflexion is the mechanism of injury. An individual's age can influence the type of fracture that occurs. In elderly persons, extra-articular fractures are more common because these patients have a thinner metaphyseal cortex. Young adults are prone to complicated intra-articular fractures because of both a stronger metaphyseal cortex and a propensity for greater forces associated with athletic activities.

Examination

Localized pain and swelling are noted over the distal radius. Often, a gross **dinner fork deformity** results from dorsal angulation. The median nerve may be compressed in the carpal tunnel, producing paresthesias and thenar muscle weakness. An examination of the elbow and shoulder can exclude likely associated injuries.

Radiography

On the PA view, the cortex of the radial metaphysis is disrupted, and shortening may be observed. Intra-articular fractures may extend into the radioulnar or radiocarpal joints. These Colles variants typically have an inverted-T appearance on the PA view. So-called **die-punch fractures** through the lunate fossa may be present, so named because of the visible step-off and depression of the articular surface. These fractures often are comminuted and involve the distal radioulnar joint. Ulnar styloid fractures also may be present. The lateral view confirms the extent of dorsal angulation and comminution.

Treatment

Colles fractures are classified as stable or unstable depending on their radiographic appearance. In general, unstable fractures have more than 20 degrees of angulation, shortening of 1 cm or more, sig-

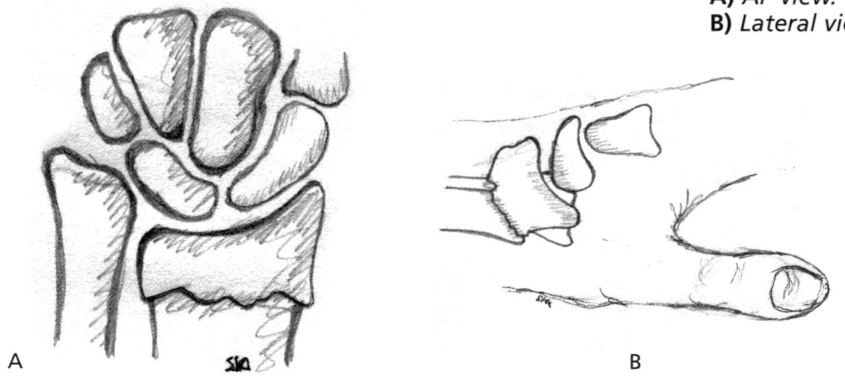

Figure 12-7.

Colles fracture. Note dorsal angulation.
A) *AP view.*
B) *Lateral view.*

nificant comminution, or intra-articular involvement.[9,10] Unstable fractures typically require open reduction, although some respond well to closed reduction. Orthopedic consultation is warranted. Stable fractures are treated with a volar splint or by closed reduction using finger traps and arm counterweighting followed by immobilization with a short arm splint past the MCP joints.[9] The goal of restoring the normal length and volar tilt to the radius is critical for future wrist function. Any question regarding adequate reduction and immobilization of a stable Colles fracture should be referred to an orthopedic consultant.

Complications

Loss of reduction, malunion, nonunion, median nerve compression, carpal instability patterns, and early degenerative arthritis are possible complications.

Smith Fracture

Anatomy

Refer to the information provided for Colles fracture.

Mechanism

A Smith fracture results from a direct blow or fall on the dorsum of the hand or from a fall on an outstretched hand with the hand moving from a supinated to a pronated position.

Examination

Local swelling and tenderness are noted over the distal radius, as is a **garden spade deformity** with palmar displacement of the hand. Examination of the shoulder and elbow excludes associated injuries.

Radiography

On the PA view, the radius shows a metaphyseal fracture and appears shortened. The lateral view is a mirror image of a typical Colles fracture, hence the often-used term **reverse Colles fracture**. The distal fragment is displaced volarly and angulated dorsally (Figure 12-8). The fracture may be intra-articular or extra-articular.

Treatment

Unstable fractures (see "Colles Fracture") may require open reduction and external or internal fixation.[11] Stable fractures are managed with closed reduction and a long arm splint for 6 to 8 weeks. Emergency treatment of stable fractures consists of pain medication, ice, elevation, immobilization in a posterior mold, and prompt orthopedic consultation.

Complications

As with a Colles fracture, complications include median nerve injury, malunion, and posttraumatic arthritis.

Barton Fracture

This is an intra-articular fracture that involves either the dorsal or volar rim of the radius. Dislocation or subluxation of the carpus in the direction of the fracture segment produces a fracture-dislocation injury (Figure 12-9).

Anatomy

See "Colles Fracture."

Mechanism

A Barton fracture-dislocation is the result of high-energy trauma and should be considered unstable. Volar and dorsal Barton fractures actually are intra-articular variants of Smith and Colles fractures, respectively, with the dorsal being the more common of the two.

Examination

Tenderness over the distal radius and marked edema with an obvious deformity are noted. Median nerve compression is possible and should be sought.

Radiography

On the PA view, there is a metaphyseal fracture with overlap of the carpals and the distal radius. On the lateral view, carpal subluxation or dislocation overshadows the radius fracture, which involves either the dorsal or volar lip of the distal radius.

Treatment

Barton fractures require orthopedic consultation for reduction and stabilization. Unstable fractures are those that involve more than 50% of the articular surface and those with associated carpal subluxation or dislocation. These require either external fixation or open reduction and internal fixation.[11,12]

Figure 12-8.

Smith (reverse Colles) fracture. Note volar angulation.

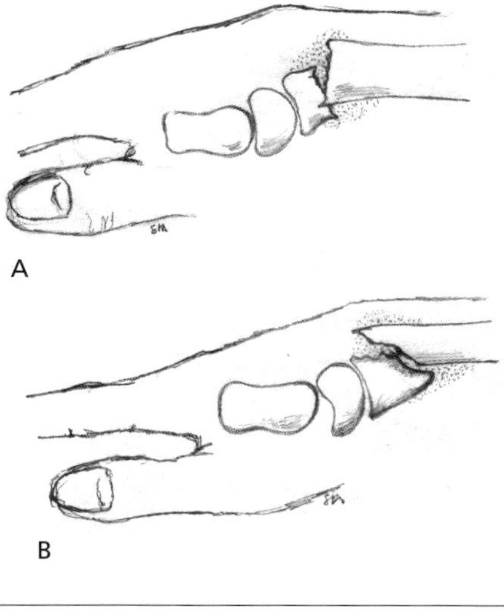

Figure 12-9.

Barton fracture. Note significant displacement of entire hand.

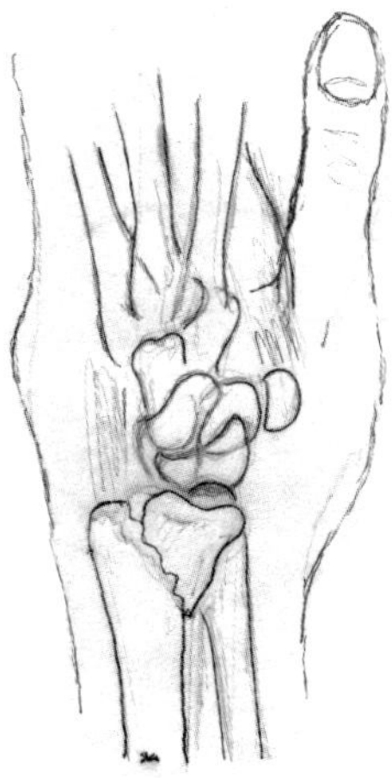

Complications

Posttraumatic arthritis and delayed carpal instability are common with inadequate reduction.

Chauffeur (Hutchinson) Fracture

Anatomy

The radial styloid is the key point of attachment of the extrinsic carpal ligaments. These link the radius to the carpal bones.

Mechanism

The chauffeur fracture got its name from the wrist twist or torque that was produced when a hand-cranked automobile backfired while being started, thus reversing direction. This caused sudden traction on the radial styloid, which resulted in avulsion of the radial styloid. Today this injury typically is the result of a fall or trauma such as a motorcycle crash.

Examination

Mild swelling and point tenderness are noted over the bony prominence of the radial styloid.

Radiography

The PA view shows a lucent line that crosses the base of the radial styloid (Figure 12-10).

Treatment

A radial gutter splint is satisfactory pending orthopedic followup care. Closed reduction and percutaneous pinning are required for some displaced fractures. Definitive treatment for nondisplaced fractures is wrist immobilization for 4 to 6 weeks.

Complications

Carpal instability and posttraumatic arthritis may occur.

Ulnar Styloid Fracture

Anatomy

The ulnar styloid is attached to the triangular fibrocartilage complex that stabilizes the distal radioulnar joint. This complex supports the extrinsic ligaments and acts as a shock absorber between the carpals and the ulna.

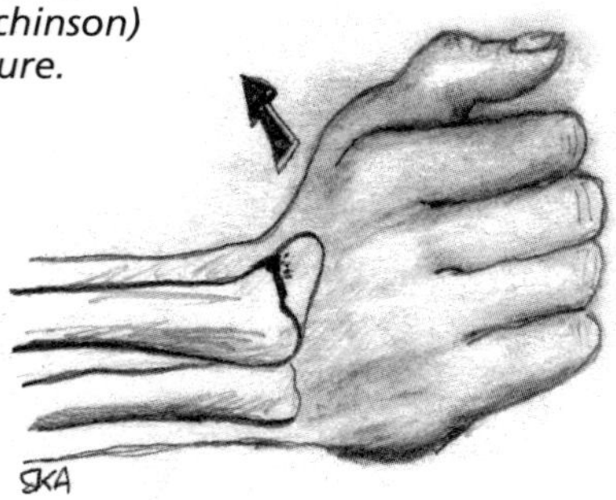

Figure 12-10.

Chauffeur (Hutchinson) fracture.

Mechanism

The mechanism of injury is a fall on an outstretched hand with forced dorsiflexion (often in combination with a Colles fracture), radial deviation, or rotation of the wrist.

Examination

There is local tenderness over the ulnar styloid. Tears of the fibrocartilage complex may produce pain or a click with wrist rotation.

Radiography

The PA view shows a lucent line or, more often, displacement of the ulnar styloid. The fracture looks rather benign, but more significant tears of the triangular fibrocartilage complex may be present.

Treatment

Isolated ulnar styloid fractures may be splinted in neutral position or ulnar deviation with good results. Fractures associated with distal radius fractures or triangular fibrocartilage complex tears may require open repair. Painful nonunion may require excision of the bony fragment.

Complications

Nonunion and distal radioulnar joint instability may occur.

Radioulnar Joint Dislocation

Anatomy

The distal radioulnar joint is a trochlear joint that assists forearm rotation. Volar and dorsal ligaments and the triangular fibrocartilage complex support it.

Mechanism

Isolated injury is rare. When it occurs, it typically is caused by a fall on an outstretched hand with hyperpronation of the wrist. More often, this injury accompanies intra-articular fractures of the distal radius or a Galeazzi fracture-dislocation.

Examination

There is pain on the ulnar aspect with increased prominence of the ulnar styloid dorsally (volar dislocation is almost nonexistent). There may be pain or a clicking sensation with wrist movement. Joint laxity can be detected by grasping the distal radius and ulna separately and moving them in opposite directions, known as the **piano keys sign**.

Radiography

The PA view may reveal that the distal radius and ulna overlap at the joint instead of revealing the normal space. The lateral view shows the dorsal displacement of the ulna.

Treatment

This dislocation is easily reduced, and the wrist must be immobilized with a long arm splint in supination for 4 weeks. Open reduction and internal fixation is sometimes necessary in the event of a delay in diagnosis or failure of closed reduction.[13]

Complications

Dorsal dislocations have a high recurrence rate and may require open repair.

References

1. Ritchie JV, Munter DW. Emergency department evaluation and treatment of wrist injuries. *Emerg Med Clin North Am.* 1999;17:823-842.
2. Waeckerle JF. A prospective study identifying the sensitivity of radiographic findings and the clinical efficacy of clinical findings in carpal navicular fractures. *Ann Emerg Med.* 1987;16:733.

3. Terry DW, Ramin JE. The navicular fat stripe: a useful roentgen feature for evaluating wrist trauma. *AJR Am J Roentgenol.* 1975;124:25-28.
4. Murphy D, Eisenhauer M. The utility of the bone scan in the diagnosing of clinical scaphoid fracture. *J Emerg Med.* 1994;12:709-712.
5. Barton NJ. Twenty questions about scaphoid fractures. *J Hand Surg.* 1992;17B:289-310.
6. Leslie IJ, Dickson RA. The fractured carpal scaphoid. *J Bone Joint Surg.* 1981;63B:225.
7. Frankel VH. The Terry Thomas sign. *Clin Orthop.* 1978;135:311.
8. Colles A. On the fracture of the carpal extremity of the radius. *Edinb Med Surg J.* 1814;10:182.
9. Cooney WP, Dobyns JH, Linscheid RL. Complications of Colles fractures. *J Bone Joint Surg.* 1980;62A(4):613.
10. Rettig ME, Dessa GL, Raskin KB, et al. Wrist fractures in the athlete. *Clin Sports Med.* 1998;17:469-489.
11. Louis DS. Barton's and Smith's fractures. *Hand Clin.* 1988;4(3):399.
12. Mehara AK, Rastogi S, Bhan S, et al. Classification and treatment of volar Barton's fractures. *Injury.* 1993;24(1):55.
13. Buterbaugh GA, Palmer AK. Fractures and dislocations of the distal radioulnar joint. *Hand Clin.* 1988;4:361.

Additional Reading

Cohen MS. Ligamentous injuries of the wrist in the athlete. *Clin Sports Med.* 1999;17:533-552.

Greenspan A, ed. *Orthopedic Radiology: A Practical Approach.* Philadelphia, Pa: Lippincott; 2000:151-195.

Nguyen DT, McCue FC, Urch SE. Evaluation of the injured wrist on the field and in the office. *Clin Sports Med.* 1998;17:421-432.

Schreibman KL, Freeland A, Gilula LA, et al. Imaging of the hand and wrist. *Orthop Clin North Am.* 1997;28:537-582.

Tiel-van Buul MMC, van Beek EJR, Nooitgedacht EA, et al. Diagnosing scaphoid fractures: radiographs cannot be used as the gold standard! *Injury.* 1992;23:77-79.

Waizenegger M, Barton NJ, Davis TRC, et al. Clinical signs in scaphoid fractures. *J Hand Surg.* 1994;19B:743-747.

CHAPTER 13

Flexor Tendon Injuries

Madonna Fernández-Frackelton, MD

Flexor tendon injuries of the hand most often occur with lacerations secondary to sharp objects. Blunt trauma and rheumatoid arthritis also can cause injury but much less frequently. The correct diagnosis of flexor tendon injuries is vital for appropriate emergency department treatment and is helpful for predicting future hand function. The emergency physician must accurately identify tendon injuries and provide wound management and appropriate referral.

Anatomy

The flexor tendons of the hand originate from the muscle bellies of the volar forearm and extend to the distal phalanges. Any injury that occurs between these two points can damage flexor tendons. All of the flexor tendons except the palmaris longus run under fibrous bands at the wrist called the **palmar carpal ligament** and the **flexor retinaculum**. The **palmaris longus** tendon is contiguous with the palmar carpal ligament and the **palmar aponeurosis** (Figure 13-1). The flexor retinaculum lies just deep to the palmar carpal ligament and, with the carpal bones, forms the **carpal tunnel**.

The flexor tendons are surrounded by tendon sheaths, or **bursae**, which allow for smooth range of motion. The index, middle, and ring fingers and the thumb typically have individual bursae, and the bursa of the little finger communicates with the ulnar bursa. There are variations in this anatomy (Figure 13-2). The bursae are composed of a series of pulleys that tether the tendons close to the bone to prevent bow-stringing and to allow for smooth motion. In the index through little fingers, there are five annular pulleys (A1 to A5) and three cruciate pulleys (C1 to C3) (Figure 13-3). The tendon sheath of the thumb is composed of two annular pulleys and one oblique pulley. The motor function of each of the flexor tendons is listed in Table 13-1. Of note, the tendons of the flexor digitorum superficialis (FDS) insert at the base of the middle phalanx of all four fingers. The tendons of the flexor digitorum profundus

(FDP) run deep to the FDS in the hand and proximal finger. They split the tendons of the FDS and insert at the base of the distal phalanx of all four fingers (Figure 13-4).

The tendons are divided into anatomic zones according to location, treatment options, and prognosis. These zones are shown in Figure 13-5.

Zone I

Zone I extends from just distal to the insertion of the FDS at the proximal portion of the middle phalanx to the insertion of the FDP. By definition, injuries here involve only the FDP. Damage to tendons in zone I are most frequently caused by sharp objects. Blunt force avulsion of the FDP from its insertion is commonly a sports injury referred to as **jersey finger** because of its occurrence in football players. The ring and little fingers are most often involved.

There are four types of avulsion. **Type I avulsion** occurs when the tendon retracts into the palm beneath the A1 pulley. The blood supply to the tendon is essentially lost. **Type II avulsions** are the most common, and they occur when the tendon rests at the PIP level. The blood supply remains largely intact in these cases. **Type III avulsions** are associated with a fracture fragment that is attached to the tendon, and the tendon does not retract past the A4 pulley. **Type IV avulsions** involve bony avulsion from the distal phalanx along with avulsion of the tendon from the bone fragment; these avulsions are rare.[1]

Figure 13-1.

Wrist, palmar view.

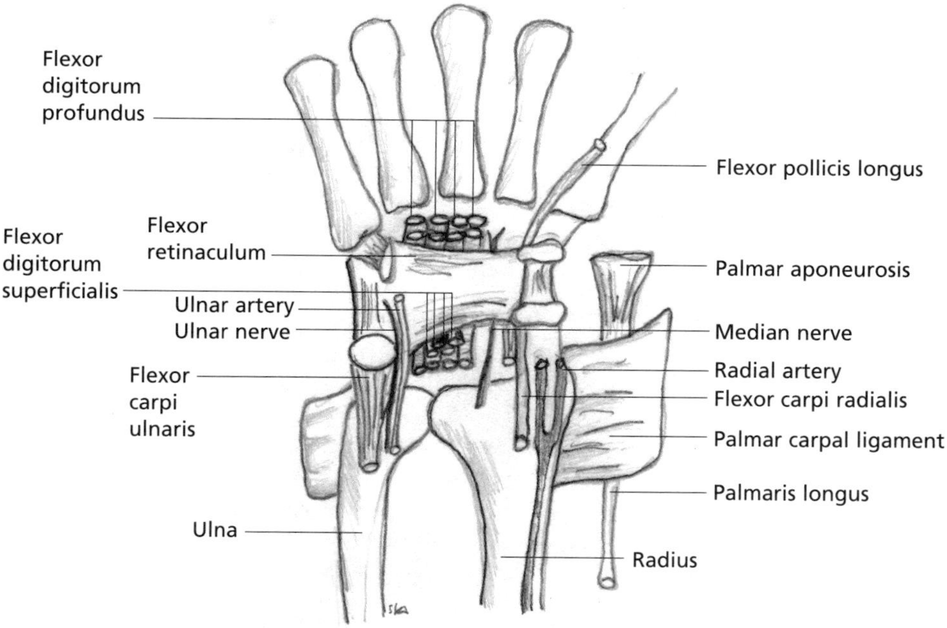

Zone II

Zone II encompasses the area in the digital canal occupied by both the FDP and the FDS. It extends from the distal palmar crease to the proximal portion of the middle phalanx. Injuries in this area are common, and outcomes are frequently poor. At this level, the FDP and the FDS have a precarious blood supply through the vinculum longum (the fibrous bands that connect tendons), which is fed by the digital arteries.

Zone III

Zone III extends from the distal edge of the carpal tunnel to the proximal end of the flexor sheath in the digits. Outcomes of injuries in this area usually are good.

Zone IV

Zone IV consists of the carpal tunnel. Injuries in this area are unusual because of the depth of the well-protected carpal tunnel. When zone IV injuries occur, however, they frequently involve multiple structures. Damage to the median nerve is common, and a careful examination for thumb opposition (intrinsic motor branch) and palmar sensation (palmar sensory branch) should be performed.

Figure 13-2.

Tendon sheaths, palmar view.

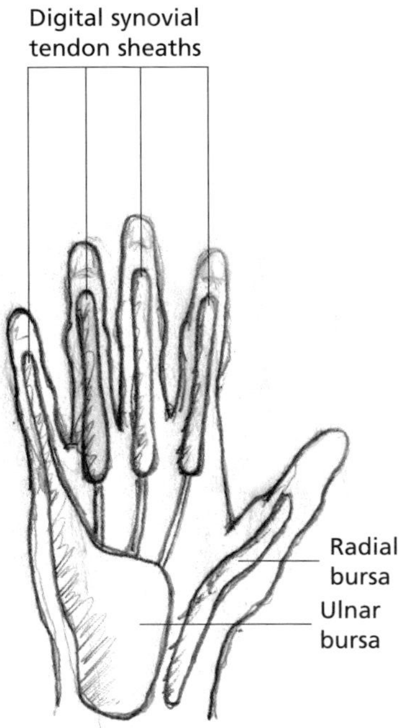

Figure 13-3.

Pulleys of the flexor tendon sheaths, lateral view (A, annular pulley; C, cruciate pulley).

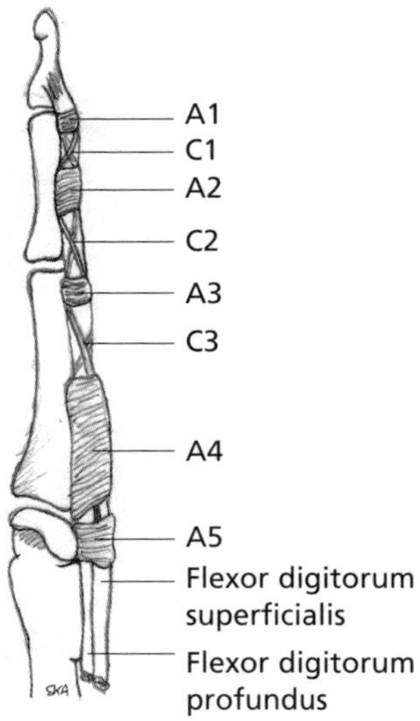

Zone V

Zone V encompasses the area proximal to the carpal tunnel. Injuries in this area frequently involve multiple tendons (**spaghetti wrist**), as well as the median or ulnar nerve, or both. Injuries in this zone are typical of suicide attempts, and profuse hemorrhage is common.

Injuries to the **flexor pollicis longus (FPL)** present a unique problem. The neurovascular bundles are closer to the volar aspect of the thumb than are those in the fingers, so concomitant and iatrogenic injuries are more likely. The zones in the thumb are similar to those in the fingers (Figure 13-5). Spontaneous rupture of the flexor pollicis longus can occur in patients with rheumatoid arthritis due to erosion of the tendon against the arthritic scaphoid carpal bone; this is known as **attritional rupture**, or **Mannerfelt syndrome**.[2]

Examination

History

The mechanism of injury, causative object, and time and location of injury should all be documented. Flexor tendon injuries are most often caused by knives or glass with the digit in a flexed position. As noted, blunt injuries can result in tendon rupture. The patient should be questioned about foreign body sensation and the possibility of a retained foreign body. Chemical exposure should be assessed in occupational and high-pressure injection injuries. The patient's age, handedness, occupation, and hobbies are important in the assessment and treatment of all

Table 13-1.

Tendon motor function and physical examination.

Tendon	Function	Physical Examination
Flexor digitorum superficialis	Flexion of digits at PIP and MCP joints	Hold MCP in neutral position and have patient flex PIP
Flexor digitorum profundus	Flexion of digits at DIP, PIP, and MCP joints	Hold MCP and PIP straight and have patient flex DIP
Flexor carpi radialis	Flexion and radial deviation of hand at wrist	Have patient flex and radially deviate wrist
Flexor carpi ulnaris	Flexion and ulnar deviation of hand at wrist	Have patient flex and ulnarly deviate wrist
Flexor pollicis longus	Flexion of thumb at IP and MCP joints	Hold MCP straight and have patient flex IP; then, have patient flex thumb across palm
Palmaris longus	Tightening of palmar aponeurosis/flexion of hand at wrist	No specific examination to test this tendon function; not necessary for normal hand function

hand injuries. Any medical problems, medications, and allergies should be documented, as well as tetanus immunization status. Any treatment rendered in the field or before presentation also should be noted. All patients with zone V injuries should be questioned about suicidal intent.

Physical Examination

Inspection

The physical examination should be performed with adequate lighting and preferably in a bloodless field. Direct pressure and elevation usually are adequate to control bleeding. If necessary, a blood pressure cuff can be placed and inflated to a pressure about 10 to 20 mm Hg above the patient's systolic blood pressure to help control bleeding. The cuff should be left in place for no longer than 20 minutes. The use of blind clamping and suturing to control bleeding is contraindicated and may cause serious damage to underlying structures. The position (or attitude, or lie) of the hand should be noted. In a resting position, the affected finger does not assume its normal graduated, cascading position compared with the other digits if a complete flexor tendon injury is present. The wound should be examined for the presence of foreign bodies and injury to underlying structures.

Palpation

If a complete tendon laceration has occurred, the retracted proximal portion of the tendon may be identified as a tender area. This tenderness may be more proximal to the laceration than initially suspected.

Figure 13-4.

Tendons at the distal digits, palmar view.

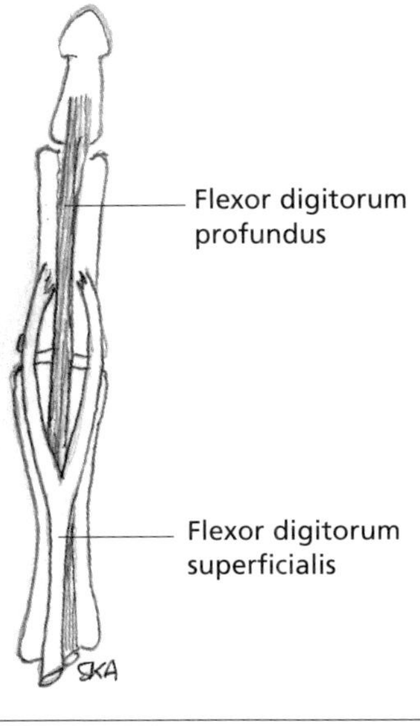

Figure 13-5.

Zones of the flexor tendons, palmar view.

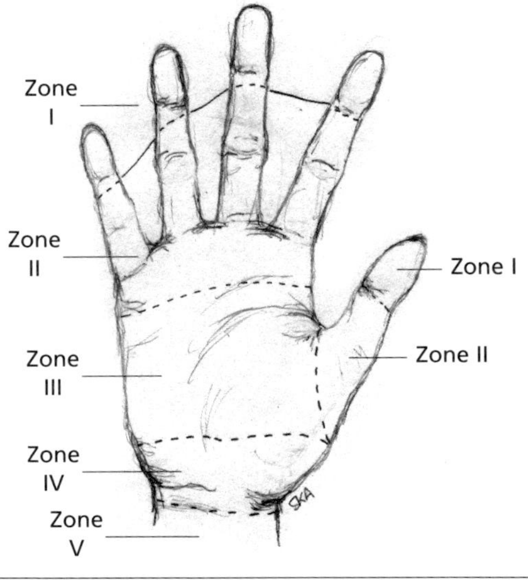

Nerve Function

Regional anesthesia often is necessary for adequate wound inspection and motor examination but should be administered only after a complete neurovascular examination. Nerve function is assessed by checking sensation to light touch and two-point discrimination (normal, less than 6 mm) in the distribution of the digital nerves and superficial nerves of the hand (Figure 13-6).

Circulation

Capillary refill time (normal, less than 2 seconds), hand temperature compared with that of the unaffected hand, and radial and ulnar pulses should be determined, and the Allen test should be performed. Circulation is especially important in zone V injuries. Completely lacerated arteries may contract and spasm. As a result, hemorrhage may be

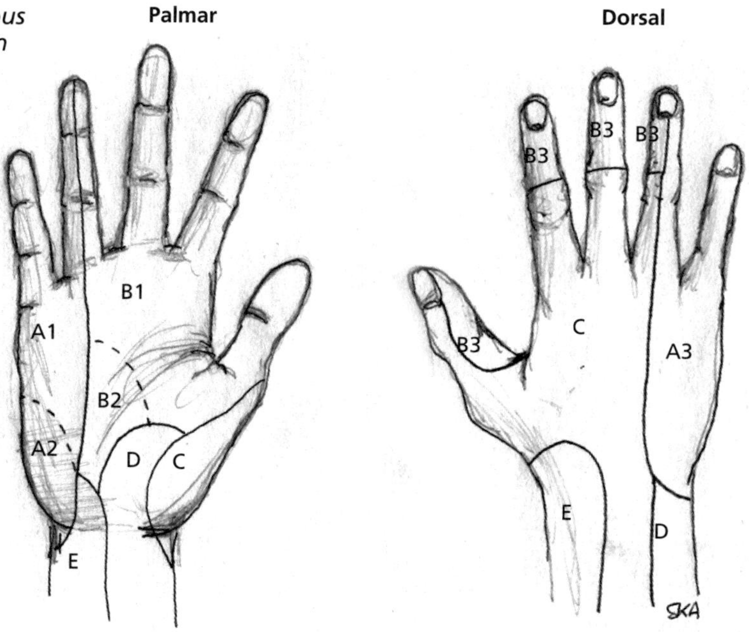

Figure 13-6.

Peripheral innervation to the hand. **A)** *Ulnar nerve: 1) palmar digital branch; 2) palmar branch; 3) dorsal branch.* **B)** *Median nerve: 1) palmar digital branch; 2) palmar branch; 3) proper palmar digital branch.* **C)** *Radial nerve.* **D)** *Musculocutaneous nerve.* **E)** *Median antecubital cutaneous nerve.*

less impressive on emergency department presentation than the multiple tendon and nerve injuries, but there undoubtedly is significant blood loss. If circulation to the hand is compromised, emergent vascular repair by a surgeon takes precedence over tendon and nerve repair.

Motor Function

The motor function of each tendon should be noted (Table 13-1). Partially lacerated tendons frequently maintain function. Because tendons slide freely in the sheaths, a complete or partial laceration that occurs while the hand is flexed may not be visualized if the hand is examined in extension. The entire excursion of the tendon must be examined to determine whether there is a laceration; a partial tendon laceration may not initially be visualized in the wound site. If a laceration occurs while the digit is flexed, the tendon injury will be distal to the skin injury when the digit is extended. For this reason, all hand lacerations should be assessed through their entire range of motion. Any partial lacerations should be graded in terms of the percentage of involved tendon.

Imaging

Plain radiographs should be obtained for all injuries that involve glass, possible retained radiopaque foreign bodies, high-pressure injection injuries, possible underlying fractures, and infection. Many foreign bodies are not radiopaque (wood, plastic, other organic matter), so the possibility of a missed foreign body should be discussed with the patient when it is relevant. If there is a high index of suspicion, MRI should be considered.

Treatment

General Guidelines

Pain Control

Anesthesia may be necessary for adequate examination (see Chapter 4). If a patient is anxious or uncomfortable, adequate wound management will be difficult. Children and anxious adults may require systemic analgesic agents (narcotics) or anxiolytics (benzodiazepines), or both, for proper wound management. A limited examination of a patient that includes neurovascular function should always be conducted before local or regional anesthesia is administered.

Irrigation and Débridement

With anesthesia and a careful examination, the wound *must* be cleansed and prepped. This begins with the removal of foreign material (including rings) and débridement of necrotic tissue, followed by irrigation with copious amounts of sterile water or normal saline at 15 psi of continuous nonpulsatile pressure (with an 18-gauge Angiocath or Zerowet splash guard on a 30-mL syringe). Povidone-iodine solution (Betadine) is not recommended because it has been shown to impair wound healing and has no demonstrated benefit over irrigation with normal saline or sterile water.

Skin Closure

After the wound is cleansed and hemostasis is achieved, the skin should be closed in the emergency department. Patients with flexor tendon injuries should be referred to a hand surgery specialist for primary repair. Although the emergency physician does not perform the tendon repair, proper wound care provided initially in the emergency department improves overall outcome.

Skin overlying flexor tendon lacerations should be loosely approximated with as few sutures as necessary to achieve tissue approximation. Simple interrupted sutures of 5-0 nylon or polypropylene are adequate. The entire pass of each needle throw should be directly visualized to avoid grasping underlying tendons, nerves, and blood vessels. A nonadherent material should be placed over the closed wound and a fluffy dressing applied.

Immobilization

In flexor tendon injuries, immobilization is indicated. The hand is splinted in a position of function with the wrist in a neutral position and the MCP joint at 90 degrees of flexion. The patient should be instructed to elevate the injured hand to prevent further swelling. For flexor tendon lacerations of the thumb, a thumb spica splint is applied with the MCP and IP joints in flexion.

Tetanus

All patients 7 years old and older who have tetanus-prone wounds should receive 0.5 mL of tetanus and diphtheria toxoid (Td) intramuscularly if they have not been vaccinated in the past 5 years. (Patients younger than 7 years should receive the pediatric preparation DTaP, or DT if the pertussis vaccine is contraindicated.) All other patients should receive a booster if they have not been vaccinated in the past 10 years. In patients with tetanus-prone wounds who have never been vaccinated, tetanus immune globulin (TIG) and Td (or DTaP or DT for children younger than 7 years) should be administered at separate sites on the body, with followup at 1 and 6 months for the complete tetanus vaccine series (see Table 5-1, page 52).

Prophylactic Antibiotics

There are no prospective data on the use of prophylactic antibiotics in simple open injuries of the hand that specifically involve the flexor tendons. Prophylactic antibiotics have questionable value in simple lacerations of the hand and in various soft tissue injuries of the hand.[3,4] In a retrospective review of 140 patients with open flexor tendon injuries, Stone and Davidson[5] found no difference in the infection rate between patients who received antibiotics and those who did not. Only three of the patients developed infection, and two of these were in the antibiotic-treated groups. Prophylactic antibiotics are recommended only for large or grossly contaminated wounds and for wound-associated open fractures and animal (including human) bites. Meticulous wound care with irrigation and early skin closure is the best way to prevent infection.

Laboratory Evaluation

Any patient who requires flexor tendon repair in the operating room should undergo preoperative laboratory tests based on his or her age and coexisting medical conditions.

Admission Indications

All patients with wounds that are grossly contaminated after emergency department débridement should be admitted for débridement in the operating room. Patients with complex crush injuries, open fractures, open joints, and high-pressure injection injuries also should be hospitalized. Patients who present to the emergency department with infection and postoperative infections frequently require hospitalization for intravenous antibiotic administration and possible drainage in the operating room.

Need for Referral

Hand surgery consultation and referral are indicated for all flexor tendon injuries. Whether the surgeon must see the patient immediately or in followup depends on the injury.

Emergent Referral

Emergent referral (while the patient is still in the emergency department) to a hand surgeon is required for the following flexor tendon injuries:

- Acute injury with open joint or open fracture
- Acute injury with arterial laceration with or without vascular compromise
- Any open wound over a flexor tendon injury that cannot be closed in the emergency department (If the wound can be closed in the emergency department, this becomes an urgent referral.)
- Grossly contaminated wounds, including animal (and human) bites
- High-pressure injection injuries

Urgent Referral

Urgent referral (within 24 to 76 hours) is appropriate for all acute flexor tendon injuries that do not fall into the emergent category, including flexor tendon lacerations after skin closure, closed avulsion injuries, tendon lacerations with associated nerve lacerations, and attritional rupture of the FPL. Repair should occur within the first week because scarring and tendon retraction make repair more difficult after 10 to 14 days. In zone II, the annular pulleys contract, and blood supply to the proximal tendon may be compromised. In zone III, substantial bleeding is common and can result in significant scarring, making repair more difficult. An exception is the type II FDP avulsion; because the blood supply from the vinculum is usually intact and the tendon is not significantly retracted, successful repair can be performed up to 3 months after the injury.

Routine Referral

Patients with chronic flexor tendon injuries receive routine (within weeks to months) followup care. The decision to repair chronic flexor tendon injuries is difficult; these patients present late and may be noncompliant. The rehabilitation necessary to obtain a good outcome from surgery requires strict compliance to the regimen, and the decision to operate must be made on an individual basis.

Specific Surgical Repairs Based on Zones of Injury

Several techniques are used by hand specialists to repair tendon injuries. Most involve a core suture of 3-0 to 4-0 braided synthetic material placed through the center of the tendon and running parallel to the tendon fibers. A grasping stitch is required to hold on to the fiber bundles; this is achieved by ensuring that the transverse pass of the suture is in a different plane than that of the longitudinal pass. An epitendinous running suture of 6-0 to 7-0 monofilament nylon is then placed to prevent snagging of the free edge of the tendon on other structures. This usually is necessary only for repairs within the digital sheath/zone II (Figure 13-7). The type of repair that the surgeon chooses depends on the location of injury and the technique with which he or she is most comfortable.

Zone I Repairs

Repairs in zone I involve the FDP. The proximal tendon is retrieved with a tendon passer or an alligator forceps. A counterincision in the palm may be necessary to retrieve the proximal tendon, which is then repaired just proximal or just distal to the A4 pulley. If the bone of the distal phalanx is avulsed or insufficient tendon is present distally, holes can be drilled through the distal phalanx and out through the nail bed. The tendon is anchored and tied over a button on the nail bed. If the distal end of the tendon is less than 1 cm, the suture also can be passed through the pulp of the finger with a hypodermic needle as a guide. The suture is then tied externally (Figure 13-8). A good to excellent outcome can be achieved in up to 75% of patients.[6]

Figure 13-7.

Technique of tendon repair. **A)** *Core suture.* **B)** *Epitendinous suture.*

A

B

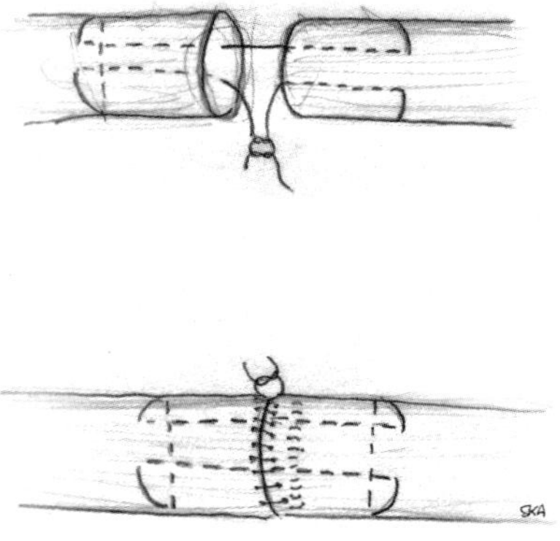

Zone II Repairs

Zone II is referred to as “no man’s land” because of the difficulty involved in repairing two tendons in the same sheath to ensure that they glide smoothly. A zigzag incision is used, incorporating the initial laceration when possible. The retrieval of proximal and distal tendons can result in tendon injury. Primary repair is preferred in this zone to minimize the amount of adhesions before surgery. Outcomes used to be much worse, but with current surgical techniques and early repair, good to excellent outcomes are reported in 70% to 75% of patients.[6]

Zone III Repairs

In zone III, adequate exposure is necessary to identify tendon ends. These injuries are repaired with core sutures, and favorable outcomes are the rule. Epitendinous sutures usually are not necessary here. The superficial palmar arch and major branches of the median and ulnar nerves also may require repair.

Zone IV Repairs

Repair in zone IV is similar to repair in zone V. Tendons are matched by their function, size, and expected anatomic positions. The median nerve and other structures also may require repair.

Zone V Repairs

The most important aspect of repair in zone V is the assurance of adequate hand perfusion. The radial and ulnar arteries in this area can be easily lacerated. Fractures should be stabilized. Adequate exposure of all injured tendons should be obtained before beginning the repair. The flexor carpi ulnaris, flexor carpi radialis, palmaris longus, and the most superficial tendons usually are easily opposed (see Figure 13-1). Repair of the palmaris longus is not necessary because it provides no additional motor function to the hand or wrist. The FPL has its own sheath and is the deepest tendon in zone V. The four tendons of the FDP and the four tendons of the FDS are aligned on the basis of caliber and expected anatomic location. Tendons to the middle and ring fingers are more superficial than are tendons to the index and little fingers. The prognosis for repair in zone V is good. Psychiatric consultation is indicated for patients whose injuries resulted from suicidal intent.

The FPL has a less-complicated tendon sheath, and primary repair is less difficult than that for other flexor tendon injuries. Injuries in the thenar web space can be confused with FPL injuries because the thenar muscle has a broad fascia and ligamentous attachment. When lacerated, the thenar muscle may look like visible tendon in the wound. If the use of adequate local anesthesia and wound exploration in the emergency department confirm there is no tendon injury, the muscle can be repaired by the emergency physician with deep absorbable sutures and the skin closed

Figure 13-8.

Repair in zone I if the proximal tendon segment is less than 1 cm. **A)** *Sutures can be pulled through a needle and tied at the tip of the finger.* **B)** *Sutures can be passed through the distal phalanx and tied over a button. The proximal fragment is sutured to the newly repaired distal segment.*

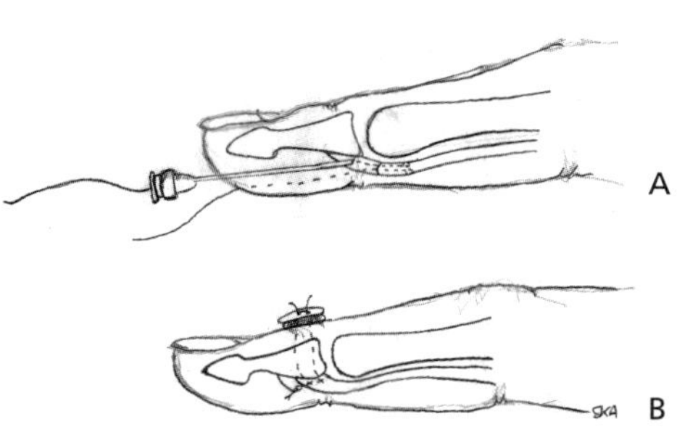

with 5-0 nonabsorbable suture. If the motor branch of the median nerve is damaged, the patient should be referred to a hand surgeon.

Partial Tendon Laceration Repairs

As previously noted, a partially lacerated tendon can maintain motor function, so visual inspection is as important as determining motor activity. The wound should be examined through an entire range of motion, with particular attention paid to the tendons in the position at the time of injury. As a general rule, flexor tendon lacerations that are less than 20% to 30% of the diameter of the tendon may not require a formal repair, but tattered tendinous tissue must be "tidied up" by a hand surgeon to prevent snagging on other tissue during movement. Lacerations of 20% to 60% of the tendon diameter may require only a running epitendinous suture. Lacerations of more than 50% to 60% require repair with a core suture and a peripheral suture. These percentages vary among hand surgeons; the decision regarding repair ultimately is that of the consultant. The literature supports a surgeon's preference regarding repair versus nonrepair of lacerations of 30% to 60% of the tendon diameter.[1]

If an injured tendon cannot be repaired with these techniques, tendon-lengthening procedures and tendon grafting may be necessary. A description of these techniques is beyond the scope of this chapter.[7]

Splinting

After surgery, a dorsal splint should place the wrist in a flexed position at about 40 degrees and extend over the digits to hold the MCP joints in flexion at about 55 degrees.

Complications

Infection

Infection rates vary depending on the type of injury and coexisting injuries. Simple lacerations that involve flexor tendons have an infection rate of approximately 2% regardless of whether prophylactic antibiotics are administered.[5] As noted, there is no role for prophylactic antibiotics in these patients. Open fractures and crush injuries are associated with a higher infection rate (up to 30%), and animal bite injuries become infected in more than half of patients.[8,9] Infections of the flexor tendon sheath may require emergency surgical drainage, and all patients should be hospitalized for parenteral antibiotic therapy.

Tetanus is a rare infection that results in spastic paralysis secondary to toxins synthesized by the bacterium *Clostridium tetani* and must be prevented with standard vaccinations.

Retained Foreign Body

Foreign bodies and chemicals from high-pressure injection injuries can result in serious infection and tissue necrosis. Both of these delay wound healing and can result in long-term disability, especially if the dominant hand is involved. A missed foreign body is a major source of liability for emergency physicians.

Rupture

Tendon rupture is a common complication of flexor tendon repair and usually occurs within the first 3 months after surgery. The patient usually presents with a sudden loss of active flexion and a popping sensation. The tendon is tender where it has retracted proximally, and motor function of that tendon is completely lost. The rate of rupture of repairs is reported to be 3% to 6% in zone I and 3% to 20% in zone II. There are little data on the rupture rate of repairs in zones III to V.[6] In a study of 526 zone I and II repairs, Harris and colleagues[10] reported a rupture rate of 5% and 4%, respectively. Ninety-one percent of ruptures occurred within the first 5 weeks after repair. The causes of rupture were secondary to patient non-compliance with instructions in half of the cases.[10] Patients who present with an acute rupture after a recent repair should be splinted as appropriate for the original injury and referred back to the specialist.

Loss of Function

Adhesion formation is the most common complication of tendon injury and repair.[6] Definitions of "excellent" and "good" outcomes and need for tenolysis are poorly defined in the literature and are patient dependent. Significant adhesion may form in 1% to 25% of patients depending on the zone of injury and the extent of damage. Concomitant injury to surrounding structures (fractures, nerve and blood vessel injuries) increases the risk of adhesion formation. It is important to note that adhesions lend strength to the tendon repair. Early mobilization through dynamic traction after surgical repair decreases adhesion formation and improves mobility. Early mobilization increases the risk of rupture but also improves future tendon function. If adhesions significantly impair motion, tenolysis may be required.[1] Joint contractures and pulley failures are complications that may limit hand function. They are best avoided with early rehabilitation and careful attention to preservation of the pulley mechanism during surgery.

High-Pressure Injection Injury

High-pressure injection injuries represent a special situation for emergency physicians and hand surgeons. These injuries can result in compartment syndromes, flexor tenosynovitis, and extensive tissue necrosis. Oil-based solvents (grease, paint, paint thinner) are particularly dangerous, with associated amputation rates of 16% to 48%.[11] The initial injury often is unimpressive, and if the history of high-pressure injection injury is not obtained by the emergency physician, the outcome can be even more devastating. Emergent wide débridement, drainage, and open wound packing by a hand surgeon, along with prophylactic antibiotics, represent the standard of care for these injuries.[12] This injury is described in more detail in Chapter 24.

Long-Term Care and Rehabilitation

Early mobilization should be initiated at 3 to 5 days after surgery to improve outcome. Movement should first be passive in flexion and active in extension to allow for tendon movement without increased tension on the repair. This can be accomplished with a pulley-and-elastic mechanism that holds the involved digit in flexion and requires the intact extensors to straighten the digit (Figure 13-9). Over several weeks, tension is added to the repair by slowly allowing the wrist to extend. By 7 to 8 weeks, flexion against mild resistance and strengthening exercises begin. When active motion peaks at about 2 to 3 months, therapy can be discontinued.[13] Patients with repairs that involve less than 50% laceration of the tendon can begin rehabilitation with active motion. The most critical aspect of rehabilitation is patient compliance.

References

1. Ingari JV, Pederson WC. Update on tendon repair. *Clin Plast Surg.* 1997;24:161-173.
2. Lester B, ed. *The Acute Hand.* Stamford, Conn: Appleton & Lange; 1999:245-257.
3. Haughey RE, Lammers RL, Wagner DK. Use of antibiotics in the initial management of soft tissue hand wounds. *Ann Emerg Med.* 1981;10:187-192.
4. Grossman JA, Adams JP, Kunec J. Prophylactic antibiotics in simple hand lacerations. *JAMA.* 1981;245:1055-1056.
5. Stone JF, Davidson JSD. The role of antibiotics and timing of repair in flexor tendon injuries of the hand. *Ann Plast Surg.* 1998;40:7-13.
6. Blair WF, ed. *Techniques in Hand Surgery.* Baltimore, Md: Williams & Wilkins; 1996.
7. Tubiana R, Gilbert A, Masquelet AC, eds. *An Atlas of Surgical Techniques of the Hand and Wrist.* Philadelphia, Pa: Lippincott Williams & Wilkins; 1999.
8. Sloan JP, Dove AF, Maheson M, et al. Antibiotics in open fractures of the distal phalanx? *J Hand Surg.* 1987;12:123-124.
9. Aghababian RV, Conte JE Jr. Mammalian bite wounds. *Ann Emerg Med.* 1980;9:79-83.
10. Harris SB, Harris D, Foster AJ, et al. The aetiology of acute rupture of flexor tendon repairs in zones 1 and 2 of the fingers during early mobilization. *J Hand Surg.* 1999;24B:275-280.
11. Schnall SB, Mirzayan R. High-pressure injection injuries to the hand. *Hand Clin.* 1999;15:245-248, viii.
12. Pinto MR, Turkula-Pinto LD, Cooney WP, et al. High-pressure injection injuries of the hand: review of 25 patients managed by open wound drainage. *J Hand Surg.* 1993;18A:125-130.
13. Martin DS, Weeks DM. Tendon congruity. In: Martin DS, Collins ED, eds. *Manual of Acute Hand Injuries.* St Louis, Mo: Mosby–Year Book; 1998:251-261.

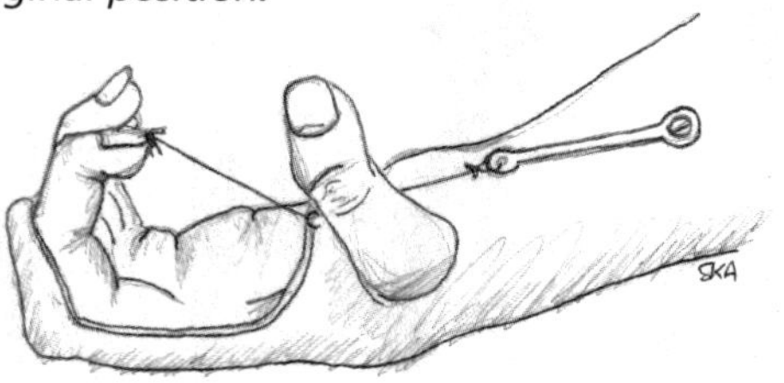

Figure 13-9.

Kleinert dynamic splinting for postoperative rehabilitation. The finger is held in flexion by a pulley system attached to a rubber band. Active extension is possible, and passive flexion then returns the digit to its original position.

Additional Reading

Hart RG, Kutz JE. Flexor tendon injuries of the hand. *Emerg Med Clin North Am.* 1993;11:621-636.

Strickland JW. Flexor tendon injuries, I. foundations of treatment. *J Am Acad Orthop Surg.* 1995;3:44-54.

Strickland JW. Flexor tendon injuries, II. operative technique. *J Am Acad Orthop Surg.* 1995;3:55-62.

CHAPTER 14

Extensor Tendon Injuries

Robert W. Wolford, MD, FACEP, and Jason M. White, MD, FACEP

The superficial location of the extensor tendons of the hand makes them particularly susceptible to injury. Injuries frequently are associated with open wounds (typically lacerations) but also occur with blunt trauma or overuse.

Extensor tendon injuries are commonly diagnosed in the emergency department, but the complexity of the injuries is frequently underestimated. This chapter reviews the anatomy of the extensor mechanism of the hand and the management of common injuries.

Anatomy

The musculature that produces extension of the fingers and hand is either **intrinsic** (located completely within the hand) or **extrinsic** (located in the forearm with tendons that extend into the hand).

Intrinsic Musculature

The intrinsic musculature is composed of the lumbrical and interosseous muscles and is innervated by the median and ulnar nerves.

The **lumbricals** originate from one or two of the tendons of the FDP, pass radially along the digit, and insert into the extensor hood and the base of the proximal phalanx. The ulnar two lumbricals are innervated by the ulnar nerve, and the radial two lumbricals are innervated by the median nerve. They flex the MCP joint and extend the IP joints. Their most important role is adjustment of the motion of the digits.

The **interossei** are identified by their origin. The four dorsal interossei originate from the dorsal aspect of adjacent metacarpals in the intermetacarpal spaces. The three palmar interossei originate from the palmar aspect of single metacarpals in the medial three intermetacarpal spaces. The ulnar nerve innervates all interossei. The dorsal interossei abduct the digits, and the palmar interossei adduct them. Like the lumbricals, the interossei have an important role in adjusting the motion of the digits.

Extrinsic Musculature

The extrinsic muscles originate in the forearm and are innervated by the radial nerve. The extensor tendons of the extrinsic muscles pass dorsally over the wrist through six compartments. These compartments form a synovium-lined fibro-osseous tendon sheath, or retinaculum. The six compartments are numbered beginning on the radial side (Figure 14-1).

The **first compartment** contains two tendons: the abductor pollicis longus and the extensor pollicis brevis. Deep branches of the radial nerve innervate both muscles.

- The **abductor pollicis longus** originates from the shafts of the ulna and radius and inserts into the base of the first metacarpal. It abducts and extends the thumb and radially deviates the wrist, and it is palpable just distal to the radial tubercle.
- The **extensor pollicis brevis** originates from the shaft of the radius and the interosseous membrane and inserts into the base of the proximal phalanx of the thumb, forming the radial side of the

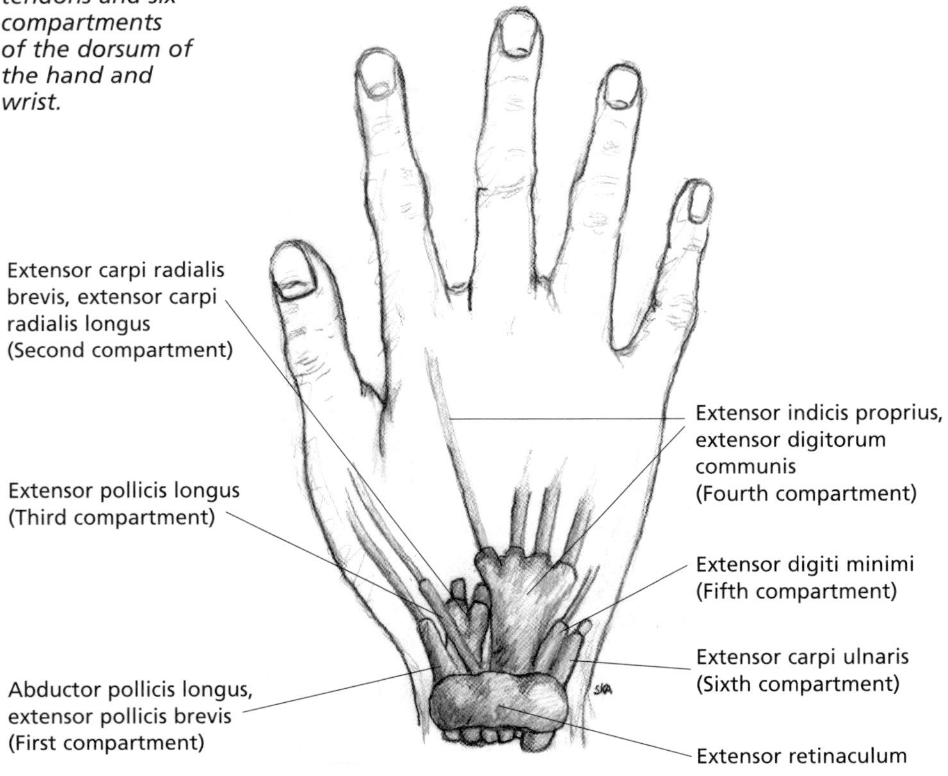

Figure 14-1.

The extensor tendons and six compartments of the dorsum of the hand and wrist.

anatomic snuffbox. This tendon extends the MCP joint of the thumb.

The **second compartment** contains two tendons: the extensor carpi radialis brevis and the extensor carpi radialis longus. Both are innervated by the radial nerve and work to extend the hand at the wrist. Wrist extension is functionally important for optimal grip strength.

- The **extensor carpi radialis brevis** originates from the lateral epicondyle of the humerus and inserts into the base of the third metacarpal.
- The **extensor carpi radialis longus** originates from the lateral supracondylar ridge of the humerus and inserts into the base of the second metacarpal.

The **third compartment** contains only one tendon: the **extensor pollicis longus**, which originates from the shaft of the ulna and the interosseous membrane. It crosses over the extensor carpi radialis brevis and longus tendons to insert into the base of the distal phalanx of the thumb. The extensor pollicis longus tendon forms the ulnar border of the anatomic snuffbox, and the extensor pollicis brevis tendon from the first compartment forms the radial side. The extensor pollicis longus is innervated by the radial nerve and acts to extend the distal phalanx of the thumb at the IP joint.

The **fourth compartment** contains four extensor digitorum communis tendons (one each for the index, middle, ring, and little fingers) and the extensor indicis proprius tendon to the index finger. These function to extend the hand and fingers and are innervated by the radial nerve.

- The **extensor digitorum communis** originates from the lateral epicondyle of the humerus and inserts into the middle and distal phalanges of the index, middle, ring, and little fingers.
- The **extensor indicis proprius** originates from the ulna and interosseous membrane and inserts into the extensor expansion of the index finger formed by the extensor digitorum communis tendon at the level of the MCP joint.

The **fifth compartment** contains the **extensor digiti minimi**, which originates from the lateral epicondyle of the humerus and inserts into the extensor expansion of the little finger. It extends the MCP joint and is innervated by the radial nerve.

The **sixth compartment** contains the **extensor carpi ulnaris**, which originates from the lateral epicondyle of the humerus and inserts into the base of the fifth metacarpal. It is innervated by the radial nerve and is involved in wrist extension and ulnar deviation.

Over the dorsum of the hand and proximal to the MCP joint, the four extensor digitorum communis tendons are connected by the obliquely running **juncturae tendinum**. The juncturae tendinum allows these tendons to assist each other in extension of the fingers. This is clinically important; extensor tendon injuries may be missed because some function of extension may be maintained even in the presence of complete disruption of an extensor digitorum communis tendon.

Extensor Hood

The extensor expansion, or hood, is formed by the extensor digitorum communis tendons with participation from the tendons of the lumbrical and interosseous muscles (Figure 14-2). This hood-like mechanism extends over the proximal and middle phalanges and holds the extensor tendon centrally over the metacarpal head at the MCP joint. The sagittal bands of the transverse metacarpal ligaments form the proximal portion of the extensor hood. These sagittal bands are circumferential and merge with the transverse metacarpal ligament and the volar plate to keep the extensor digitorum communis tendon centered over the MCP joint. The extensor digitorum communis tendon inserts at the base of the proximal phalanx with both a loose dorsal insertion, just past the MCP joint, and an attachment to the volar plate through the sagittal bands. The extensor digitorum communis divides into three portions over the proximal phalanx. Its major central slip inserts onto the base of the middle phalanx. The lateral slips of the extensor digitorum communis tendon join with the lateral bands from the interosseous and lumbrical muscles to form the conjoined lateral bands. The two conjoined lateral bands fuse over the middle phalanx to form the **terminal extensor mechanism**, which inserts into the base of the distal phalanx. The **triangular ligament** connects the two conjoined lateral bands to keep

Figure 14-2.

The extensor hood of the finger.
A) *Lateral view.*
B) *AP view.*

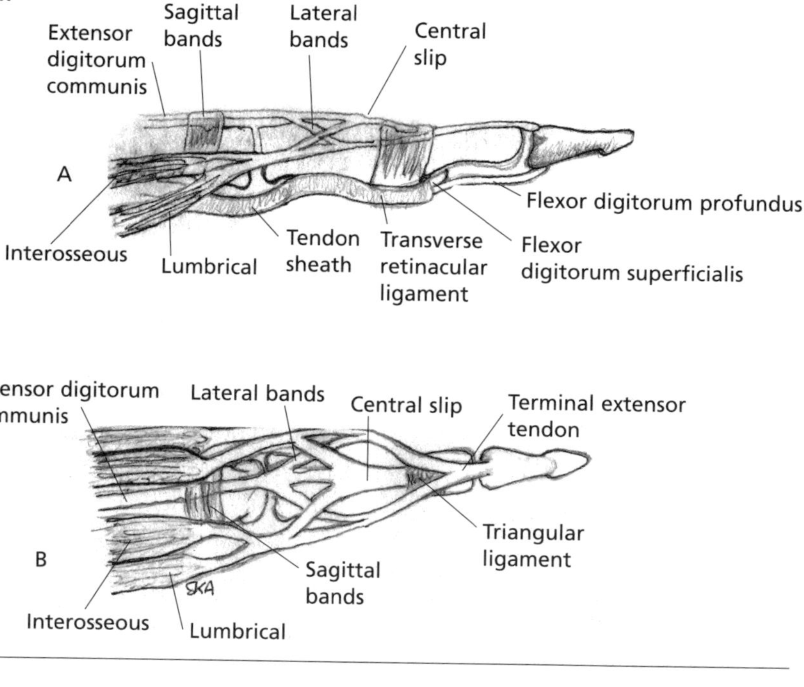

them over the dorsal aspect of the digit. The extensor indicis proprius tendon joins the extensor digitorum communis tendon of the index finger at the level of the second MCP joint. The extensor digiti minimi tendon parallels the course of the extensor digitorum communis tendon of the little finger.

The intrinsic muscles of the hand, the lumbricals, and the dorsal and volar interossei act to flex the MCP joints, thereby assisting extension at the proximal and distal IP joints. Extension of a digit is the result of complex interactions of intrinsic and extrinsic muscles.

History and Physical Examination

History

The assessment of potential extensor tendon injuries of the hand begins with a detailed history. The position of the hand at the time of injury is important to understand the mechanism and likely location of injury. In addition, the examiner must determine the potential for foreign material or bacterial contamination from a bite or contact with a tooth. Lacerations of the dorsum of the hand should be treated as a bite wound until proved otherwise. Prophylactic antibiotic treatment should be considered when a potentially unreliable historian denies oral contact. Patients should be questioned regarding the loss of motor or sensory function. Particular attention should be given to painful movement, both with and without resistance; this may indicate a partially or completely disrupted tendon, even in the presence of intact skin. The patient also should be questioned about the possibility of and location of dislocation and of subsequent relocation before presentation in the emergency department. Such information may indicate a serious tendinous or ligamentous injury. In addition, general historical information such as dominant hand, time of last meal, allergies, medications, tetanus immunization status, past medical history, time of injury, and first aid measures provided should be obtained.

Physical Examination

The physical examination should begin with a general observation of the contours and positioning of the hand. Unopposed flexion of a finger may indicate disruption of the extensor mechanism. Although the focus may be on the hand itself, general examination of the entire extremity is appropriate. Careful inspection is necessary to determine the status of skin integrity and to check for the presence of any type of wound. All wounds on the dorsum of the hand should be considered potential extensor tendon injuries.

The extensor tendons should be palpated. This is best accomplished by positioning the hand palm down on the examining table with the fingers extended and checking for signs of step-off, laxity, tenderness, or swelling associated with any tendon. Motor function should be assessed by having the patient extend the fingertips against resistance. Pain during movement may indicate a partial or complete disruption of the extensor tendon. The sensory-impaired patient is less reliable during this portion of the examination. It is important to note that patients may possess normal strength with up to 90% disruption of an extensor tendon. The sensory examination should focus on evaluation of the radial, median, and ulnar nerves.

Direct examination and exploration of the wound may reveal unexpected or underappreciated injuries. This should be performed using sterile technique and appropriate anesthesia with optimal lighting. The extensor tendon is a relatively mobile structure and should be observed in the position of injury and throughout its full range of motion. Wound exploration, débridement, irrigation, and examination for foreign bodies should be conducted simultaneously. Radiographic evaluation may demonstrate unsuspected fractures.

The uncooperative or impaired patient may not be able to allow a thorough evaluation and definitive care at the time of initial emergency department presentation. This situation necessitates primary skin closure, splinting, and referral for definitive examination and treatment.

Classification and Treatment

The hand, wrist, and forearm can be divided into eight anatomic zones to facilitate classification and treatment of extensor tendon injuries (Table 14-1). Injuries to the extensor tendons of the thumb are treated in a similar manner as injuries to the analogous level of the extensor tendons of the other digits and are not discussed further here.

Repair of extensor tendons in the emergency department requires meticulous preparation, including adequate anesthesia, good lighting, a bloodless field, and exposure of the injury, which often requires extension of the original laceration. Complete tendon lacerations are repaired with a colorless, nonabsorbable, synthetic suture (4-0 or 5-0 polyester). Incomplete tendon lacerations may be repaired with a similar-sized absorbable suture.

Complications from the repair of extensor tendon injuries, even when proper technique was used, may result in significant impairment of function. In addition, most tendon repairs may be delayed up to 72 hours. Therefore, in most cases, a discussion with a hand surgeon should occur before repairs are attempted in the emergency department. Injuries in zones IV and VI usually are the most amenable to repair by experienced emergency physicians.

Table 14-1.

Zones of extensor tendon injury.

Zone	Finger	Thumb
I	DIP joint	IP joint
II	Middle phalanx	Proximal phalanx
III	PIP joint	MCP joint
IV	Proximal phalanx	Metacarpal
V	MCP joint	CMC joint
VI	Metacarpals	
VII	Carpals	
VIII	Proximal wrist and distal forearm	

Zone I Injuries

Injury over the distal phalanx or the DIP joint results in disruption of the terminal extensor tendon. The classic deformity is known as **mallet finger**, **drop finger**, or **baseball finger**.

Mechanism of Injury

This is commonly a closed injury caused by a direct blow to the tip of the finger, as might occur while playing baseball, forcing the distal phalanx into flexion while the extensor is contracting, causing the tendon to stretch, rupture, or avulse from the base of the distal phalanx. This injury also may be caused by a direct blow to the dorsum of the DIP joint (rupturing the tendon), forced hyperextension of the tip of the extended finger (shearing off a large portion of the base of the distal phalanx), or laceration over the dorsum of the DIP joint. Mallet finger injuries may be identified (type I, II, or III) according to the structure involved (Figure 14-3).

Physical Examination

Classically, if a patient presents with an acute injury, swelling and tenderness are noted over the DIP joint. The distal phalanx is flexed, and the patient is unable (or demonstrates reduced ability) to actively extend, although passive extension is possible. Volar subluxation of the DIP joint may be noted if more than 50% of the articular surface is involved in a fracture fragment. Lateral stability of the DIP joint should be assessed to detect injuries of the collateral joint ligaments.

Radiography

A true lateral view is necessary to detect the presence of fracture fragments and subluxation of the joint.

Emergency Department Management

Management of mallet finger is controversial. For closed injuries, splinting generally is preferred. The DIP joint is splinted in extension

Figure 14-3.

Types of mallet finger injuries.

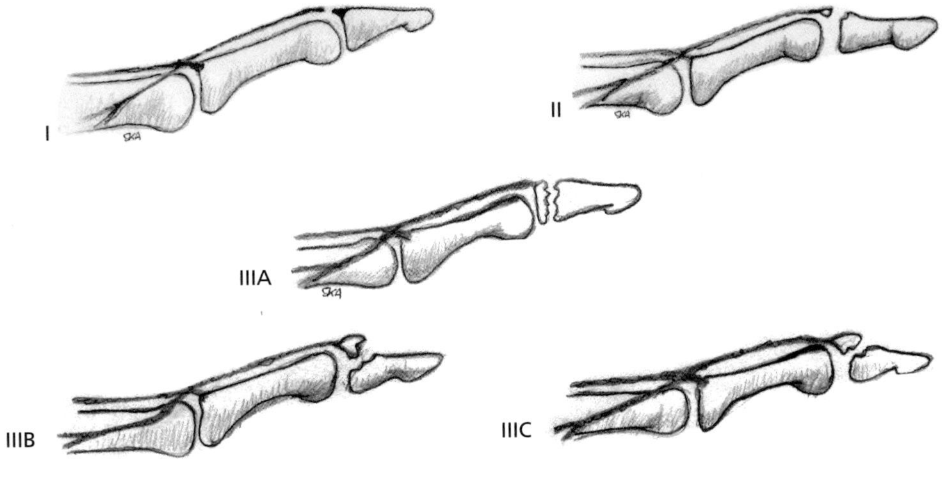

with either a commercially available splint (Stack splint, Bird & Cronin, Inc, Eagan, Minn) or an aluminum-foam splint (applied to either the dorsal or volar surface). Displaced fractures should be reduced before splinting. The PIP joint should not be included in the splint. Hyperextension is avoided due to the potential for blistering and loss of skin over the dorsum of the joint. Open mallet injuries may be repaired with a figure-of-eight or running roll–type suture, which approximates both the skin edges and the tendon (Figure 14-4). The finger is then splinted in the same manner as closed injuries.

Patients should be instructed to wear the splint for 6 weeks. If the splint is removed, the finger must be kept in extension (place the involved hand palm down, with the fingers extended, on a table and slip off the splint) until the splint is replaced. Patients who may require surgical fixation and repair include those who are unreliable and those with a transepiphyseal fracture, large fracture fragments, subluxation of the DIP joint, loss of overlying skin or tendon, or an inability to wear the splint.

Referral

Outpatient followup care should be arranged with a hand surgeon before discharge from the emergency department. Patients with complicated or open mallet injuries may require surgical management, and the hand surgeon should be contacted early in the patient's emergency department course.

Complications

Skin maceration associated with the splint is common. Hyperextension of the DIP joint can lead to skin ischemia and sloughing and is to be avoided. Increasing age and degree of extensor lag are associated with decreasing recovery of function. A **swan-neck deformity** (hyperextension at the PIP joint and hyperflexion at the DIP joint) may occur with untreated mallet injuries (Figure 14-5).

Figure 14-4.

Repair of the extensor tendon in open mallet finger injuries. **A)** *Figure-of-eight suture.* **B)** *Running roll suture.*

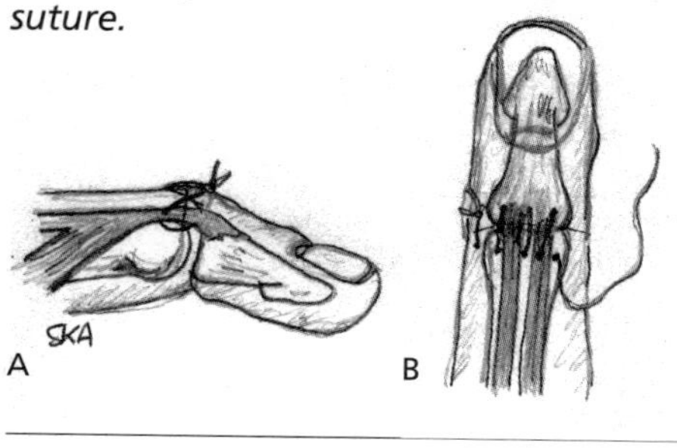

Figure 14-5.

Swan-neck deformity.

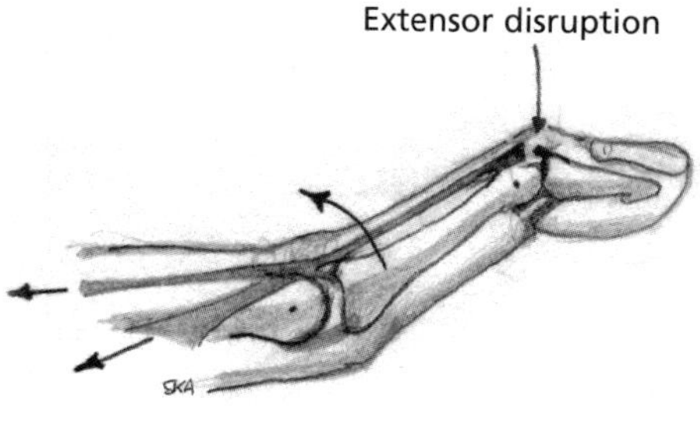

Zone II Injuries

These injuries occur over the middle phalanx and result in injury to the extensor tendons.

Mechanism of Injury

This type of injury is most commonly caused by a laceration or a crush injury.

Physical Examination

The typical mallet finger deformity is found, as is evidence of injury over the dorsum of the middle phalanx. Careful exploration of all lacerations is required to determine whether a partial or complete laceration of the extensor tendon is present.

Radiography

Radiographs should be obtained for injuries that may also have caused a fracture.

Emergency Department Management

Partial tendon lacerations that involve less than 50% of the tendon can be managed with simple closure of the overlying skin and splinting (as described for zone I injuries) for 7 to 10 days. Tendon lacerations of more than 50% should be repaired primarily, followed by splinting as for zone I injuries, for 6 weeks.

Referral

Outpatient followup care should be arranged with a hand surgeon before discharge from the emergency department. Patients with complicated or open injuries may require surgical management, and the hand surgeon should be contacted early in the patient's emergency department course.

Complications

Skin maceration associated with the splint is common. Hyperextension of the DIP joint can lead to skin ischemia and sloughing and is to be avoided. A swan-neck deformity may occur with untreated injuries.

Zone III Injuries

These injuries occur over the PIP joint, with the central slip of the extensor tendon most commonly injured.

Mechanism of Injury

In athletes, this common type of injury is caused by a direct blow to the dorsum of the PIP joint or an acute flexion force while the PIP joint is actively extended. If the injury is caused by a laceration, it is most commonly found over the dorsum of the PIP joint. Again, the most common injury to the extensor mechanism is a disruption of the central slip of the extensor tendon.

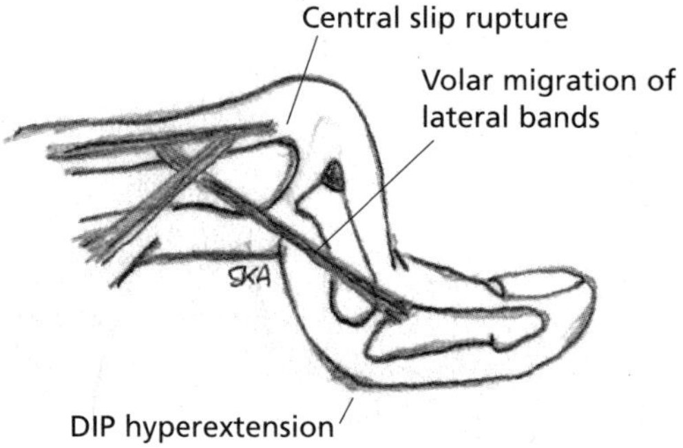

Figure 14-6.

Boutonnière deformity.

If unrecognized and untreated, the classic **boutonnière deformity** (flexion of the PIP joint with hyperextension at the DIP and MCP joints) results (Figure 14-6) from the unopposed flexion of the FDS, forcing the PIP joint dorsally through the defect in the extensor tendon. With time, the triangular ligament stretches, allowing the lateral bands to move volarly and become flexors of the PIP joint, contributing to the deformity. The disrupted central slip portion of the extensor tendon retracts proximally with resultant redistribution of its forces to the remaining extensor mechanism. This redistribution results in increased tension in the sagittal bands (hyperextension of the MCP joint) and lateral bands (flexion of the PIP joint and hyperextension of the DIP joint).

Physical Examination

In acute, closed injuries, the rupture of the central tendon slip is difficult to detect and may be misdiagnosed as a sprain. Patients typically present with pain and swelling over the PIP joint, with slight flexion at the PIP and slight extension at the DIP joint. Often, the patient lacks 15 to 30 degrees of active extension at the PIP joint. If the finger is extended at the PIP joint, the lateral bands are able to maintain extension and the injury is missed. If the PIP joint is flexed to 90 degrees, the lateral bands are volar to the joint axis and are unable to extend. The **tabletop test** can help make the diagnosis. To perform this test, the patient's hand is placed flat on a table with the PIP joint flexed 90 degrees over the edge, then the patient attempts to extend the finger against resistance.

Open injuries should be explored thoroughly to detect the injury as well as any violation of the PIP joint capsule. Partial central tendon slip injuries are frequently missed because the patient is able to actively extend at the PIP joint against resistance. Zone III injuries frequently are missed on initial presentation and are not noted until the patient presents 10 to 14 days later with the classic deformity.

Radiography

Radiographs should be obtained to detect any associated fractures.

Emergency Department Management

Multiple techniques have been suggested for the management of these injuries.

Closed injuries. Splinting generally is preferred for any suspected injury using a variety of commercial splints or a custom-made splint. In all designs, the PIP joint is splinted in extension and the DIP joint is allowed full mobility. The splint should be worn for several weeks until full passive extension at the PIP joint and near-normal flexion at the DIP joint are obtained. Dynamic splinting of the finger (not typically done in the emergency department) may result in an improved outcome.

Indications for surgical repair include a large displaced avulsion fracture at the base of the middle phalanx and a central slip rupture associated with volar PIP joint dislocation.

Patients who present weeks to months after the initial injury and with the classic deformity should be referred. If passive extension at the PIP joint is possible, the involved finger should be splinted as previously described.

Open injuries. The tendon laceration may be repaired primarily, or the laceration may be closed with a figure-of-eight suture that simultaneously approximates the skin margins and tendon ends. Splinting as previously described for closed injuries should be performed.

Referral

Outpatient followup care should be arranged with a hand surgeon before discharge from the emergency department. For open injuries, the hand surgeon should be contacted before attempted repair because some advocate internal fixation as well as primary tendon repair.

Complications

Unrecognized injuries may result in permanent loss of function. Skin maceration associated with the splint is common. Diminished function may occur as a result of scarring or adhesion formation.

Zone IV Injuries

These injuries occur over the proximal phalanx.

Mechanism of Injury

Typically, this type of injury is caused by a laceration over the proximal phalanx with a partial laceration of the extensor mechanism. The lateral bands usually are not involved due to the protective curvature of the phalanx.

Physical Examination

Direct examination of the laceration often is the only way to diagnose the injury.

Radiography

A radiograph should be obtained if an underlying fracture or the presence of radiopaque foreign bodies is suspected.

Emergency Department Management

The central tendon or lateral bands may be repaired with fine nonabsorbable suture. The PIP joint should be splinted as described for zone III injuries.

Referral

In general, a hand surgeon should be consulted before repair of these injuries is attempted. Outpatient followup care should be arranged with a hand surgeon before discharge from the emergency department.

Complications

Local wound infections are possible, and loss of function may occur due to scarring or adhesions.

Zone V Injuries

These injuries are caused by trauma over the dorsum of the MCP joint.

Mechanism of Injury

Human bite wounds should be suspected as the cause of any laceration in this area. Wounds may result in lacerations of the extensor tendon or extensor hood. The proximal end of the extensor tendon does not often retract in this location. Simple lacerations, blunt trauma, or a forceful flexion or extension injury of the finger may result in a tear of the radial sagittal band and oblique fibers of the extensor hood with resultant ulnar dislocation of the extensor tendon. These patients often are boxers or football players, and the middle finger is most commonly involved.

Boxer knuckle is a direct injury to the extensor hood with a longitudinal rent of the dorsal joint capsule, with or without dislocation of the extensor tendon. These injuries typically present as pain over the metacarpal head. A defect in the extensor hood may be palpable.

Physical Examination

Lacerations should be explored thoroughly to identify injuries to the extensor tendon and joint capsule and to locate any foreign bodies. This frequently requires extension of the laceration. The finger should be moved through full flexion and extension to identify any injury to the extensor tendon that is not seen initially with the hand in a neutral position.

Patients with an acute blunt mechanism of injury and rupture of the extensor hood or traumatic dislocation of the extensor tendon present with pain and swelling over the MCP joint and decreased ability to fully extend at the MCP joint. If the finger is passively extended, the patient usually is able to maintain extension actively because the extensor tendon may reduce spontaneously. Delayed presentation is common, with main complaints of chronic pain over the MCP joint, weak extension at the MCP joint, and ulnar deviation of the finger. The extensor tendon may be palpable along the ulnar aspect of the joint.

Emergency Department Management

The management of these injuries is based on the mechanism of injury.

Bite wounds. In general, these injuries should be referred to a hand surgeon for surgical exploration and copious irrigation. Cultures of the wound frequently are recommended. Typically, these wounds are left open, with tendon repair and closure (if done) performed secondarily in 5 to 7 days. The hand is splinted with the wrist in 40 to 45 degrees of extension and the MCP joints in 15 to 20 degrees of flexion.

Simple lacerations. Lacerations of the extensor tendon should be repaired with simple, nonabsorbable sutures. Dynamic splinting (usually performed by the hand surgeon) after repair is often used. Lacerations of the extensor hood or sagittal bands must be repaired (using buried interrupted nonabsorbable sutures) to keep the extensor tendon centered and to prevent subluxation of the tendon. Extension and flexion exercises are used. Buddy-taping with an adjacent finger is used to prevent adduction or abduction movements.

Traumatic dislocation of extensor tendon. Primary surgical repair frequently is recommended. If this injury is diagnosed early, splinting of the MCP joint in 0 degrees of extension for 4 to 6 weeks may be attempted. Injuries that present late usually require surgical repair.

Radiography

Radiographs should be obtained to detect fractures and foreign bodies.

Referral

In general, a hand surgeon should be consulted before repair of these injuries is attempted. Outpatient followup care should be arranged with a hand surgeon before discharge from the emergency department.

Complications

Wound infections of lacerations are a major concern. Dislocation of the extensor tendon with the resulting impairment of extension may also occur.

Zone VI Injuries

These injuries are caused by trauma to the extensor tendons over the metacarpals. The prognosis for these injuries is better than that for zone II to V injuries.

Mechanism of Injury

The extensor tendons are very superficial and poorly protected over the metacarpals. Injuries are typically secondary to lacerations, and wounds that appear to be minor may result in multiple tendon lacerations.

Physical Examination

All wounds must be explored thoroughly while the patient moves the fingers through full extension and flexion. Intact extension may be found despite complete tendon disruption as a result of the transmission of extension forces from adjacent extensor tendons via the juncturae tendinum.

Emergency Department Management

Primary repair of the tendon injury with nonabsorbable suture may be made by an experienced emergency physician. Initially, splinting with the wrist in 30 degrees of extension, the MCP joint in extension, and the PIP and DIP joints free is recommended. Dynamic splinting (usually done by the hand surgeon) beginning 3 to 5 days after tendon repair frequently is recommended.

Radiography

Generally, radiographs are not required unless a fracture or the presence of a foreign body is suspected.

Referral

In general, a hand surgeon should be consulted before repair of this type of injury is attempted. Outpatient followup care should be arranged with a hand surgeon before discharge from the emergency department.

Complications

Infection is the major concern. Failure of the repair and skin adhesions, with resultant loss of function, may occur.

Zone VII Injuries

These injuries occur over the dorsum of the carpal bones.

Mechanism of Injury

This type of injury typically is caused by lacerations. Tendon injuries are complicated by associated lacerations of the extensor retinaculum. Extensor tendon rupture may occur associated with a closed fracture (extensor pollicis longus and extensor digitorum communis tendons and Colles fractures) or dislocation with disruptions of the extensor retinaculum.

Physical Examination

All wounds must be explored thoroughly while the patient moves the fingers through full extension and flexion. On exploration, puncture wounds may be found to have caused significant tendon injury. Retraction of the proximal end of the severed tendon may occur. Careful examination of the function of all extensor tendons is required.

Emergency Department Management

Primarily, management is focused on the detection or suspicion of injury. These injuries should be referred to a hand surgeon for management. Skin wounds may be closed after routine wound care if immediate surgical repair is not anticipated. After closure of the skin, the hand and wrist are splinted with a volar splint with 35 to 45 degrees of wrist extension and 15 to 20 degrees of MCP flexion.

Radiography

Radiographs are indicated if a fracture or the presence of a foreign body is suspected.

Referral

All patients with zone VII injuries should be referred to a hand surgeon.

Complications

Adhesions that result in loss of function and wound infections may occur.

Zone VIII Injuries

These injuries occur over the dorsum of the proximal wrist and distal forearm.

Mechanism of Injury

Typically, this type of injury is caused by lacerations, although crush injuries also may result in disruption of the musculotendinous junction.

Physical Examination

Exploration of all lacerations is required, and it is often necessary to extend the initial wound to allow adequate visualization. Retraction of the proximal portions of the tendon or muscle belly is common.

Emergency Department Management

As for zone VII injuries, patients with zone VIII injuries should be referred to a hand surgeon. Nonabsorbable sutures are used to approximate the tendon and muscle belly. Splinting is the same as for zone VII injuries.

Radiography

Radiographs are indicated if a fracture or the presence of a foreign body is suspected.

Referral

Referral to a hand surgeon is required for all except minor injuries.

Complications

Wound infections and failure of surgical repairs are the most common complications.

Other Conditions

Peritendinous Fibrosis (Secrétan Disease)

Peritendinous fibrosis presents as persistent edema over the dorsum of the hand. It is associated with work-related injuries and may represent a factitious disorder. Multiple management techniques have been recommended, including expectant neglect. Generally, emergency department management is not required beyond appropriate referral.

Posttraumatic Subluxation of the Extensor Carpi Ulnaris Tendon

This injury is caused by hypersupination and associated palmar flexion or ulnar deviation, which results in rupture of the tendon sheath with ulnar and palmar subluxation of the extensor carpi ulnaris tendon. Patients present with localized pain and tenderness over the ulnar styloid and a history of "clicking" with forearm rotation. On physical examination, the extensor carpi ulnaris tendon is often felt subluxing over the distal ulna. In acute injuries, a 6-week trial of splinting in a long arm cast with midsupination may be appropriate. Referral to hand surgeon is recommended.

de Quervain Disease

de Quervain disease (tenosynovitis) is seen frequently in persons who participate in sports that require repetitive radial and ulnar wrist deviation and forceful grasp (tennis, golf). It is the result of stenosing tenosynovitis of the extensor tendons (abductor pollicis longus and extensor pollicis brevis) passing through the fibro-osseous tunnel on the radial styloid (first compartment). Patients complain of pain over the radial styloid that is exacerbated by movement of the thumb or wrist. Examination reveals localized tenderness and swelling over the radial styloid and a positive **Finkelstein test** (pain is reproduced by the patient making a fist around the flexed thumb, then ulnar deviation is passively applied at the wrist). Pain also can be produced by resisted thumb extension with the wrist in maximum radial deviation. Initial treatment is with NSAIDs and a thumb spica splint. Pain frequently responds to a local steroid injection (usually performed by a hand surgeon). Surgery may be required for patients who do not respond to initial treatment. Tenosynovitis of other extensor tendons (including the extensor pollicis longus [**drummer boy palsy**], common digital extensors, extensor digiti minimi, and extensor carpi ulnaris) may occur.

Intersection Syndrome

This symptom complex is seen frequently in persons who participate in activities that require repetitive wrist extension (canoeing, weightlifting). Patients complain of pain, swelling, and crepitus on the dorsal surface of the distal radial forearm. Examination reveals tenderness and swelling 4 to 6 cm proximal to the radial carpal joint on the dorsum of the forearm (crossing point of the abductor pollicis longus, extensor pollicis brevis, extensor carpi radialis longus, and extensor carpi radialis brevis). The cause is unknown. Initial management consists of stopping the activity that elicits the condition and applying a splint and the use of NSAIDs. If symptoms persist, a hand surgeon may consider a steroid injection in the second extensor compartment or surgery.

Additional Reading

Aronowitz ER, Leddy JP. Closed tendon injuries of the hand and wrist in athletes. *Clin Sports Med.* 1998;17:449-467.

Doyle JR. Extensor tendons—acute injuries. In: Green DP, ed. *Operative Hand Surgery.* 3rd ed. New York, NY: Churchill Livingstone; 1993:1925-1954.

Fulcher SM, Kiefhaber TR, Stern PJ. Upper-extremity tendinitis and overuse syndromes in the athlete. *Clin Sports Med.* 1998;17:433-448.

Hart RG, Uehara DT, Kutz JE. Extensor tendon injuries of the hand. *Emerg Med Clin North Am.* 1993;11:637-649.

Kleinert HE, Verdan C. Report of the committee on tendon injuries. *J Hand Surg.* 1983;8:794-798.

Snell RS, Smith MS. *Clinical Anatomy for Emergency Medicine.* St Louis, Mo: Mosby; 1993;582-583, 656-657, 665-666.

Sokolove PE. Extensor tendon injuries in the hand and wrist. In: Roberts JR, Hedges JR, eds. *Clinical Procedures in Emergency Medicine.* 3rd ed. Philadelphia, Pa: WB Saunders; 1998:805-818.

Woodburne RT. *Essentials of Human Anatomy.* 5th ed. New York, NY: Oxford University Press; 1973;95-127.

CHAPTER 15

Nail Bed and Fingertip Injuries

Lance K. Freeman, MD, FACEP

As the most functional part of the hand, the fingertips also are the most vulnerable to injury. Emergency physicians are likely to see patients with a wide spectrum of injuries to this area. This chapter reviews trauma to the fingertips, including subungual hematoma, lacerations, fractures, crush injuries, and amputations.

Anatomy

The **fingertip** is defined as the area distal to the insertion of the flexor profundus and extensor tendons. This region can be divided into two major anatomic structures: first, the tuft, and second, the nail and its supporting structures (Figure 15-1).

The **tuft of the distal phalanx** is well padded by adipose tissue and covered by highly innervated skin, which is tethered to the distal phalanx through a series of fibroseptae. The pulp is the tissue of the fingertip between the volar skin and the distal phalangeal bone.

The **nail plate** (commonly called the **fingernail**) consists of compacted scales that originate from keratinized epithelium cells. The proximal, hidden end of the nail plate is called the **root**, and the visible portion is called the **body**. The white crescent near the root is called the **lunula** or the **germinal matrix** and is where the nail substance is made. The nail grows from the germinal matrix along the nail bed, to which it is firmly adherent.

The **nail** lies on the surface of the nail bed and is surrounded laterally and proximally by a thick fold of tissue called the **nail fold**. The sides of the nail fold are called the **paronychium**, and at the base, the fold is called the **eponychium**. Between the nail fold and the nail bed is the **nail groove**. At the distal end of the finger, under the free edge of the nail, the thickened epithelium is called **hyponychium**. In the nail bed, the dermis is directly attached to the periosteum of the distal phalanx, with a rich capillary bed that provides the blood supply to this complex.

Initial Evaluation and Management

History

Before an injury is evaluated, a detailed history must be taken. Important aspects of the history include mechanism of injury, hand dominance, occupation, previous injuries, and patient age. In trauma patients, the history also should include answers to the following specific questions[1]:

- How much time has elapsed since the injury?
- Where did the injury occur, and was the environment clean or dirty?
- How did the injury happen, and what was the exact posture of the hand at the time of injury?
- What treatment has been administered?

Physical Examination

When inspecting the fingertip to assess circulation, both color and the more proximal radial and ulnar pulses should be observed. The presence of swelling or edema should be noted, as well as any abnormal posture or position of the finger at rest. Skin moisture, localized tenderness, and sensation must be evaluated. The range of both passive and active motion of the DIP and IP joints of each digit should be measured and recorded. Grip and pinch strength, as well as the patient's ability to use the finger during simple tasks, should be documented.

Sensation is exceedingly important for a fully functional hand. The insensate hand is poorly used even when the tendons and joints are nor-

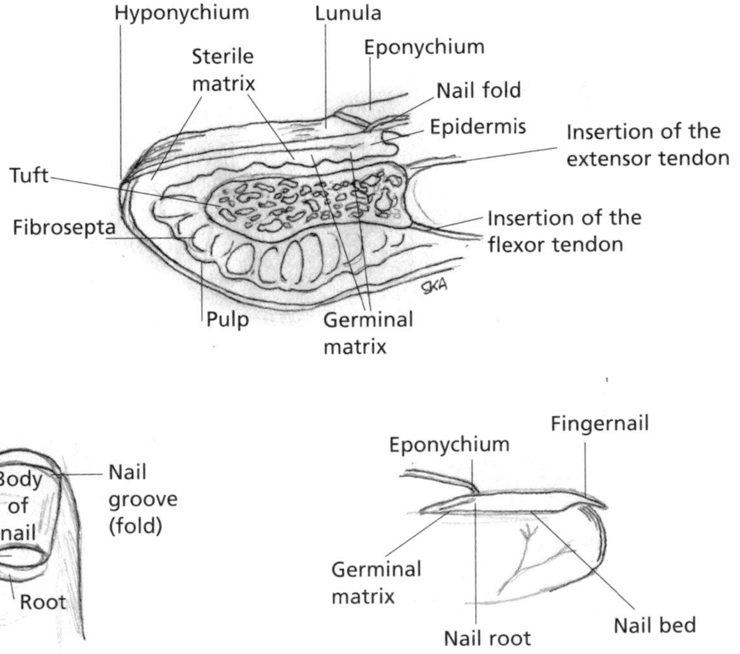

Figure 15-1. *Anatomy of the fingertip–nail complex.*

mal. Two-point light touch discrimination is the most important sensory test for the fingertip. Vibratory perception also is lost with nerve division. With a mild or moderate degree of nerve compression, two-point discrimination is preserved, but sensory threshold changes such as diminished perception of tuning fork stimulation and abnormal cutaneous pressure sensation are noted.

The circulation of the hand is evaluated by noting the color of the skin and fingernails and the blanching and flush of the nail bed. The radial and ulnar arteries supply the hand with blood. There is an arterial arch system that provides the hand and fingers a generous collateral blood supply; only the vessels that are end arteries travel to the fingertip.

Examination of the involved digit should include an assessment of the extent of damage to the soft tissue, the nail, and the nail bed; the level and angle of amputation; the presence or absence of exposed bone; and the vascular status, including capillary refill. The ability to flex and extend at the DIP joint should be evaluated; normal function suggests that the integrity of the flexor and extensor tendons is at least partially intact.

Radiographic evaluation with AP, lateral, and oblique views of the involved finger is necessary to assess for bone injury and to exclude retained radiopaque foreign bodies.

Wound Care

Cleansing

To facilitate adequate exploration and irrigation, anesthesia is necessary, usually in the form of a digital block. Once adequate anesthesia is achieved, the wound should be irrigated to remove debris, reduce bacterial contamination, and lessen the risk of wound infection. Irrigation through an 18- to 20-gauge needle attached to a 30- to 60-mL syringe generates a peak pressure of about 30 psi, which usually is adequate to dislodge foreign material from wounds. Unless there is a significant amount of contamination, the irrigation of fingertip wounds usually can be accomplished with a total of 250 to 500 mL of normal saline, or approximately 60 mL/cm of wound length adjusted to the condition and location of the wound.

Tourniquet Use

For thorough exploration and repair of a fingertip wound, a bloodless field is required. Several types of tourniquets may be used, including the use of a pneumatic blood pressure cuff placed around the upper arm or a digital tourniquet with a Penrose drain or a surgical glove. In the latter, the patient wears a glove that has a cut fingertip that corresponds to the injured digit. As the glove is rolled from distal to proximal, a tight band is produced that acts as a tourniquet around the base of the digit. The disadvantage of using this technique in the emergency department is that different glove sizes, varying thicknesses of the glove material, and varying numbers of rolls may generate a wide range of pressures.

A simple and safe method of achieving hemostasis is the use of a digital Penrose tourniquet. With a 1/4- to 1-inch Penrose drain, the finger is wrapped carefully from distal to proximal, thereby exsanguinating the digit. The drain then is removed carefully from distal to proximal, placed around the base of the finger, and secured with a hemostat. The stretch of the drain should be limited to no more than 50% of the original length.

Regardless of the type of constricting device that is used, it is imperative not to leave the tourniquet in place for more than 30 minutes at a time after repair to avoid neurovascular damage.

Adjunct Therapy

Care of the involved digit must begin with meticulous attention to wound care. In addition to active tetanus toxoid immunization, a patient who has an incomplete primary tetanus vaccination or whose status is unknown at the time of presentation and who has a severely contaminated wound (a wound that has been in contact with soil, feces, or organic material) may require passive immunization with tetanus immune globulin (see Table 5-1, page 52).

Broad-spectrum antibiotics are not routinely recommended but may be considered for patients with wounds that are contaminated or more than 12 hours old, in the presence of exposed bone, or in patients with concurrent medical illness that may affect wound healing, such as diabetes, renal disease, or peripheral vascular disease. Antibiotics should be chosen to cover suspected pathogens and contaminants, which include *Staphylococcus aureus*, streptococci, Gram-negative bacilli, and/or anaerobes.

Specific Injuries

Most fingertip injuries are isolated and can be managed appropriately by the emergency physician. However, early consultation with a hand or plastic surgeon is necessary when the injury is extensive or complex, when the function of the finger is vital to the patient's occupation, or when the injury requires skin grafting. Special attention should be paid if the involved digit is the thumb or index finger. The goal of repair of the index finger is to preserve pinch, whereas with the thumb, it is crucial to establish a functional, sensate tip with preservation of as much length as possible.

Subungual Hematomas

Diagnosis

Subungual hematomas result from blunt trauma or crush injury to the nail bed that results in disruption of the blood vessels. The nail bed is predisposed to injury because it is interposed between the firm nail and the distal phalanx. The injury typically presents with pain and dark red to black discoloration of the nail bed and is classified by the percentage of the total nail area that is involved. The area of the hematoma is directly proportional to the degree of vascular damage. A radiograph should be obtained to identify possible associated fractures.

Treatment

If the hematoma covers less than 50% of the area under the nail, treatment can be accomplished with the creation of a hole or trephination of the nail to allow for adequate decompression and drainage. Various tools can be used, including a heated paper clip, electric nail drill, electrocautery, 18-gauge needle, and scalpel. Anesthesia usually is unnecessary for decompression, and pain relief is immediate. If a significant fracture is present, the digit should be splinted.

It was recommended previously that, for a subungual hematoma that occupies more than 50% of the nail bed area, the nail must be removed to evaluate the nail bed and to repair any associated laceration.[2,3] Patients with a subungual hematoma that is more than 50% of the nail have a 60% incidence of nail bed lacerations; if there is an associated fracture of the distal phalanx, the incidence is 95%. However, in two recent prospective studies, trephinating alone produced a good to excellent outcome in about 85% of patients regardless of hematoma size, the presence of fracture, or infection.[4,5] Therefore, simple trephination is adequate treatment for most subungual hematomas, with nail removal recommended if there is associated nail avulsion or surrounding nail fold disruption.

Nail Bed Injuries

Lacerations

Nail bed lacerations should be repaired to minimize aesthetic deformity and the duration of functional impairment. These injuries generally do well after primary repair, but late reconstruction of the nail bed is unpredictable, and usually little improvement is obtained.

Nail removal can be accomplished easily after adequate anesthesia is provided. Digit exsanguination and elevation of the nail from the nail bed can be accomplished by spreading and advancing a small hemostat or iris scissors (Figure 15-2). The eponychium is separated similarly from the nail edges. Then, complete nail removal is accomplished with gentle longitudinal traction with a hemostat. Lacerations of the nail bed should be repaired carefully with 6-0 or 7-0 absorbable sutures (Figure 15-3).

The nail should be cleansed gently with saline and, with care taken to avoid damage to the germinal matrix, a 5-0 nylon suture placed through the proxi-

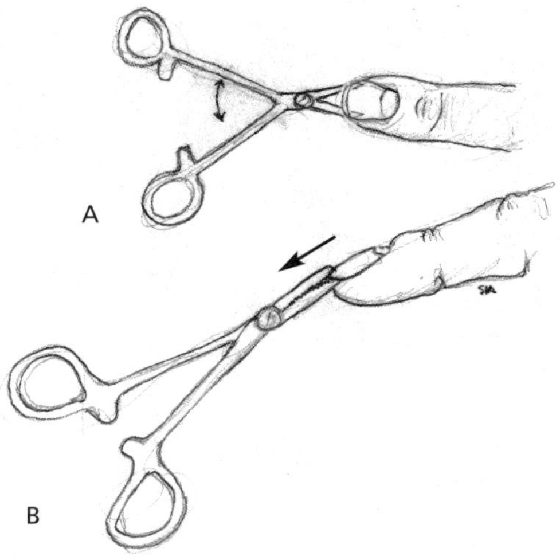

Figure 15-2.

Elevation of the nail from the nail bed.
A) *Displace nail bed from nail with iris scissors.*
B) *Remove from nail fold with hemostat.*

mal end of the nail plate. The suture then is passed under and through the center of the eponychial fold, avoiding the nail bed. Once the nail is returned to its anatomic position, the suture should be tied down over the nail (Figure 15-4). The replaced nail acts as a natural splint to the terminal phalanx and protects the sensitive nail bed. After the nail bed is accurately approximated, a separate hole should be burned through the nail to allow adequate drainage from the subungual area. If the nail cannot be replaced, nonbiological stents of Silastic or silicone may be used. If neither is available, the sterile piece of aluminum foil that is used to wrap suture materials or Adaptic gauze material may be cut into the shape of the avulsed nail and inserted into the eponychium to maintain an open nail fold to allow new nail growth. This helps prevent the formation of synechiae and scarring (which lead to nail deformity), protects the nail bed, and acts as a splint (Figure 15-4).

The fingertip should be dressed in nonadherent gauze and placed in a volar splint to limit movement of the DIP joint. Wound care instructions should include hand elevation and neurovascular checks, and adequate analgesia should be provided. The dressing should be left undisturbed for 5 to 7 days unless obvious purulence is noted. After this, the site should be examined for new hematoma formation. The suture attached to the nail may be removed after 3 weeks. The existing nail is dislodged by the new ingrowing nail after 1 to 3 months.

Avulsion

Nail bed avulsion commonly leaves fragments of the nail bed attached to the undersurface of the avulsed nail. In such cases, optimal results are obtained if the nail is replaced as accurately as possible onto the avulsion site. Repair should be made with mattress sutures without an attempt to separate the nail from the nail bed. If tissue is not available and the defect is small, it heals effectively by secondary intention. If the defect is large, consultation with a hand surgeon is appropriate for full-thickness nail bed grafting, which is accomplished by harvesting a graft from the patient's toe and suturing it into the nail bed of the affected finger.

Figure 15-3.

Nail bed repair.

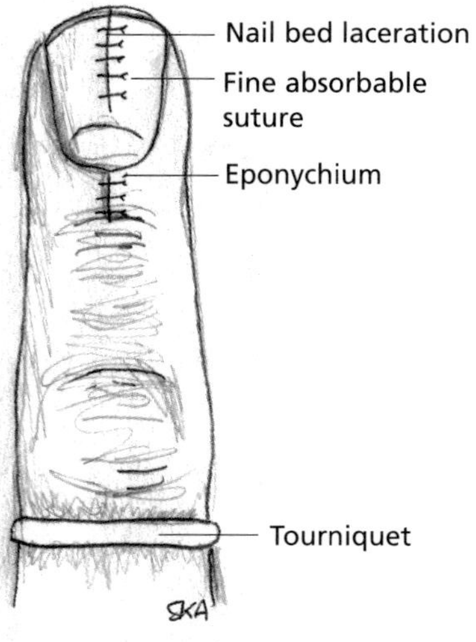

Open Fractures

Diagnosis

Distal phalanx fractures are the most common fractures of the hand, accounting for more than half. Most of these tuft fractures are produced by crush injuries and appear as **crushed eggshell fractures**. Soft tissue avulsion or disruption results in open fracture. Longitudinal and transverse fractures of the shaft, which usually are caused by a direct blow, are less common and are seen as lucencies that transect the bone.

Treatment

When there is significant angulation, transverse fractures require pin fixation. Shaft fractures should be assessed for intra-articular extension because this alters management. Surgical consultation should be obtained.

If an associated distal phalanx fracture coexists with a nail bed laceration, it usually manifests as an avulsion of the nail out of the proximal eponychial fold. When this happens, the nail is removed, the fracture is stabilized with manual reduction, and the nail bed is repaired as previously described. Unstable fractures require consultation with a plastic surgeon or hand surgeon for internal fixation using K-wires to prevent deformity of the nail. Although a distal phalangeal fracture with a subungual hematoma technically is an open fracture, such injuries usually heal without problems, and ungual tuft fractures are not associated with osteomyelitis. A patient with a significant hematoma should be informed that he or she might lose the nail.

The risk of infection with an open fracture of the phalanx proper must be considered, and broad-spectrum antibiotic coverage and close followup care are recommended. Antibiotics also may be considered for wounds that are contaminated, for injuries that are more than 12 hours old, and in patients with concurrent medical problems that may affect wound healing, such as diabetes, renal disease, or peripheral vascular disease. Antibiotics should be chosen to cover the suspected contaminants and pathogens, including *S. aureus*, streptococci, Gram-negative bacilli, and/or anaerobes. One common choice is cephalexin. Antibiotics should be given early and by a route to achieve high blood and tissue levels, often intravenous.[6]

Figure 15-4.

Replacement of nail over injured nail bed.
A) *Suture through nail, avoiding germinal matrix.*
B) *Suture through eponychium.*
C) *Attach foil in place of nail.*

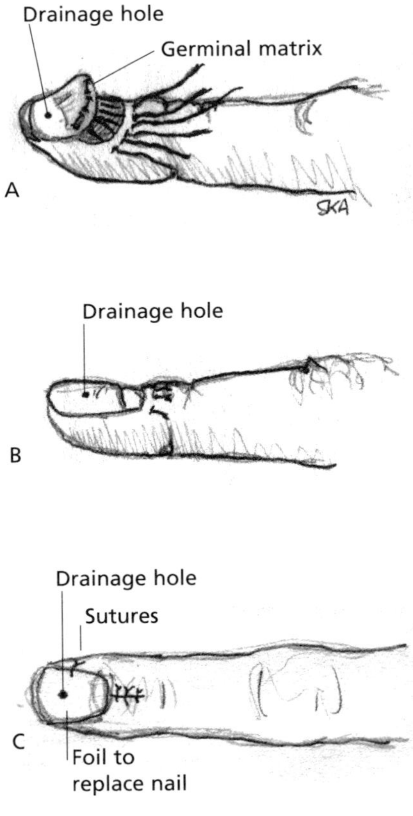

Fingertip Amputations

Fingertip amputations are the most common type of amputation of the upper extremity. They can be classified into zones of injury (Figure 15-5), as follows:

- Zone I injury—Proximal two thirds of the nail bed is preserved.
- Zone II injury—Bone is exposed.
- Zone III injury—Entire nail bed is lost.

Zone I Injury

Distal fingertip amputations that are 1 cm^2 or less in size without exposed bone usually can be treated conservatively in the emergency department, with serial dressing changes and close followup care.

The patient must be made aware that wound care is vital to the success of this approach to treatment. Such care must be described accurately to the patient and documented with clearly written discharge instructions. Initial management should include careful and meticulous wound cleansing, a nonadherent dressing, appropriate tetanus prophylaxis, and splinting to protect the tip. The patient should be instructed to soak the injured fingertip once a day for 10 minutes in warm water to which an antibiotic soap has been added, followed by tap water irrigation and the application of a sterile nonadherent dressing. This procedure is performed daily for the first 10 to 15 days and every other day thereafter. Close followup care should be arranged within 2 days for a wound check. Complete healing by secondary intention may take 4 to 8 weeks. Both the cosmetic appearance and the sensation of the fingertip are quite satisfactory using this conservative approach. It is advocated in children younger than 12 years because they have greater regeneration potential.

If the severed fingertip is available, an alternative approach to treatment is to use the amputated portion as a **full-thickness skin graft**. To accomplish this, the amputated tissue should be cleansed and débrided of nonviable tissue and the undersurface of the skin defatted with sharp scissors and sutured to the defect with nylon sutures. Sutures should be left long and tied over a 2 × 2-cm gauze stent dressing to compress the graft firmly against the fingertip. Followup care with a hand surgeon in 2 to 3 days should be arranged. Unless obvious purulence ensues, the stent dressing should be left in place for 7 to 12 days.

Figure 15-5.

Fingertip amputations, zones of injury.

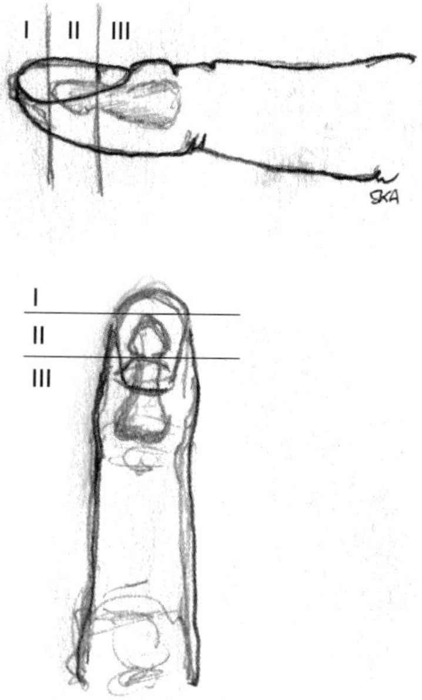

Skin grafting can be used to treat fingertip amputations that have significant avulsed tissue. It can provide a repair that is both functional and cosmetically acceptable. A split- or full-thickness skin graft harvested from a distant site may be indicated in situations where the severed skin tip is either not available or nonviable or there is significant pulp tissue loss. If the patient wants to have full use of the hand before the 4 to 8 weeks necessary to heal by secondary intention, this also may be an option. In these cases, consultation with a specialist is appropriate.

Zone II Injury

Many agree that conservative management of fingertip injuries, even with some initial bone exposure, is superior in terms of cosmetic appearance, improved function, and sensation. In cases where a small protuberance of phalangeal bone (less than 0.5 cm) is exposed, it may be trimmed back with a rongeur to just below the skin level and allowed to heal by secondary intention. In most cases, the wound heals through a process of granulation, wound contracture, and reepithelialization within a few weeks. Amputations that involve the distal phalanx usually are treated as contaminated open fractures with an initial intravenous dose of a cephalosporin followed by an oral course.

Zone III Injury

Fingertip injuries that involve significant soft tissue (especially volar) or bone loss usually require the expertise of a hand surgeon. The size and geometry of the injury, the angle of the tip amputation, and the availability of the amputated tip are factors that determine which options are available for wound closure. A dorsal obliquely angulated wound may be treated in the emergency department by a hand specialist with bone shortening followed by primary closure of the wound using adjacent volar tissue. An injury of this type has a favorable prognosis because the sensate volar skin is intact. Fat from the local tissue may have to be trimmed to allow wound closure without tension. The nail should be removed, with attention paid to associated injuries to the nail bed and surrounding structures. If a hand surgeon is unavailable, the repair may be made by the emergency physician, but the patient must be informed that complete functional recovery is unlikely with even the most meticulous repair. Although the results are comparable to those after conservative management, shortcomings include loss of length, tenderness of the fingertip, and some degree of functional disability.

Amputations that are angled in either a transverse or a volar direction have less favorable outcomes. They do not always have adequate soft tissue and skin coverage to allow for primary closure and preservation of length. Consultation with a plastic surgeon or hand surgeon is necessary because these injuries often require the use of sophisticated local V-Y advancement or pedicle flaps to maintain length and provide tissue coverage, a technique that is beyond the scope of practice and time constraints of most emergency physicians.

Incomplete digital tip amputations are defined by the retention of the neurovascular bundles and a portion of the underlying bone. These may be replaced as a composite graft, but these injuries are among the most difficult to repair and require consultation with a specialist. If adequate circulation is retained in the tip, the injury is treated with fracture reduction, internal pin fixation, and repair of the soft tissue injury. This procedure is optimally performed in the operating room.

In all patients with complete amputations that occur proximal to the lunula, consultation with a hand surgeon or plastic surgeon is recommended for possible replantation in the operating room. This amputation injury commonly leaves the patient with a painful, cold-intolerant fingertip. This complication occurs after primary closure, coverage with grafts or flaps, and healing by secondary intention. Skin grafting may result in induration, fissuring, and diminished sensation. Nail deformity is common, particularly if there is considerable loss of volar tissue.

References

1. American Society for Surgery of the Hand. *The Hand, Examination and Diagnosis.* 3rd ed. Edinburgh, UK: Churchill Livingstone; 1990.
2. Hart RG, Kleinert HE. Fingertip and nail bed injuries. *Emerg Med Clin North Am.* 1993;11:755.
3. Chudnofsky CR, Sebastian S. Special wounds: nail bed, plantar puncture, and cartilage. *Emerg Med Clin North Am.* 1992;10:801.
4. Seaberg DC, Angelos WJ, Paris PM. Treatment of subungual hematomas with nail trephination: a prospective study. *Am J Emerg Med.* 1991;9:209-210.
5. Meeks S, White M. Subungual hematomas: is simple trephining enough? *J Accid Emerg Med.* 1998;15:269.
6. Louis DS. Amputations. In: Green DP, ed. *Operative Hand Surgery.* New York, NY: Churchill Livingstone; 1993.

Additional Reading

Brown EZ Jr. Complication of fingertip injuries. *Hand Clin.* 1994;10:125.

Dalsey WC. Management of amputations. In: Roberts JR, Hedges JR, eds. *Clinical Procedures in Emergency Medicine.* Philadelphia, Pa: WB Saunders; 1991.

Guy RJ. The etiologies and mechanisms of nail bed injuries. *Hand Clin.* 1990;6:9.

Stevenson T. Fingertip and nail bed injuries. *Orthop Clin North Am.* 1992;23:149.

CHAPTER 16

Neurovascular Injuries

Scott M. Benson, MD, and Janet M. Williams, MD, FACEP

Impairment of hand function as a result of nerve or vessel injury can be devastating and can compromise a patient's ability to perform normal daily activities. For this reason, accurate assessment and proper treatment of acute hand injuries are vital to reduce associated complications and optimize outcome. This chapter reviews how to perform a neurovascular examination of the hand and how to recognize and treat acute neurovascular hand injuries appropriately.

Anatomy

The hand is innervated by three nerves that originate from the brachial plexus and enter the hand at the wrist (Figure 16-1). The **median nerve** originates from C5-T1 and runs through the upper arm near the brachial artery. It enters the wrist through the carpal tunnel and innervates the thenar muscles responsible for thumb flexion, abduction, and opposition. Sensory innervation includes the volar thumb and the second, third, and lateral fourth digits. The median nerve also innervates the dorsal second, third, and lateral fourth distal digits. Isolated sensory innervation is assessed at the second or third fingertip.

The **ulnar nerve** originates at C7-T1 and courses along the posterior humerus into the forearm, where it is responsible for wrist flexion and ulnar deviation. The nerve then goes through Guyon's canal and divides into a superficial branch that is responsible for sensory function and a deep branch that is responsible for motor function. The deep motor branch provides finger flexion, adduction, and abduction, as well as MCP flexion and IP extension. The superficial branch provides sensation to both volar and dorsal fifth and medial fourth digits.

The **radial nerve** originates at C5-T1; at the elbow, it divides into the superficial branch and posterior interosseous branch. The superficial branch provides sensory innervation to the lateral three fourths of the dorsal hand, and the posterior interosseous branch provides motor innervation, resulting in wrist and finger extension (including the thumb) and both radial and ulnar deviation.

The **digital nerves** arise from the median, ulnar, and radial nerves. They divide into dorsal and palmar branches and are found on both medial and lateral sides of each digit (Figure 16-2).

The **vascular supply** to the hand lies contiguous to the nerves (Figure 16-3). Particular care must be taken when evaluating obvious vessel injury because nerve injury probably also exists. The radial and ulnar arteries branch to form the superficial and deep arches, which give rise to the common digital arteries. A complete palmar arch exists in approximately 80% of patients.[1]

Initial Evaluation and Management

History

An accurate history of the traumatic event is crucial for appropriate diagnosis and management. The mechanism of injury and the amount of time elapsed since the injury dictate whether débridement, suturing, and antibiotics are indicated. The position of the hand at the time of injury is helpful in detecting neurovascular injury. Elements of the past medical and social histories are important to consider and should include questions related to bleeding diatheses, tetanus immunization status, prior hand injuries, and smoking status.

Figure 16-1.

Innervation of the hand.
A) *Palmar.*
B) *Dorsal.*

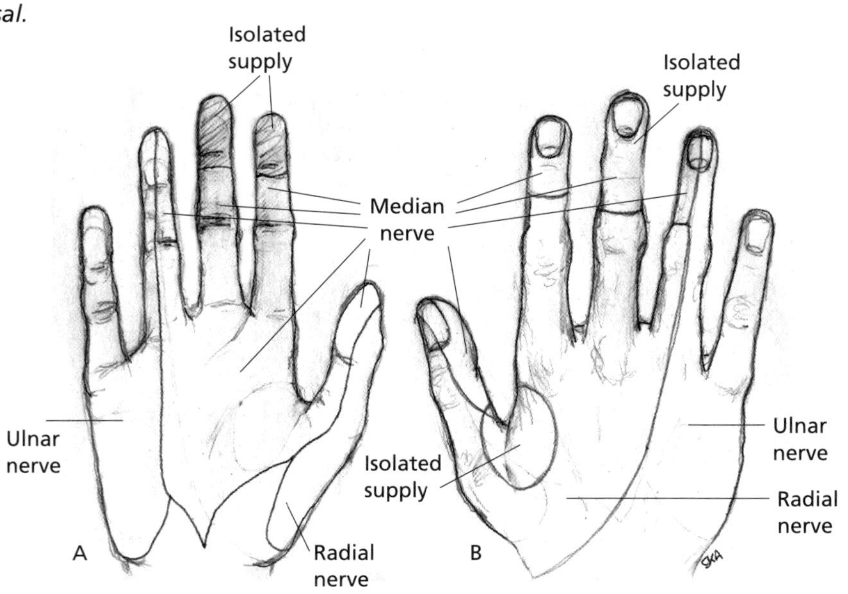

Physical Examination

On physical examination of the hand, the appearance and location of soft tissue injuries, amount and type of bleeding, obvious tendon or muscular injury, and position of the hand held at rest should be noted. Capillary refill, presence and strength of pulses, and the Allen test are vital in assessing vascular status. A neurologic examination should be performed before anesthesia is provided and should include an assessment of both sensory and motor modalities.

Sensory Examination

Light touch and two-point discrimination tests should be performed to assess sensory function. **Light touch** assesses proximal nerve function and is performed by lightly stroking regions of the hand (see Figure 16-1) depending on the nerve being tested. It is very important to tell the patient to look away during the test to avoid false localization.

Static two-point discrimination is used to assess digital nerve function and may be tested with ECG calipers or a paper clip that has been bent into a V shape. Two-point discrimination is intact (with 80% accuracy) if the patient can feel two points separated by less than 6 mm at the fingertip.[2] When performing this test, it is important to place the two points in the axial plane of the finger without crossing the midline to assess the individual digital nerves and to allow 3 to 4 seconds between each subsequent test so that the patient experiences a new stimulus each time.

Motor Examination

The motor function of each nerve should be tested. The radial nerve provides extension of the fingers. The median nerve supplies muscles of opposition and flexion of the index and middle fingers. The ulnar nerve supplies the intrinsic muscles of the hand and flexion of the ring and little fingers. Table 16-1 provides a review of the motor function test for each nerve.

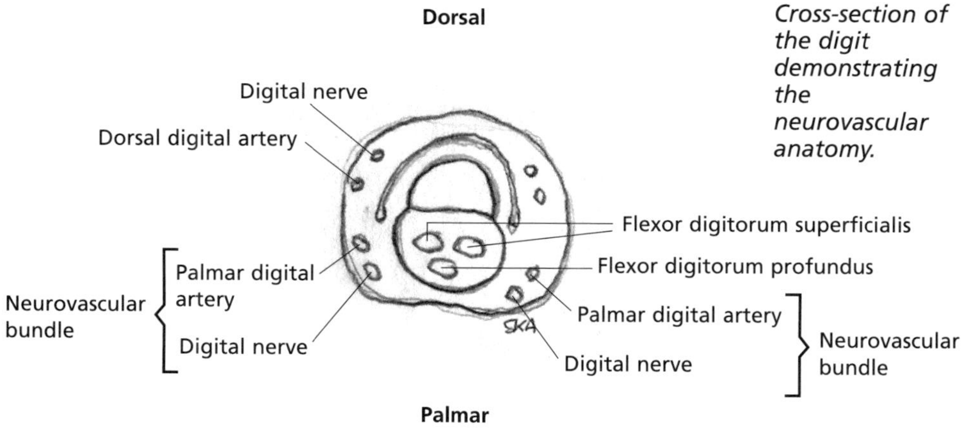

Figure 16-2.

Cross-section of the digit demonstrating the neurovascular anatomy.

Testing should include graded muscle strength. First, the patient should perform the motor function without resistance (against gravity), and then increasing resistance is added. Muscle strength should be documented according to the following scale (normal muscle strength is 5/5):

- Grade 0—No muscle movement
- Grade 1—Fasciculations visible only
- Grade 2—Moves but not against gravity
- Grade 3—Moves against gravity
- Grade 4—Moves against minimal resistance
- Grade 5—Normal strength

Vascular Examination

Because the vascular supply of the hand is highly duplicated through a network of collateral circulation, isolated vascular injuries seldom result in vascular compromise. Ischemic pain is the most common complaint suggestive of vascular insufficiency. Skin color and capillary refill are used to assess the vascular status of the hand.

The Allen test should be performed to determine the integrity of the radial and ulnar arteries. To perform the Allen test, the physician should instruct the patient to make a fist to exsanguinate the hand. Next, while the physician uses the index and middle fingers to occlude the ulnar and radial arteries, the patient opens his or her hand. The physician releases the ulnar artery, assesses vascular refill into the hand, and then repeats the test to assess the radial artery contribution. The test is positive (abnormal) if there is no flush into the hand within 5 seconds.[1]

Figure 16-3.
Vascular supply.

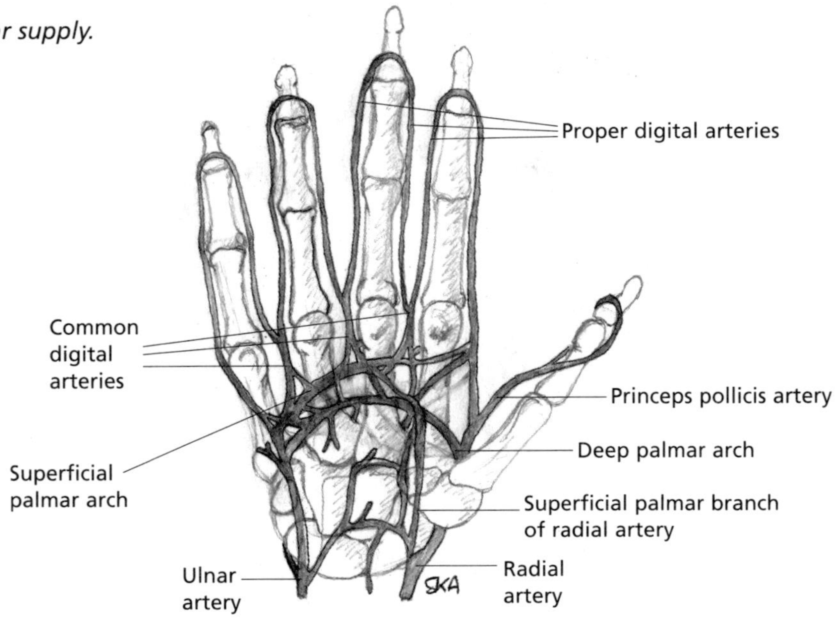

Wound examination is best performed with a bloodless field. This can be accomplished with the application of a tourniquet with a blood pressure cuff or Penrose drain. The blood pressure cuff should be inflated on the upper arm to 30 mm Hg above the patient's systolic pressure but for no longer than 30 minutes. If more time is needed for the examination, the pressure should be relieved for a few minutes and then the cuff reinflated.[3] For the examination of a digital injury, a bloodless field can be achieved by tightly wrapping a Penrose drain around the digit base and securing it with hemostats.

General Management

Tetanus toxoid should be administered in fully immunized patients with open wounds if it has been more than 10 years since the last booster. Tetanus immune globulin should be administered only if a patient has had fewer than three tetanus vaccinations in his or her lifetime. If tetanus immune globulin is indicated, it should be administered in the contralateral arm before débridement because of potential exotoxin release.

All wounds should be considered contaminated and be irrigated.

Table 16-1.

Motor and sensory neurologic examination of the hand.

Nerve	Motor Examination	Sensory Examination
Median	**"OK" sign:** Have the patient make the "OK" sign, then assess the patient's ability to maintain the position while trying to pry the fingers apart. **Thumb abduction:** Place the patient's dorsal hand on a flat surface, then have the patient abduct the thumb and point to the ceiling, apply resistance.	Volar fingertip of the index finger
Ulnar	**Finger abduction:** Have the patient spread the fingers apart forcefully against resistance. **Index finger abduction:** Place the patient's ulnar forearm on a flat surface, then have the patient abduct the index finger against resistance.	Volar fingertip of the little finger
Radial	**Wrist/hand extension:** Place the patient's volar forearm on a flat surface, then have the patient extend the wrist, hand, and fingers against resistance.	Dorsal web space between the thumb and index fingers

Obviously contaminated wounds (a crush injury that occurred in a barnyard) may require copious irrigation and débridement of nonviable tissue. Saline irrigation with a 19-gauge needle and a 35-mL syringe achieves the recommended pressures of 5 to 8 psi to rid the wound of bacteria.[4] Higher irrigation pressures can distend tissue planes and drive bacteria deeper into a wound, potentially increasing the risk of infection. At least 60 mL of irrigant/cm length of laceration should be used.

A wound that is more than 6 to 12 hours old or heavily contaminated (especially with human saliva) is at high risk for infection, and a sutured repair is relatively contraindicated. However, in patients who require delayed surgical repair of an acute nerve injury, the wound may be loosely closed.

Nerve Injury Patterns

General Patterns

Nerve injuries usually result from contusions, lacerations, and puncture wounds of the hand. There are three classifications of nerve injury: neuropraxia, axonotemesis, and neurotemesis. Neuropraxia and axonotemesis generally are associated with contusion and crush injuries; neurotemesis is primarily associated with soft tissue lacerations that include the nerve itself.[5]

Neuropraxia

Neuropraxia is defined as a localized conduction block with intact axons, Schwann cells, and endoneurium, and it most commonly results from contusions. Patients may present with abnormal sensation (paresthesias) and possibly mild motor weakness. On examination, light touch is intact but altered, and the patient notices a difference in sensation compared with the uninjured side. Neuropraxias usually resolve spontaneously within days or weeks, and return of function is complete.

Axonotemesis

Axonotemesis resulting from crush injury occurs when the axon is severed but the endoneurium remains intact. Although presenting complaints are similar for neuropraxia and axonotemesis, the latter condition is more likely if the Tinel sign is present. The **Tinel sign** exists if light percussion of the nerve proximal to the injury elicits paresthesias distally. Recovery is complete but prolonged due to axonal regeneration (approximately 1 inch per month).

Neurotemesis

Neurotemesis refers to complete transection of the nerve. Recovery is unlikely unless the nerve is reapproximated. Distal regeneration does occur, but without formal nerve repair, the axons do not properly align for reinnervation to occur.

Specific Nerve Injuries

Median Nerve

Injury to the median nerve at the wrist impairs both motor and sensory function, but injury at the thenar region impairs only motor function.

Motor testing of the median nerve focuses on movements of the thumb. One method to assess abduction of the thumb is to have the patient rest his or her dorsal hand on a table and point the tip of the thumb toward the ceiling. Strength against resistance should be documented. Thumb opposition can be tested two ways. In the first method, the patient is asked to grasp a piece of paper tightly between the thumb and index finger, and then the physician attempts to pull the paper from the patient's grasp. If the patient can resist removal of the paper, the median nerve is most likely intact. Another method of assessing opposition is to ask the patient to make the "OK" sign; the physician then assesses whether the patient can resist separation of the thumb and index finger.

Ulnar Nerve

Injury to the ulnar nerve near the wrist results in both sensory and motor impairment. Injury near the MCP joint impairs finger abduction/adduction, but sensory and hypothenar function remain intact. Light touch and two-point discrimination of the fifth fingertip should be used to assess ulnar nerve sensation. To test motor function, the patient is instructed to spread (abduct) his or her fingers, and the physician then assesses the strength of the patient's fingers against resistance.

Radial Nerve

Injury to the superficial branch at the anatomic snuffbox results in only sensory loss. Posterior interosseous branch injury usually occurs at the proximal forearm and is associated with deep lacerations and proximal radius fracture. To test motor function, the patient is instructed to extend the wrist and fingers against resistance. The physician then assesses sensation at the dorsal thumb and index finger web space.

Digital Nerve

The digital nerves provide sensory innervation and should be assessed with light touch and two-point discrimination. Intact light touch in the absence of normal two-point discrimination indicates digital nerve injury due to compensation by proximal nerves. Digital artery lacerations often are associated with digital nerve injuries because of their close anatomic proximity.

Treatment

Surgical repair of a transected nerve may be indicated depending on which nerve is lacerated and its contribution to overall hand function. For example, the thumb and fifth digit are always repaired because of their vital function in everyday activities. The patient's occupation and hobbies should be reflected in the decision of whether a repair is desirable. Most nerve injuries can be repaired primarily, are associated with a more desirable outcome, and subject the patient to only one procedure. Delayed repair is reserved for patients with complex crush injuries that are contaminated. Delayed repair can occur up to 3 months after injury and provides the surgeon with a much cleaner soft tissue environment.

With complete transection, the surgeon may elect to tie the nerve ends together pending delayed repair. This maintains normal tension on the nerve and may eliminate the need for nerve grafting at the time of repair. If delayed repair is needed, laceration repair probably is not indicated. Lacerated skin can be loosely approximated with adhesive tape or sutures to allow adequate wound drainage, but care should be taken not to close the skin completely. After a proper dressing is applied, the hand should be splinted in a functional position. Patients with closed nerve injuries should always be referred to a hand specialist.

Prognosis

Not all patients achieve complete recovery after surgical repair of a nerve laceration, and maximal functional recovery may take as long as 3 to 5 years.[6] As a general rule, sensory function returns before motor function. Also, sensory function usually returns closer to the preinjured state than does motor function. Younger patients tend to have better outcomes because of increased nerve plasticity, which leads to improved sensory reeducation after rigorous rehabilitation. Patients with contusions (neuropraxias) can expect resolution of symptoms within days or weeks.

Complications

Paresthesias may complicate nerve injury, and resolution of symptoms is dependent on the type of injury and treatment. After surgical repair of a transected nerve, paresthesias may persist for months or longer; in some cases, it may never resolve.

A mass of irregularly arranged nerve tissue, or neuroma, may form at the site of nerve injury. Neuromas may result in pain or paresthesias and should be resected if symptoms do occur.

Reflex sympathetic dystrophy is a disabling condition that occurs in up to 15% of patients with nerve injuries. This condition is characterized by severe pain, burning, swelling, or stiffness of the previously injured extremity. The treatment is pain control through the use of oral analgesia or sympathetic nerve blocks.

Nerve injuries of the hand also can lead to muscle atrophy. Denervation reduces or eliminates stimulus to the muscle, and in turn, muscle cells and spindles atrophy. After approximately 2 years, the muscle fragments and disintegrates.[6]

Vascular Injuries

General Principles

Serious vascular injuries of the hand are rare due to abundant collateral circulation. Most arterial injuries occur from penetrating trauma. Many arterial lesions do not require surgical repair due to the duplication in vascular supply to the hand. The presence of an arterial lesion should raise suspicion of an accompanying nerve injury because the two structures travel in close proximity.

Treatment

Direct pressure is the initial treatment for any bleeding wound and often is sufficient to halt bleeding. Pressure may have to be applied with increased force or for extended periods if bleeding persists. Vascular clamps should never be used to stop bleeding in the hand because of possible injury to nearby tendons and nerves. A hand specialist should be consulted immediately for surgical repair in cases of vascular compromise due to an arterial injury.

Large vessel lacerations such as those involving the palmar arches and radial or ulnar arteries are best explored in the operating room, where repair can be made if needed. If there is no vascular compromise and a hand surgeon deems repair to be unnecessary, the ends of the lacerated vessel can be ligated with nonabsorbable suture. Repair or reanastomosis also should be considered with arterial injuries that are at or proximal to the PIP joints; a hand specialist should be consulted. Digital arteries often are repaired only when both arteries are compromised or if there is evidence of significant vascular compromise (poor capillary refill).

Because vascular reanastomosis can be complicated by thrombosis, the patient should not be subjected to this risk unless there is definite vascular compromise. If a patient presents to the emergency department with complaints of pain or cyanosis after reanastomosis, the patency of the artery should be checked. Blood flow can be checked by testing distal capillary refill, by using a small Doppler device to hear flow over the anastomosis site, or by comparing fingers on the basis of readings with a pulse oximeter. A review of the patient's symptoms and an examination by the patient's hand specialist are recommended.

Complications

Arterial thrombosis or the development of a false aneurysm may complicate blunt trauma to the hand. These entities present with pain, swelling, and varying degrees of vascular compromise. In either case, appropriate followup care with a hand surgeon should be arranged. If vascular compromise is present with thrombosis, emergency consultation should be sought.

References

1. Newmeyer WL. Vascular disorders. In: Green DP, ed. *Operative Hand Surgery.* Vol 2. New York, NY: Churchill Livingstone; 1988.
2. Overton DT, Uehara DT. Evaluation of the injured hand. *Emerg Med Clin North Am.* 1993;11:585-600.
3. Antosia R, Lyn E. The hand. In: Rosen P, Barkin R, eds. *Emergency Medicine: Concepts and Clinical Practice.* 4th ed. St Louis, Mo: Mosby; 1998.
4. Simon B. Principles of wound management. In: Rosen P, Barkin R, eds. *Emergency Medicine: Concepts and Clinical Practice.* 4th ed. St Louis, Mo: Mosby; 1998.
5. Mackinnon S. Peripheral nerve injuries. In: Light TR, ed. *Hand Surgery Update 2.* Rosemont, Ill: American Academy of Orthopaedic Surgeons; 1999.
6. Wilgis EFS, Brushart TM. Nerve repair and grafting. In: Green DP, ed. *Operative Hand Surgery.* Vol 2. New York, NY: Churchill Livingstone; 1988.

CHAPTER 17

Amputations

Brian N. Aldred, MD, FACEP

The care of amputations, specifically of the parts of the hand, has changed dramatically in recent years. Three factors have contributed to these changes.

The first factor is technologic advances in the procedures themselves, which were brought about by the triumphs and failures of a few innovative physicians. The microvascular and replantation procedures performed routinely today were rarely if ever attempted 30 or 40 years ago. For example, microsurgical techniques were used in the first arm replantation in 1962; the first successful thumb replantation was performed in Japan in 1965.[1-3] Along with improvements in replantation techniques and instrumentation developed a second factor: specialized training programs, which groom hand surgeons (who today staff most urban medical centers) in microsurgical techniques, and the subsequent advent of hand surgery teams, which now are becoming commonplace.

A third factor is increased community awareness with improvements in emergency care. Emergency care personnel today are trained in the proper recognition and treatment of patients in prehospital and emergency department settings, and they have a better understanding of the indications and contraindications for replantation. The key to an emergency physician's care of a patient who has an amputated or nearly amputated part is the understanding that ***all*** amputated parts must be considered for replantation and prepared accordingly, and a surgeon must be consulted promptly.

Together, these factors create an opportunity for hand surgeons to have replantation success rates as high as 90% with patients who sustain amputation injuries.[1,2,4-11]

Initial Assessment and Management

Amputations involve five tissue structures: integument, bone, vasculature, tendons, and nerves. For a replantation to be successful, all of these structures must be evaluated and be reparable to attain viability and, more important, functionality. Based on historical observations,[12] when three of the five tissue structures are severely damaged, repair has been inadequate or has failed. Standards for preserving injured parts now must surpass the functionality of surgical amputation and revision procedures.[1,13,14]

As always, in emergency care, the ABCs and life-threatening injuries must be addressed first. Many patients with amputated parts have sustained multisystem trauma that requires emergency resuscitation, but during initial stabilization, emergency department personnel can be directed to care for the amputated part and to begin preparations for possible replantation or revascularization. Careful evaluation for concomitant injuries and resuscitation are necessary, including control of bleeding. Direct pressure and elevation are recommended for bleeding from extremity injuries. The history can provide the emergency physician with information on the mechanism of injury (crushing, lacerating, or distracting forces); knowledge of preexisting medical and surgical conditions such as diabetes mellitus and vascular disease is helpful for predicting surgical outcomes. A secondary survey should be performed with special attention to the five tissue structures and contamination at the injury site. Neurovascular and tendon function should be tested and pain management instituted.

Physical Examination

The initial examination should identify bleeding sites from the proximal stump of the amputated part. Arterial hemorrhage can be devastating and must be managed emergently. If the bleeding is not controlled by the intrinsic mechanism of retraction of the blood vessels and local vasoconstriction, direct pressure bandaging usually suffices. Alternatives include regional control with direct point pressure of the affected vessels or proximal control with a tourniquet. In most circumstances, pressure bandaging and elevation of the extremity are adequate. Care must be taken not to apply pressure bandaging improperly and unknowingly apply a tourniquet. The proximal stump may sustain irreversible ischemic damage within 3 hours. Conversely, inadequate pressure may lead to continued hemorrhage in a bulky dressing and unnecessary blood loss and hemodynamic instability. Both situations may occur in the prehospital setting or during transport between institutions.

Ligation with sutures or instruments across an amputated part or to visible vessels generally should not be performed in the emergency department. Irreversible damage to vital neurovascular structures may lead to complications and replantation failure. If a tourniquet is needed in an emergency attempt to control significant bleeding, it should be replaced with point pressure control techniques once the site is identified.

Wound Care

Wound contamination is a problem with many complete or partial amputations. After the neurovascular status of the injury has been assessed and the patient stabilized, wound irrigation and débridement should be performed. Appropriate anesthesia (local, regional, or general) should be achieved before wound care. Limitation of movement and splinting of partial amputations in the emergency department can prevent further tissue injury, promote hemostasis, and improve patient comfort. Irrigation can gently remove most debris without further tissue damage. Care must be taken with any débridement to preserve tissue for replantation or grafting. Radiography can reveal the extent of bony injuries and may identify foreign bodies that were not visible on inspection.

If the patient's tetanus immunization status is not current (within 5 years), a booster should be administered. Contaminated wounds are more susceptible to tetanus infection; a patient whose immunization history is questionable should receive both the tetanus booster and tetanus immune globulin. Antibiotics should be administered to patients with amputations or near-amputations. Coverage for staphylococcal and streptococcal organisms is warranted, usually with a first-generation cephalosporin (cephalexin or cefadroxil for outpatients; cefazolin for inpatients). Some mechanisms of injury may require more targeted prophylaxis. Human bite wounds, for example, may be contaminated with *Eikenella corrodens* in approximately 15% of patients. Cat and dog bites have a propensity for inoculation of *Pasteurella multocida* sp. Broader coverage with a β-lactamase inhibitor such as amoxicillin/clavulanate orally or parenteral ampicillin/sulbactam parenterally is recommended. In penicillin-allergic patients, a combination of clindamycin and a fluoroquinolone (levofloxacin or gatifloxacin) can be used.

Antibiotics should be administered parenterally in the emergency department before salvage procedures are performed by the hand surgeon. Dosages should be adjusted appropriately for age and renal function. In all of these injuries, proper wound irrigation and decontamination is of utmost importance.

Care of the Amputated Part

Prehospital personnel must locate and preserve all amputated parts at the scene. Mutilated parts may not be salvageable, but this decision should be made in consultation with a surgeon in the emergency department; tissue may still be harvested for grafting to another injury.

Cooling

Cooling the amputated part (without freezing it) can enhance tissue survival and improve the patient's functional recovery. Multiple studies have shown that cooling an amputated part to 4°C is beneficial.[1,2]

First, the part should be gently cleansed of gross debris with sterile saline, then wrapped in saline-soaked sterile gauze and enclosed in a dry plastic bag. The bag should then be placed on ice (Figure 17-1). Care should be taken to avoid direct tissue contact with ice, thus preventing freezing. Dry ice can cause permanent tissue injury and should never be used.

Ischemia Times

Limitation of warm ischemia times promotes successful replantation. To avoid myonecrosis, warm ischemia times should not be longer than 12 hours for digits and 6 hours for parts that contain significant muscle. With cooling, major limb parts such as those proximal to the wrist can maintain viability for up to 12 hours, and digits may withstand up to 24 hours.[1,2] Major muscle injuries such as those that occur with crushing forces may cause serious complications, such as myoglobinuria and acute renal failure.

Preparation for Replantation or Revascularization

All amputations and partial amputations should be considered for replantation or revascularization. In fact, emergency physicians should always prepare patients and amputated parts for replantation regardless of what decision a surgeon makes regarding definitive care. By definition, **replantation** is the reattachment of a complete amputation, and **revascularization** is the repair of a partial amputation. Revascularization procedures usually have better functional outcomes than replantation attempts.

Evaluation

A hand surgeon must weigh multiple variables when considering and attempting a repair. As many as 90% of amputated parts can be viably replanted with current surgical techniques.[1,2,4-11] However, a chronically painful or insensate, dysfunctional, or malaligned digit is not a successful outcome; the ultimate goal is functional recovery. When multiple digits are injured, the goal of replantation is to provide the best possible functionality. The thumb is of most importance; the little finger provides the least function. Mutilating injuries that involve two or more adjacent digits may require the salvage of one digit with the use of "spare parts" from the others. A patient who can oppose the thumb with two other digits usually can reacquire adequate function, but a replantation of a single amputated finger is less likely to improve function significantly.

In children, any amputated part should be replanted if possible. Children have much better recoveries of form and function than do adults if viability is attained, although performing the procedure is more technically difficult. Children sustain more crush and avulsion-type injuries and have smaller structures to repair.

Figure 17-1.

The cleansed, amputated part should be wrapped in sterile, saline-soaked gauze and placed in a waterproof plastic bag. The bag should be placed on ice, avoiding direct contact of the tissue with the ice.

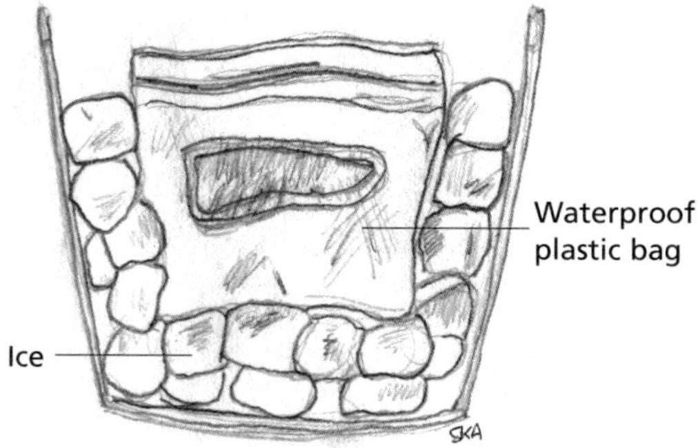

Finally, extensive damage to three or more of the five tissue structures may lead the surgeon to decide to perform a revision amputation rather than risk an unsuccessful replantation.

Mechanism of Injury

The mechanism of injury is an important factor for consideration. Clean, guillotine-type amputations are much more feasible to repair than contaminated crush injuries. With advances in machinery safety in the workplace, fewer hand injuries are occurring. Crush and avulsion injuries have become relatively more common and require more expertise for repair. Multiple levels of injury to the same digit may prevent neurovascular anastomosis and, thus, viability.

The environment in which the patient was injured also is important. Gross contamination of a wound may result in a much higher incidence of infection and loss of viability. Also, significant tissue damage hinders success and may lead to an increased chance of vascular thrombosis and infection in the replanted part.

Medical History

Patients with prior medical illnesses such as cardiovascular disease or microvascular compromise (diabetes mellitus, connective tissue disease) have a poorer prognosis. Age is a factor at both extremes. Even with newer surgical techniques and field magnification, small structures in very young patients are technically very difficult to repair. Older patients who have underlying disease have less successful outcomes and potentially devastating complications, including rhabdomyolysis and severe infection or sepsis. The hand surgeon also must consider concomitant injuries of a more life-threatening nature. The patient's hemodynamic stability must be ensured before replantation. Ischemia times must be minimal to ensure optimal outcomes, especially in parts with significant muscle mass. Technically, longer parts may be more easily replanted or reanastomosed, but the procedure must be performed more promptly (less than 6 hours of warm ischemia or 10 to 12 hours of cold ischemia).

Social History

Although a patient's social history is sometimes difficult to determine in the emergency department, it is important to document. Smokers have poorer outcomes in digit replantations. Occupational history may have a bearing on the aggressiveness of repair, with hand dominance a minor but relevant factor. The patient's ability to follow through with rehabilitation is critical, and psychological issues may be of concern. This is especially true if the amputation is self-inflicted, which is a relative contraindication to replantation. Some patients, when given the option, choose to undergo a revision amputation rather than endure a rigorous, lengthy rehabilitation for little functional benefit. Economic constraints also are a factor. The preference of the patient, after informed consent of alternatives, guides the hand surgeon's decision making.

Risks

The multiple surgical risks include blood loss, infection, and complications of anesthesia. Risks more specific to amputations are compartment syndrome, rhabdomyolysis, and consequent metabolic derangements. With prolonged warm ischemia times, irreversible myonecrosis ensues and can lead to myoglobinuria, renal damage, and resultant acidosis and electrolyte abnormalities. Patients who have underlying disease may be more susceptible. These complications compromise the viability of the replantation and can be devastating to the patient. Above all, if the outcome of an adequately functional and cosmetically acceptable digit or extremity is likely, the surgeon will undertake replantation after considering the risks.

Indications

The goal of replantation, again, is to achieve the best possible function. The thumb is necessary for pinch function, so replantation of an amputated thumb is an absolute indication. When injuries occur to multiple adjacent digits, the restoration of as many digits as possible ensures best pinch function. In children, aggressive attempts should be made to replant all amputated parts to prevent lifelong functional impairment and poor cosmesis. Children have better healing, remodeling, and adaptive capacities, as well as fewer complicating illnesses.[15] For proximal injuries such as palmar, wrist, or forearm amputations, prompt replantation can have good functional results and is highly indicated. With injuries that are more proximal, the risks of more extensive tissue damage are higher; complications such as infection and compartment syndrome are more prevalent. Preservation of the FDS tendon in injuries distal to the PIP joint is a marker for better functional recovery (Figure 17-2).

Figure 17-2.

Indications and relative contraindications for replantation.[1,2]

Indications
- Thumb
- Multiple adjacent digits
- Pediatric patient
- Wrist and forearm
- Sharp, guillotine-type

Relative Contraindications
- Severe crush or avulsion injury
- Multilevel amputation
- Severe premorbid medical illness
- Single digit proximal to the FDS tendon insertion
- Severely contaminated wounds
- Severe premorbid dysfunction to the area
- Prolonged warm ischemia
- Inadvertent cold injury resulting from poor preparation
- Severe psychiatric illness
- Concomitant life-threatening illness

Contraindications

Irreparable devascularization is the only absolute contraindication to replantation, although it may not be noted until after a failed replantation attempt. Relative contraindications include a single index or little finger amputation (border digits), severe crush or avulsion injury, and prolonged warm ischemia. Inadvertent cold injury resulting from poor preparation of the amputated part also is a contraindication. The utmost care must be provided for patient stabilization, tissue preservation, and preparation for replantation. Even for border digits and significant crush injuries, emergency department staff must prepare the patient for definitive treatment, with the surgeon making the ultimate decision regarding care. The crush or avulsion injury or a multilevel digit amputation may be found by the surgeon to have irreparable tissue injury. Revision of the amputation will be attempted and may necessitate grafting tissue from the damaged parts. Again, proper preservation of the parts without freezing or prolonged warm ischemia is critical. Freezing of the tissue leads to ice crystal formation and irreversible tissue and capillary damage, with resultant thrombosis.

The level of injury in an amputated digit is important. Amputations at the middle phalanx proximal to the insertion of the FDS tendon are zone II injuries, which have a much poorer prognosis with limited functional recovery of PIP joint motion. The replanted digit becomes a hindrance, and thus this injury is a relative contraindication.

Other relative contraindications include the following:

- Severely contaminated wounds
- Severe premorbid medical illness
- Severe anesthetic risks
- Severe psychiatric illness
- Significant premorbid dysfunction to the injured area
- Multilevel amputation

Concomitant life-threatening injuries must always take precedence over a limb injury. Whenever possible, emergency department staff should begin preparation for replantation while the emergency physician and trauma services personnel are providing resuscitative efforts (see Figure 17-2).

Functional Outcomes

Advanced microsurgical techniques have made replantation much more common, with viability as high as 90% of digit amputations.[1,2,4-11] Functionality varies, especially in patients at the extremes of age, crush and avulsion injuries, and multilevel amputations.

Measurements of functional outcomes have varying results. Range of motion as high as 80% of normal can be attained in digit amputations.[1,8] Poor range of motion to the PIP joint has been documented in amputations proximal to insertion of the FDS tendon, leaving those patients with a hindrance rather than improved outcome. These injuries constitute a relative contraindication.[1,8] The same results are likely for function, both with range of motion and sensation, following significant crush and avulsion injuries of the digits. More than 50% of patients overall have discernible two-point discrimination of 7 to 15 mm.[1,16] Results regarding the ability to return to work and perform daily functions adequately are less discernible. Studies have shown that as many as 80% of patients with thumb replantations perform activities of daily living capably, although pinch function is variably less in many replantation versus revision amputees.[1,17] This is especially true for single border digit amputations, when grip may even become hindered with a dysfunctional replantation. Children usually remodel in a manner superior to adults, with better outcomes functionally. Bony growth must be followed closely in children, although problems are uncommon.[15]

Results are not as good among patients with premorbid medical illnesses. Vascular compromise, bleeding, and infection are more likely. Psychiatric patients have been noted to have less optimal outcomes.[1] These factors and the inability to follow through with rigorous postoperative rehabilitation are relative contraindications of replantations.

References

1. Boulas HJ. Amputations of the fingers and hand: indications for replantation. *J Am Acad Orthop Surg.* 1998;6:100-105.
2. Schlenker JD, Koulis CP. Amputations and replantations. *Emerg Med Clin North Am.* 1993;11(3):739-753.
3. Komatsu S, Tamai S. Successful replantation of a completely cut-off thumb: case report. *Plast Reconstr Surg.* 1968;42:374-377.
4. Goldner RD, Stevanovic MV, Nunley JA, et al. Digital replantation at the level of the distal interphalangeal joint and the distal phalanx. *J Hand Surg (Am).* 1989;4:214-220.
5. Kleinert HE, Jablon M, Tsai TM. An overview of replantation and results of 347 replants in 245 patients. *J Trauma.* 1980;20:390.
6. Morrison WA, O'Brien BM, MacLeod AM. Evaluation of digital replantation—a review of 100 cases. *Orthop Clin North Am.* 1977;8:295.
7. Tamai S. Twenty years' experience of limb replantation—review of 293 upper extremity replants. *J Hand Surg (Am).* 1982;7:549.
8. Urbaniak JR, Roth JH, Nunley JA, et al. The results of replantation after amputation of a single finger. *J Bone Joint Surg (Am).* 1985;67:611-619.
9. Velanovich V, McHugh TP, Smith DJ Jr, et al. Digital replantation and revascularization: factors affecting viability, prognosis, and pattern of injury. *Am Surg.* 1988;54:598-601.
10. Ward WA, Tsai TM, Breidenbach W. Per primam thumb replantation for all patients with traumatic amputations. *Clin Orthop.* 1991;266:90-95.
11. Weiland AJ, Villareal-Rios A, Kleinert HE, et al. Replantation of digits and hands: analysis of surgical techniques and functional results in 71 patients with 86 replantations. *Clin Orthop.* 1978;133:195.
12. McCormack RM. Reconstructive surgery and the immediate care of the severely injured hand. *Clin Orthop.* 1959;13:75-82.
13. Arellano AO, Wegener EE, Freeland AE. Mutilating injuries to the hand: early amputation or repair and reconstruction. *Orthopedics.* 1999;22(7):683-684.
14. Kleinert JM, Graham B. Macroreplantation: an overview. *Microsurgery.* 1990;11:229-233.
15. Dautel G. Fingertip replantation in children. *Hand Clinics.* 2000;16(4);541-546.
16. Glickman LT, Mackinnon SE. Sensory recovery following digital replantation. *Microsurgery.* 1990;11:236-242.
17. Goldner RD, Howson MP, Nunley JA, et al. One hundred eleven thumb amputations: replantation versus revision. *Microsurgery.* 1990;11:243-250.

CHAPTER 18

Infections

Dean E. Wolanyk, MD, FACEP, FACP

The human hand is capable of a wide variety of complicated and intricate movements. The underlying anatomy of the hand is equally complicated and intricate. An infection can destroy this underlying anatomy and permanently impair hand function. Hand infections are caused by bacteria, mycobacteria, viruses, and fungi. Physicians must diagnose infections accurately and initiate treatment promptly to obtain the best possible outcomes. The appropriate management of hand infections requires an understanding of hand anatomy, mechanism of injury, environment to which the hand is exposed, and immune status of the patient.

In the era before modern antibiotics and surgical techniques, hand infections were associated with high morbidity and mortality rates. Individuals who did not die from their infections often were left with amputations or frozen hands. Kanavel, a surgeon in Chicago in the early 1900s, noticed that hand infections spread in specific patterns. He conducted studies of hand anatomy by injecting plaster of Paris into the spaces and potential spaces of amputated hands. By following the underlying anatomy, he determined how infections spread throughout the hand, providing insight into the best approaches to the treatment of infections while causing minimal damage to hand function. Several of his approaches for draining hand infections are still in use today. It is significant that Kanavel and other physicians of that era successfully treated hand infections by incision and drainage alone before the discovery of antibiotics.

The general management of most hand infections begins with thorough cleansing using high-pressure irrigation followed by incision and drainage when indicated, administration of antibiotics, elevation to reduce edema, and immobilization, then rapid mobilization after the inflammation has resolved. As identified in previous studies, if a wound contains fewer than 100,000 organisms/g of tissue, the body is able to clear the invading organisms and prevent an infection.[1,2] This emphasizes the need to irrigate wounds thoroughly to remove foreign material and reduce bacteria counts.

Anatomy

The hand is covered by a layer of skin that consists of the epidermis and dermis. The **fingernails**, which are specialized structures of the skin, are defined by a **nail plate** that lies on a **nail bed**, surrounded laterally by the **nail fold**. The proximal portion of the nail arises from the **paronychium**, which contains the **germinal matrix** and is covered by a thin membrane known as the **eponychium**, or cuticle (Figure 18-1).

Under the skin is the **subcutaneous fat**. Beneath that is the **aponeurosis**, a layer of connective tissue on both the palm and the dorsum to which the skin is anchored. The tendons of finger flexion and extension are deep to the aponeurosis. Beneath the tendons are the three deep potential spaces of the hand: **thenar**, **midpalmar**, and **hypothenar**. These potential spaces are important because deep infections can spread through them and their interconnections. The deepest structures of the hand consist of bones, joints, and intrinsic muscles. An infection of each structure has a unique presentation and is important to recognize because of the differences in diagnosis and management.

Infections

Paronychia

Paronychia is an infection that develops below the eponychium. When the integrity of the eponychium (see Figure 18-1) is compromised by mechanical trauma, maceration due to water exposure, or even the removal of a hangnail, bacteria are able to invade the nail fold (Figure 18-2). Paronychia presents as swollen, painful, erythematous skin adjacent to the nail.[3] The infection may extend to the other side of the nail (a runaround infection) or under the nail bed. The causative

Figure 18-1.

Schematic of the distal fingertip.

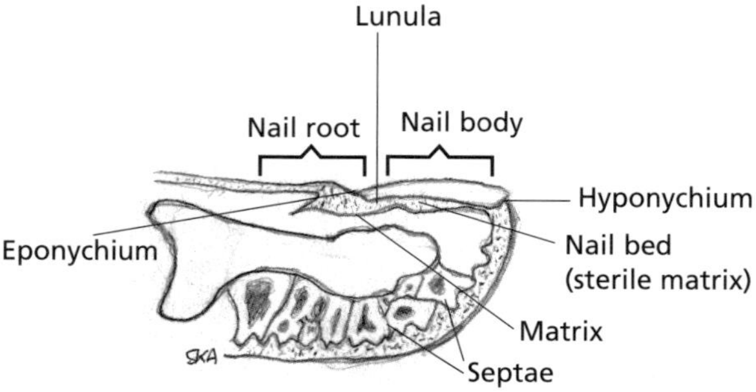

Figure 18-2.

Paronychial infection.

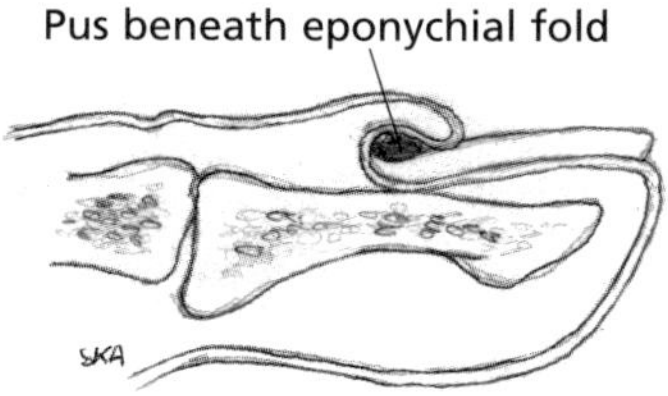

microorganisms usually are *Staphylococcus aureus, Streptococcus pyogenes,* or anaerobes; however, others can be responsible.

Treatment may include antibiotics alone, incision and drainage, or removal of the nail plate depending on the presence of pus and the extent of its spread. In early infections when there is no pus, treatment consists of oral antibiotics, warm water soaks, and followup care in 1 to 2 days. Antibiotics include dicloxacillin (250 to 500 mg PO QID for 7 to 10 days) or cephalexin (250 to 500 mg PO QID for 7 to 10 days). In the penicillin-allergic patient, erythromycin (500 mg PO QID for 7 to 10 days) is used (Table 18-1).

When pus is present, incision and drainage are indicated. A scalpel with a No. 11 blade, held parallel to the nail plate, is used to enter the abscess and lift the eponychium from the nail plate, allowing drainage of the purulent material (Figure 18-3). Oral antibiotics, warm water soaks, and followup care in 1 to 2 days are appropriate. With systemic symptoms, signs of cellulitis, or immunocompromised patients, an antistaphylococcal antibiotic is used. Treatment is with dicloxacillin (250 to 500 mg PO QID for 7 to 10 days) or cephalexin (250 to 500 mg PO QID for 7 to 10 days). Chronic infections, such as those that afflict persons who wash dishes for a living, may be caused by fungi and require antifungal treatment with topical clotrimazole.

Felon

A felon is an infection of the distal pulp space of the finger. The causative organism usually is *S. aureus* or *S. pyogenes,* which enters the pulp space following minor trauma. Patients present with exquisite pain, erythema, and swelling of the finger pad that overlies the distal phalanx. This is a suppurative infection, so an abscess may develop. By definition, a felon does not include the DIP crease. If the edema and erythema extend that far, there may be a more serious complication; the infection may have spread to the bone and joint space, invaded the tendon sheath, or formed a sinus tract to the skin.

Early infection is characterized by inflammation alone and may be treated with an oral antistaphylococcal antibiotic such as cephalexin (250 to 500 mg PO QID) or dicloxacillin (250 to 500 mg PO QID). In the penicillin-allergic patient, either clindamycin (150 to 300 mg PO QID) or erythromycin (250 to 500 mg PO QID) is used (see Table 18-1).

Typically, however, patients present for medical care after the development of

Figure 18-3.

Incision for drainage of paronychial infection.

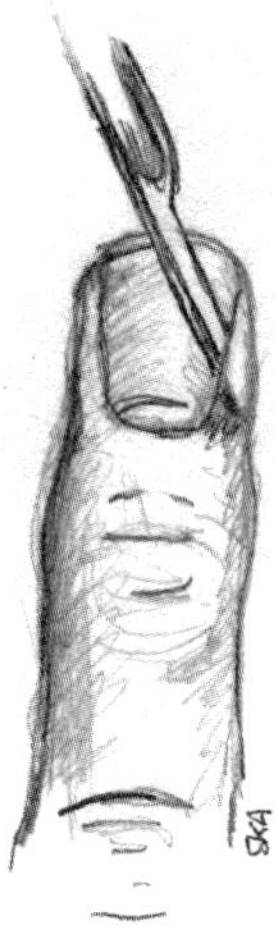

an abscess. Treatment then requires incision and drainage, but incisions of the distal finger may result in painful scars or damage to the nerves and vasculature of the distal finger pulp. The **pulp space** consists of matrix and septae that run vertically and attach the skin to the periosteum, forming compartments that serve as the nidus of infection (see Figure 18-1). When an incision and drainage procedure is performed, it is important to open these compartments to drain the abscess adequately. There are several different techniques for draining felons, with some controversy about the best approach.[3] Two techniques are thought to be most effective for controlling infection and minimizing the risk of neurovascular injury and painful scar formation: the midvolar approach and the unilateral longitudinal approach[3] (Figure 18-4). Most abscesses "point" to the middle of the finger pad, making the midvolar incision ideal.

If a sinus tract is present, the incision should include it. This facilitates complete exposure of the abscess and prevents necrosis of the skin between the incision and the sinus tract. The incision is made in the midline of the finger pad over the area of maximal swelling and tenderness (distal to the DIP crease). The incision should be long enough to allow drainage of pus and blunt dissection of the compartments of the pulp space, with care taken not to injure the underlying flexor tendon.

Some recommend the unilateral longitudinal approach when a sinus tract is not present. This incision is made on the unopposed or nonborder surface of the finger (the radial aspect of the thumb and little finger and the ulnar aspect of the index, middle, and ring fingers). The incision is made approximately 5 mm distal to the DIP crease and just volar to the nail fold, which will avoid the neurovascular bundle. This incision should extend to the subcutaneous tissue, allowing complete drainage of the abscess. Blunt dissection should be performed to break up the loculations of pus and to explore for foreign bodies, if indicated.

After either incision, the area is irrigated and packed with sterile gauze. Antibiotics are administered as discussed, and the wound is reassessed in 48 hours. Then, the gauze is removed, and the patient is instructed to soak the wound twice a day and cover it with a dry dressing after each soak. The wound is allowed to heal by secondary intention. The patient is encouraged to perform range of motion exercises to maintain mobility. If the patient is hospitalized because of comorbid or other conditions, either nafcillin (1 to 2 g IV q4-6h) or cefazolin (1 g IV q6h) is recommended.

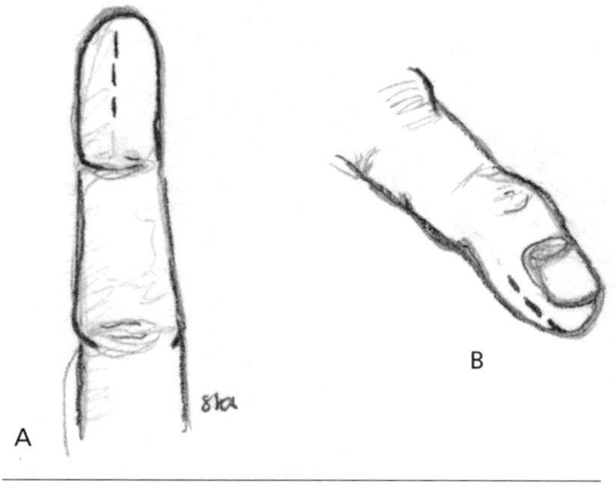

Figure 18-4.

Two techniques for incision and drainage of felons.
A) *Midvolar incision.*
B) *Unilateral longitudinal incision.*

Whitlow

At one time, whitlow was synonymous with felon. Common use of the term whitlow now refers not to a suppurative infection but rather a viral infection of the distal finger. **Herpetic whitlow** is caused by herpes virus type 1 or 2, usually of the finger but sometimes in the hand or forearm. It follows a typical course, beginning with pain and erythema 2 to 14 days after exposure.[4] The vesicular lesions then coalesce and ulcerate over the next 14 days. Herpetic whitlow is common among individuals who are exposed to oral secretions (dental hygienists, physicians, nurses, respiratory therapists, wrestlers). Until these lesions heal (grow a new layer of epithelial cells), they are contagious.

It is important for emergency physicians to recognize and differentiate herpetic whitlow from a felon for the following reasons:

- Incision and drainage are not indicated for the treatment of whitlow and may result in a superinfection.
- Antibiotics do not improve the condition, but acyclovir or another antiviral agent is indicated.
- Because herpes is very contagious, it is particularly important to keep health care workers from infecting other patients.

The diagnosis generally is made clinically, but a Tzanck prep or viral culture can help confirm a difficult diagnosis. The Tzanck prep requires unroofing a lesion and looking for giant cells under the microscope. This test can be performed while the patient is still in the emergency department, but it is not as sensitive as a viral culture, which takes several days to confirm.

The only antiviral agent approved for treatment of herpetic whitlow is acyclovir (400 mg PO TID for 10 days). Other antiviral agents such as famciclovir (250 mg PO TID for 5 to 10 days) or valacyclovir (1 g PO BID for 10 days) should also be effective (see Table 18-1).

Cellulitis

Cellulitis is an infection of the skin and subcutaneous tissue. The affected area is characterized by erythema and edema. There almost always is a break in the integrity of the skin, although on physical examination, the source may not be identifiable. The most commonly involved microorganisms are the normal flora of the skin, group A β-hemolytic *Streptococcus*, and *S. aureus*; most often, *Streptococcus* is the causative microorganism. Aspiration of the leading edge of cellulitis for culture has not been shown to be helpful.[5] By definition, there is no abscess with cellulitis.

What appears to be simple cellulitis may overlie a deep structure infection, such as one of the following:

- Subcutaneous abscess
- Suppurative flexor tenosynovitis
- Deep space infection
- Septic arthritis
- Necrotizing fasciitis

It can be difficult to distinguish simple cellulitis from one of these more serious infections, but it is important to keep them in mind during the physical examination because of their potentially severe consequences. Fluctuance indicates the presence of a subcutaneous abscess. With suppurative flexor tenosynovitis, the entire finger is swollen and flexed, with pain to palpation along the entire course of the tendon sheath and severe pain on passive extension of the finger. A deep space infection presents with severe swelling of the affected part, severe pain with movement, and possibly fluctuance to palpation. A septic joint is red and swollen, with severe pain on movement of the joint. The most important distinction to be made is with necrotizing fasciitis because it is potentially life threatening. This condition presents with severe pain, swelling and induration beyond the margins of the erythema, and sometimes crepitance but no lymphangitis or lymphadenitis. In contrast, cellulitis often has an associated lymphangitis and lymphadenitis but no crepitance.

Treatment for cellulitis involves antibiotics, elevation, and warmth. Penicillinase-producing *S. aureus* has been resistant to penicillin since the 1950s. Therefore, the antibiotics of choice are penicillinase-resistant penicillin, amoxicillin/clavulanate, first-generation cephalosporins (cephalexin), or erythromycin for the penicillin-allergic patient.

Determining which patients with cellulitis require hospitalization and which may be treated as outpatients can be difficult. Patients with large areas of skin involvement or complicating medical conditions or who are unresponsive to outpatient management usually require hospitalization.

Patients with early cellulitis may be treated as outpatients with oral antibiotics such as cephalexin (250 mg PO QID or 500 mg BID), amoxicillin/clavulanate (500 to 875 mg q8-12h). In the penicillin-allergic patient, erythromycin is used (250 to 500 mg QID) (see Table 18-1). If there is no clinical improvement in 1 to 2 days, parenteral antibiotics are required, along with reevaluation for deep structure infections.

Extensive cellulitis requires hospitalization at the onset for treatment with parenteral antibiotics such as cefazolin (1 g IV q6h), or vancomycin (500 mg IV q6h) in the penicillin-allergic patient.

Necrotizing Fasciitis

Necrotizing fasciitis is a medical emergency that is associated with high morbidity and mortality. The mortality rate can be as high as 30% to 70%. Patients with compromised immune systems and certain conditions such as intravenous drug abuse, diabetes, alcoholism, liver disease, and chronic disease are at greater risk for this infection. It requires prompt recognition, rapid initiation of antibiotics, and urgent surgical evaluation.

Necrotizing fasciitis is an infection of the subcutaneous tissue and superficial fascia. It does not involve the muscle except for those infections caused by clostridia. Generally, it starts as a break in the skin and progresses rapidly to inflammation and tissue necrosis. Thrombosis of vessels beneath the skin, which supply the subcutaneous fat and the superficial fascia, is common and accounts for the normal-appearing skin overlying the area of infection. As the infection progresses, the nutrient vessels of the skin become thrombosed and result in discoloration, bullae formation, and eventual necrosis of the overlying skin. The appearance of the surrounding skin may be normal, erythematous, or necrotic.

Early in the disease, patients most commonly complain of moderate to severe pain for what may appear to be a trivial wound. Emergency physicians ***must*** take this complaint seriously and evaluate patients thoroughly. In one study, 5 of 12 patients initially treated with incision and drainage in the emergency department were discharged home only to return with the diagnosis of necrotizing fasciitis.[6] Because the overlying skin may appear normal or only slightly erythematous, it is easy for the examining physician to underestimate the severity of the infection. One important finding on examination is swelling beyond the margins of erythematous skin. Unlike cellulitis and lymphangitis, necrotizing fasciitis causes the underlying tissue to feel hard or woody.

Necrotizing fasciitis is divided into two types: type I is caused by polymicrobial infection, and type II is caused by group A *Streptococcus.* Some suggest the use of two other categories: one for infections caused solely by *Clostridium,* and another for infections caused by the different forms of *Vibrio.*

The **polymicrobial form (type I)** of necrotizing fasciitis, which historically has been the most common type, is found on the trunk and is associated with postoperative wound infections. On average, three to five different types of microorganisms are cultured; group A *Streptococcus* is isolated from most of these wounds. Other possible microorganisms include anaerobes, aerobes, and Gram-positive and Gram-negative organisms. The necrosis and systemic effects seen with polymicrobial infections result from the synergistic action of the infecting organisms.

The **group A streptococcal form (type II)**, popularized in the lay press as "the flesh-eating bacteria," has been seen more frequently in recent years. This form most often involves the hands and legs. It is a rapidly spreading infection that results in hypotension and organ failure. Unlike other forms of necrotizing fasciitis, type II can occur in otherwise healthy individuals with no underlying medical conditions. The causative strain of group A *Streptococcus* produces several exotoxins, which accounts for its virulence.[7] One of these exotoxins, type M protein, prevents phagocytosis. Streptococcal pyogenic exotoxins act as "superantigens" that are thought to accentuate the immune response and result in the clinical picture of toxic shock and organ failure that is seen early in this type of infection. Unlike true toxic shock related to staphylococcal infections, up to 60% of patients with type II infection are bacteremic but do not experience desquamation. Individuals with recent *Varicella* infections appear to be at risk for type II necrotizing fasciitis. Patients who use NSAIDs appear to have a more aggressive course with fewer symptoms because the drugs decrease phagocytosis and pain.

Clostridial infections are the only ones that uniformly involve muscle; they have a higher mortality rate. ***Vibrio* infections** occur when salt water or marine animals contaminate a wound.

One retrospective study examined outcome based on initial therapy.[8] There were two groups: patients who underwent either delayed surgical intervention or limited excision and débridement, and patients who underwent early intervention with excision and wide débridement. Both groups received broad-spectrum antibiotics. The delayed-treatment group had a mortality rate of 38%, whereas the early treatment group had a mortality rate of 4.2%. The authors concluded that necrotizing fasciitis is best managed by rapid diagnosis, administration of broad-spectrum antibiotics, and early surgical intervention with wide débridement.

A second prospective study[9] observed the occurrence of all cases of group A streptococcal necrotizing fasciitis during a 4-year period. The study found that 21% of cases involved the upper extremity as the primary site of infection. Fifty percent of patients were bacteremic, and 50% had toxic shock syndrome. The patients were all managed by vigorous fluid resuscitation, broad-spectrum antibiotic coverage, and surgical excision and débridement. They noted that patients who received clindamycin either alone or with penicillin had better outcomes. The older the patient, the worse the outcome: for patients younger than 35 years, the mortality rate was 0%; for patients older than 70 years, the mortality rate was 65%.[9]

When managing suspected necrotizing fasciitis, emergency physicians should obtain a CBC, basic metabolic panel, clotting studies, and blood cultures. Although a radiograph is not ordinarily obtained, it may be useful in making the diagnosis if gas is present in the soft tissue. Soft tissue gas implies an anaerobic infection, although some aerobic infections also produce gas. Other modalities thought to be helpful in distinguishing necrotizing fasciitis from other nonsevere processes (simple cellulitis) and in making the diagnosis early in the disease course are CT and MRI. Computed tomography is more sensitive than plain radiography in detecting soft tissue gas. Magnetic resonance imaging shows an increased T2 signal of the superficial fasciae in necrotizing fasciitis that is not seen with cellulitis. Although CT and MRI generally are not used for the diagnosis of necrotizing fasciitis, one recent study showed the usefulness of MRI: in 33 consecutive patients, MRI helped make early diagnosis of necrotizing fasciitis by differentiating it from cellulitis.[10] This results in earlier surgical intervention and the potential for decreased mortality.

Another aid in making an early diagnosis is the use of frozen section biopsy. In a retrospective review of 19 patients,[11] eight patients who underwent a frozen section biopsy had surgical débridement an average of 21 hours after presentation and had a 12% mortality rate. A second group of 11 patients did not undergo biopsy and underwent surgical débridement an average of 6 days after presentation; this group had a mortality rate of 74%. Thus, the use of frozen section biopsy may facilitate an earlier diagnosis, resulting in earlier surgical intervention and decreased mortality.

Treatment for necrotizing fasciitis consists of broad-spectrum intravenous antibiotics, fluid resuscitation, and prompt surgical evaluation for wide débridement. For the treatment of type I infections, the following agents are appropriate: imipenem/cilastatin, ticarcillin/clavulanate, piperacillin/tazobactam, ampicillin/sulbactam, and aminoglycoside.[12] In the penicillin-allergic patient, a triple antibiotic combination of vancomycin, clindamycin, and ciprofloxacin is an alternative. For type II infections, ceftriaxone and clindamycin or penicillin and clindamycin is effective. In the penicillin-allergic patient, a combination of vancomycin and clindamycin is effective (see Table 18-1). It is worthy of note that necrotizing fasciitis caused by group A *Streptococcus* responds better to clindamycin than to penicillin. There are many possible explanations, but the most likely is that clindamycin inhibits bacterial protein synthesis, which blocks many systemic effects.

Two other treatment options are hyperbaric oxygen and intravenous immunoglobulin.[13,14] Neither of these has been studied prospectively, but there have been promising anecdotal reports of both.

To summarize, necrotizing fasciitis requires prompt recognition, initiation of antibiotics, urgent surgical evaluation for débridement, and hospitalization.

Subcutaneous Abscess

Subcutaneous abscesses present with erythema, edema, and a central area of fluctuance. The abscess usually results from a puncture wound of the hand and is most frequently inoculated with *S. aureus*, although *Streptococcus* or other pathogens are also present.

A subcutaneous abscess requires surgical drainage through an incision over the area of greatest fluctuance.[4] The wound should be cultured and irrigated with saline and all nonvital tissue débrided. The wound is packed with sterile gauze and then covered with a moist, bulky dressing, and the hand is elevated and immobilized. The hand should be reassessed in 24 to 48 hours.

A first-generation cephalosporin such as cephalexin (500 mg QID) should be used. Confounding factors require consideration. If the patient is diabetic or an intravenous drug abuser, Gram-negative organisms require coverage with an aminoglycoside such as gentamicin. In an individual at risk for an anaerobic infection, penicillin (2 to 4 million U IV q4-6h) or clindamycin (600 to 900 mg IV q8h) is used (see Table 18-1).

Suppurative Flexor Tenosynovitis

Suppurative flexor tenosynovitis is an infection of the flexor tendon sheath of the fingers. The flexor tendons are surrounded by a sheath of synovial tissue that begins at the distal metacarpal and ends at the DIP joint. The sheath is a double-walled tube consisting of an outer parietal layer and an inner visceral layer that lies close to the tendon. Between these two layers is a thin synovial space filled with synovial fluid that transports nutrients to the tendon. The flexor tendon sheath of the thumb is contiguous with the radial bursa; the flexor tendon sheath of the little finger is contiguous with the ulnar bursa (Figure 18-5). The radial and ulnar bursae sometimes communicate with each other, as well as with Parona's space in the forearm. Therefore, an infection of the flexor sheath of either of these fingers may spread throughout the hand and extend into the forearm.

Infection is caused by penetration of the tendon sheath, which introduces microorganisms into the synovial space. Synovial fluid is rich in nutrients and difficult for white cells to enter, making it an ideal location for developing infections. As infection progresses, fluid increases in the synovial space, resulting in swelling and increased pressure. This compromises the nutrition supply to the tendon, which may undergo necrosis and rupture.

Kanavel described four cardinal signs of suppurative flexor tenosynovitis,[15] as follows:

- Tenderness to palpation along the tendon sheath
- Finger held in a flexed position
- Fusiform swelling of the finger
- Pain on passive extension of the finger

Pain with passive movement is thought to be the most sensitive sign for the diagnosis of suppurative flexor tenosynovitis. Most of the signs are present 72 hours or later after the injury. All four signs of suppurative flexor tenosynovitis may not be present, especially in patients who present within 48 hours of the injury, in those treated with antibiotics,

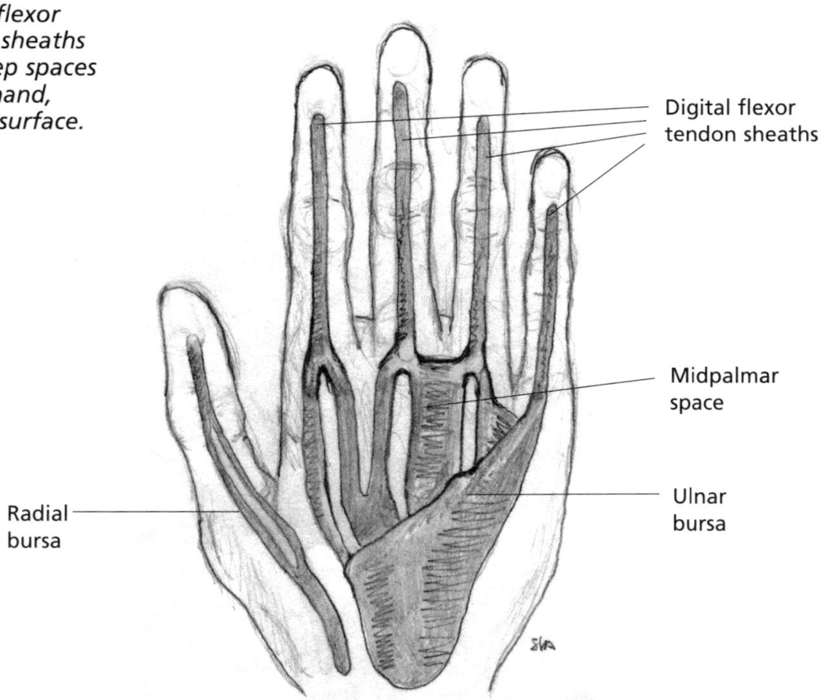

Figure 18-5.

Digital flexor tendon sheaths and deep spaces of the hand, palmar surface.

or in immunocompromised patients. Most patients present to the emergency department more than 48 hours after the initial traumatic injury. Although it is rare, untreated infection may spread into the deep hand bursae, forearm, bone, or joint space or drain through the skin.

Treatment is based on the stage of infection. In very early infection, hospital admission, intravenous antibiotics, splinting, and elevation may be sufficient.[16] If the infection does not resolve within 24 hours, surgical drainage is required. In more advanced infection, intravenous antibiotics and immediate surgical exploration are necessary. If there is no tendon necrosis, it is possible to manage the infection with local irrigation. The surgical technique requires one incision in the proximal sheath and a second incision in the distal sheath. Catheters are placed into the proximal and distal sheaths, and normal saline is irrigated into the proximal catheter with passive drainage from the distal catheter. An advantage to this approach is early mobilization of the hand 1 day after surgery.

If there is necrosis of the tendon, sheath, or pulley, the entire sheath should be opened, explored, and irrigated. Regardless of the surgical technique used, both aerobic and anaerobic cultures are obtained, and the patient is treated with antibiotics.

The microorganisms most commonly associated with a laceration or penetrating injury are *S. aureus* and *Streptococcus.* Antibiotic treatment is with cefazolin (1 g IV q6h). Bite wounds often cause anaerobic or mixed infections. In these patients, broad-spectrum coverage is recommended with nafcillin (1 to 2 g IV q4-6h) plus gentamicin, or imipenem (0.5 to 1 g IV q6h) alone (see Table 18-1).

Deep Space Infections

Kanavel identified five potential subfascial, or deep, spaces of the hand: the dorsal subaponeurotic space, interdigital web spaces, and the thenar, hypothenar, and midpalmar spaces[17] (Figure 18-6).

The **subaponeurotic space** is located on the dorsum of the hand, deep to the extensor tendons and fasciae. It is superficial to both the periosteum of the metacarpals and the fasciae of the interosseous muscles. An infection in this space usually is the result of a penetrating wound, but it may be from a contiguous structure of the hand. It results in pain, swelling, and erythema of the dorsum of the hand and is easily confused with cellulitis or a subcutaneous abscess. An important differentiating finding on physical examination is that extension of the fingers results in severe pain with a subaponeurotic space infection but minimal pain with cellulitis or subcutaneous abscesses. Treatment by the surgeon usually involves incision and drainage with the placement of two longitudinal incisions on the dorsum of the hand. One incision is made over the second metacarpal, and the second is made between the fourth and fifth metacarpals. Care must be taken not to incise the extensor tendon. The abscess is then drained and irrigated.

The **second, third, and fourth interdigital web spaces** are subfascial potential spaces distal to the bifurcation of the neurovascular bundle. The metacarpal heads form the medial and lateral borders; the distal border is the vertical septae of the palmar aponeurosis. The interdigital web space lies beneath (dorsal to) the palmar fascia and is filled with loose areolar tissue that communicates with the subcutaneous space of the dorsum of the hand.

Due to the tight attachments between the palmar fascia and the skin, an infection in the palmar interdigital web space cannot spread between these two layers, but is forced to spread into the dorsal subcutaneous space. On appearance, the dorsal and palmar aspects of the hand are swollen, so when viewing the hand from the fingertips, the involved area appears somewhat dumbbell-shaped.[4] This type of infection is often called a **collar button infection** because, in the early 1900s, collar buttons were double-sided, shaped like dumbbells.

The mechanism of infection often is a skin fissure, blister, or callus that becomes infected. Less often, it may be caused by spread from a subcutaneous abscess or a penetrating injury. On examination, there is swelling on the dorsal or palmar side of the web space, or both; typically, the swelling is worse on the dorsum. Pus in the palmar aspect results in an abducted adjacent finger, which differentiates this infection from a simple subcutaneous abscess of the dorsum of the hand. This finding is important to the treating surgeon because it requires that an incision be made on both the dorsal and palmar aspects of the hand to drain the abscess adequately.

The three deep potential spaces of the hand are the thenar, hypothenar, and midpalmar. Each of these spaces is separated by septae.

Figure 18-6.

Transverse section depicting midhand anatomy.

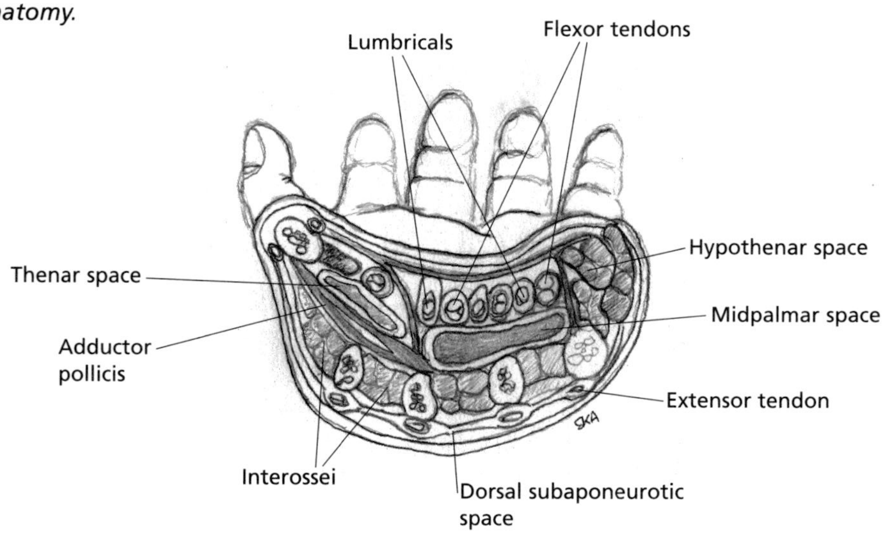

The **thenar space** lies between the adductor pollicis muscle and the FDP and the FDS tendons of the index finger. It often communicates with the first web space. The mechanism of infection can be a penetrating injury to the thenar region or the dorsum of the first web space. It also may be caused by the spread of infection from the thumb or index finger, such as an abscess or suppurative flexor tenosynovitis. An infection of this space presents as swelling, often marked, of the thenar region. On examination, the thenar region is very tender to palpation, and the thumb is held in abduction. Thumb movement, especially opposition, is limited and very painful. The infection may spread to the dorsum of the hand and require both dorsal and palmar incisions.

The borders of the **hypothenar space** are the periosteum of the fifth metacarpal, the deep hypothenar muscle fascia, and the more superficial hypothenar muscles. The mechanism of infection can be a penetrating injury or contiguous spread from a subcutaneous abscess. An infection of this space results in pain in the hypothenar region. On examination, the region is swollen and tender to palpation. An incision is made by the surgeon on the ulnar aspect of the palm, proximal to the midpalmar crease, and extending proximally to end before the wrist flexion crease. As an alternative, the incision may be made on the ulnar aspect of the hypothenar eminence.

The **midpalmar space** lies between the thenar and hypothenar spaces and is separated from them by the midpalmar (oblique) and hypothenar septae, respectively. It lies deep to the palmar aponeurosis and flexor tendons of the middle, ring, and little fingers and superficial to the fascia of the second and third interosseous muscles and the periosteum of the third, fourth, and fifth metacarpals. Likely mechanisms of infection include a penetrating wound; spread from a suppurative flexor tenosynovitis of the index, ring, or middle finger; and spread from a distal palmar abscess. An infection of this space results in pain in the midpalm area. Examination reveals loss of the normal concavity of the palm; it may appear flat or convex. Movement of the middle and ring fingers is limited in range and very painful. Drainage of the abscess requires an incision in the palm. Several approaches are available to the surgeon.

The likely pathogens for any of these infections are *S. aureus*, *Streptococcus*, and Gram-negatives. Treatment requires hospitalization for intravenous antibiotic therapy using cefazolin (1 g IV q6h) or ampicillin/sulbactam (1.5 g IV q6h). However, if the infection occurs in a patient who has a bite wound or who is at risk for a specific type of infection, broader antibiotic coverage would be appropriate, such as nafcillin (1 to 2 g IV q4-6h) and gentamicin (see Table 18-1).

All of these infections require hospitalization, administration of parenteral antibiotics, and surgical intervention to drain the abscess.

Septic Arthritis

Septic arthritis is the inflammation of a joint space due to an infectious agent. This may result from local penetration of the joint space, hematogenous spread from elsewhere in the body, bites, and contiguous spread from a hand infection.[18] A penetrating wound is the most common cause and results in direct inoculation of the joint space. The ensuing infection results in the release of bacterial toxins and enzymes into the synovial space, which destroys the articular cartilage. The immune response causes the white blood cells to migrate into the joint space, increasing fluid volume and thereby increasing pressure within the joint space. This compresses the articular cartilage, effectively decreasing blood flow and compromising vascular perfusion. Thus, the joint space cartilage is injured by the direct action of toxins and enzymes and by the compromised delivery of nutrients and oxygen. The increased pressure may force the infectious fluid through the cartilage and into the bone, resulting in osteomyelitis; through the joint capsule into the adjacent flexor tendon, resulting in suppurative flexor tenosynovitis; or through the finger, resulting in a sinus tract to the skin.

Individuals with diabetes mellitus, malignancies, cirrhosis, or chronic renal failure; elderly or alcoholic patients; and intravenous drug abusers are at a higher risk for the development of septic arthritis.

Patients usually complain of pain and swelling of the affected joint, perhaps with accompanying fever and chills. On examination, the joint is warm, swollen, and tender to palpation; often it is held in mild flexion, which allows for maximal volume of the joint space to accommodate the increased fluid volume associated with the infection. Both active and passive range of motion are painful. The erythrocyte sedimentation rate and C-reactive protein usually are elevated in immunocompetent patients; the white blood cell count often is not elevated. Radiographs are not usually helpful, except for a patient with trauma or penetrating injuries.

Aspiration of the synovial fluid is required to confirm the diagnosis. Aspirated fluid should be analyzed for cell count and differential, Gram stain, and crystals, and cultured for aerobes, anaerobes, and fungi. The white blood cell count generally is more than $50{,}000/mm^3$, with the differential showing more than 75% neutrophils.

Septic arthritis of the hand can be confused with other conditions. Crystal analysis of the fluid helps differentiate between gout and pseudogout. Cellulitis does not produce pain with passive range of motion, and suppurative flexor tenosynovitis results in tenderness to palpation along the entire tendon sheath. Septic arthritis also may coexist in joints with rheumatologic conditions or any of the previously mentioned conditions.

The most common causative bacterial agent is *S. aureus*, and the second most common are the *Streptococcus* sp. In young children, *Haemophilus influenzae* has been a common pathogen, but this probably is changing with the introduction of the HIB vaccine. The Gram-negative *Pseudomonas aeruginosa* and *Serratia* sp are seen in intravenous drug abusers and in diabetic and immune compromised patients. Animal bite infections may be caused by *Pasteurella multocida*. One third of all hand infections are caused by mixed organisms.

Emergency treatment consists of local wound care, antibiotics, and hospitalization. An appropriate initial empiric antibiotic is nafcillin (2 g IV q4-6h) plus ceftriaxone (1 g IV q24h). For septic arthritis caused by human bites, cefazolin or nafcillin can be used, adding penicillin (2 to 4 million U IV q4-6h) to cover *Eikenella corrodens*, which usually is resistant to cephalosporins. An alternative regimen is ampicillin/sulbactam (1.5 g IV q6h). The final antibiotic selection is based on Gram stain and culture results (see Table 18-1).

Septic arthritis is a surgical emergency and requires prompt treatment to preserve the joint. Destruction of the articular cartilage begins within 24 hours of onset of the infection; thus, the emergency physician must start antibiotic treatment in the emergency department and contact the surgeon for drainage of the involved joint. There is some debate over the best surgical approach for septic arthritis; two commonly used techniques are **formal arthrotomy** and **serial joint aspirations**.

Osteomyelitis

Osteomyelitis is an infection of bone that constitutes 1% to 6% of all hand infections.[19] In the hand, it involves only one bone 70% of the time, most commonly the distal phalanx. Infections are introduced by mutilating or open crush injuries, penetrating wounds, spread from a contiguous site of infection, or hematogenous spread from a distant site. Risk factors include diabetes mellitus, alcohol or intravenous drug abuse, and an immunocompromised state. The highest risk of infection occurs with mutilating or open crush injuries in a contaminated environment, such as a farm or stagnant water.

On physical examination, there is erythema, tenderness, swelling, and fluctuance. Because these findings occur in many other hand infections, making the correct diagnosis is difficult. The white blood cell count and erythrocyte sedimentation rate are seldom elevated. C-reactive protein is elevated in osteomyelitis and thought to be sensitive in both making the diagnosis and tracking response to treatment; as the infection improves, the C-reactive protein level falls. Plain radiographs may be helpful in making the diagnosis but are dependent on the age of the infection: in acute osteomyelitis (less than 2 weeks), radiographic changes are seen less than 5% of the time; in chronic cases (more than 2 weeks), radiographic changes are almost always visible. Typical changes are osteopenia, osteosclerosis, and metaphyseal rarefaction, which also are seen in healing fractures. Nuclear medicine scans, using a variety of isotopes, show visible changes before plain radiography. Magnetic resonance imaging is very accurate in making the diagnosis; abnormal marrow signals on T1 and T2 weighted images are specific for osteomyelitis.

There are many infectious agents that cause osteomyelitis. The most common is *S. aureus*, but *Staphylococcus epidermidis*, Gram-negatives (including *P. aeruginosa*), and polymicrobial infections also are causative. Certain situations increase the risk for specific pathogens. Patients with a hemoglobinopathy, especially sickle cell disease, are at increased risk

Table 18-1.

Antibiotic treatment by type of infection.[4]

Infection Type	Antibiotic	Antibiotic Alternative	Causative Organisms
Paronychia	Dicloxacillin 250-500 mg PO q6h *or* Nafcillin 1-2 g IV q4-6h *or* Cephalexin 250-500 mg PO q6h	Cefazolin 1 g IV q8h *or* Clindamycin 150-300 mg PO q6h *or* Erythromycin 250-500 mg PO q6h	*S. aureus*, anaerobes
Felon	Dicloxacillin 250-500 mg PO q6h *or* Nafcillin 1-2 g IV q4-6h *or* Cephalexin 250-500 mg PO q6h	Cefazolin 1 g IV q6h *or* Clindamycin 150-300 mg PO q6h *or* Erythromycin 250-500 mg PO q6h	*S. aureus*, oral anaerobes
Herpetic whitlow	Acyclovir 400 mg PO TID 10d	Famciclovir 250 mg PO TID 5-10d *or* Valacyclovir 1 g PO BID 10d	Herpes simplex virus
Cellulitis	Dicloxacillin 250-500 mg PO q6h *or* Nafcillin 1-2 g IV q4-6h *or* Amoxicillin/clavulanate 500-875 mg q8-12h	Cephalexin 250 mg PO QID or 500 mg BID *or* Erythromycin 250-500 mg PO q6h *or* Vancomycin 500 mg IV q6h	*S. aureus*, *Streptococcus*
Necrotizing fasciitis	Ampicillin/sulbactam 1.5 g IV q8h	Vancomycin 1 g IV q12h *plus* clindamycin 600-900 mg IV q8h	*S. aureus*, *Streptococcus*, Gram-negatives, anaerobes
Subcutaneous abscess	Cefazolin 1 g IV q8h *or* Ampicillin/sulbactam 1.5 g IV q8h *or* Cephalexin 500 mg QID	Nafcillin 1-2 g IV q4-6h *plus* gentamicin 2 mg/kg IV loading dose *or* Clindamycin 600-900 mg IV q8h	*S. aureus*, *Streptococcus*, anaerobes, Gram-negatives
Suppurative flexor tenosynovitis	Cefazolin 1 g IV q6h	Gentamicin 2 mg/kg IV loading dose *plus* nafcillin 1-2 g IV q4-6h *or* Vancomycin 1 g IV q12h *or* Imipenem 0.5-1 g IV q6h	*S. aureus*, *Streptococcus*, Gram-negatives

Infection Type	Antibiotic	Antibiotic Alternative	Causative Organisms
Deep space infections	Cefazolin 1 g IV q6h *or* Ampicillin/sulbactam 1.5 g IV q6h	Nafcillin 1-2 g IV q4-6h *plus* gentamicin 2 mg/kg IV loading dose	*S. aureus*, *Streptococcus*, anaerobes, Gram-negatives
Septic arthritis	Nafcillin 2 g IV q4-6h *plus* ceftriaxone 1 g IV q24h *(N. gonorrhoeae)*	Nafcillin 2 g IV q4-6h *or* Vancomycin 1 g IV q12h *or* Clindamycin 600-900 mg IV q8h	*S. aureus*, *Streptococcus*, *N. gonorrhoeae*
Osteomyelitis	Cefazolin 1 g IV q8h *plus* gentamicin 2 mg/kg IV loading dose	Nafcillin 2 g IV q4h *or* Vancomycin 1 g IV q12h *or* Clindamycin 600-900 mg IV q8h	*S. aureus*, *Streptococcus*, anaerobes, Gram-negatives
Human bite	Clindamycin 300 mg PO q6h *plus* ciprofloxacin 250-500 mg PO q12h *or* Cefazolin 1 g IV q8h *plus* penicillin 2-4 million U IV q4-6h	Amoxicillin/clavulanate 500 mg PO q8h *or* Ampicillin/sulbactam 1.5 g IV q6h *or* Nafcillin 1-2 g IV q4-6h *plus* penicillin 2-4 million U IV q4-6h	*S. aureus*, *Streptococcus*, *E. corrodens*, anaerobes
Animal bite	Amoxicillin/clavulanate 250-500 mg PO q8h	Cefazolin 1 g IV q8h *plus* penicillin 2-4 million U IV q4-6h *or* Ampicillin/sulbactam 1.5 g IV q6h	Gram-positive cocci, anaerobes, *P. multocida*
Intravenous drug abuse	Gentamicin 2 mg/kg IV loading dose *plus* nafcillin 1-2 g IV q4-6h *or* cefazolin 1 g IV q8h	Vancomycin 1 g IV q12h *plus* gentamicin 2 mg/kg IV loading dose	Gram-positives, Gram-negatives, anaerobes, or mixed
Diabetes related	Cefazolin 1 g IV q8h *plus* gentamicin 2 mg/kg IV loading dose	Cefoxitin 2 g IV q6h *or* Ampicillin/sulbactam 1.5 g IV q6h	Gram-positives, Gram-negatives
Traumatic/ contaminated wound	Cefazolin 1 g IV q8h *plus* gentamicin 2 mg/kg IV loading dose	Imipenem 0.5-1 g IV q6h	*S. aureus*, *Streptococcus*, anaerobes, Gram-negatives

for infection with *Salmonella.* Bite wounds are at risk for infection by α-hemolytic *Streptococcus* and *S. aureus.* Specific infections occur with specific types of bites, such as *Pasteurella* in animal bites and *E. corrodens* in human bites. *Neisseria gonorrhoeae* is a consideration in sexually active individuals with monoarticular arthritis.

Cultures are helpful in determining the course of treatment. Deep tissue samples should be obtained before antibiotics are administered. The decision to hospitalize a patient depends on the clinical presentation. For a patient with an acute course, systemic signs, or complicating medical conditions, hospitalization with surgical consultation is indicated. Recommended antibiotic therapy includes cefazolin (1 g IV q8h) plus gentamicin (2 mg/kg IV loading dose), nafcillin (2 g IV q4h), vancomycin (1 g IV q12h), or clindamycin (600 to 900 mg IV q8h) (see Table 18-1). However, a patient who has a chronic infection and is otherwise stable can be managed as an outpatient with regular, close followup care.

Bites

Bites, whether human or animal, cause injury through inoculation of infectious agents from the skin surface, oral flora, or surrounding environment and/or mechanical insults such as tearing, puncture wounds, or crush injuries. These wounds must be thoroughly inspected not only for skin lacerations but also for muscle, tendon, and neurovascular injuries. When a bite wound is near a joint, it is especially important to determine whether the joint space has been compromised. It is best to examine the hand in the position of injury because deep structures move when the hand changes position. Radiography is helpful for identifying foreign bodies such as retained teeth, fractures, and air in the joint spaces.

Treatment of bite wounds requires copious high-pressure irrigation with normal saline to remove debris and microorganisms. High-pressure irrigation reduces the number of microorganisms to a level at which the immune system can eliminate them and prevent an infection. Closure of bite wounds is problematic; the potential risk of infection versus cosmetic outcome must be considered. The consensus is that bite wounds of the hand should not be sutured. It is best to minimize débridement because of the functional role of the tissue in the hand. Consultation with a hand specialist should be considered for any bite injury that affects the deep structures of the hand. Antibiotics are a mainstay for the prevention of infection. When choosing an antibiotic, the patient's immune status, normal flora of the skin, surrounding environment, likely pathogens in the biting mouth, and resistance patterns of bacteria in the community must be considered.

Human

The human mouth contains 100 million microorganisms/mL of saliva consisting of 42 different species. Common aerobic organisms isolated from human bites are α- and β-hemolytic *Streptococcus, S. aureus, S. epidermidis, E. corrodens,* and *Neisseria* sp. Common anaerobes include bacteroides, *Fusobacterium, Peptococcus,* and *Veillonella. Eikenella* sp, found in 10% to 30% of infected human hand bites, is resistant to many common antibiotics but is sensitive to penicillin and ampicillin.

Clenched fist bite. Infections related to human bites of the hand usually are the result of violent altercations and seldom are unintentional. The mechanism of injury results in tremendous forces on a small surface area of the hand. This is especially pertinent for the **clenched fist injury**, sustained when one person punches another in the mouth, often striking the teeth with the MCP joint (Figure 18-7). The teeth not only break the surface of the skin but also may injure an underlying tendon or bone or enter the joint space.

One difficult aspect of treating a clenched fist injury may be obtaining a history. For a number of reasons, the patient may not be totally forthright in providing details of how the injury occurred. The physician must have a high degree of suspicion for any laceration on the dorsum of the hand that overlies an MCP joint. After warning the patient of the potential risk of an incorrect diagnosis (loss of hand function), the true history may be volunteered.

The hand should be assessed in the same anatomic position it was in when the injury occurred. If the injury occurred when the hand was formed into a fist but is examined while the hand is open, the site of the injured tendon may be proximal to the laceration and not visualized in the wound. It may be necessary to extend the incision to allow adequate visualization of the wound. Radiography can detect fractures, retained foreign bodies, or gas in the joint space.

When the joint space is intact, the wound is irrigated and protected with a dry dressing. The patient who is not admitted to the hospital for treatment should be discharged on antibiotics, with instructions to elevate the hand and obtain followup care in 24 hours. Appropriate antibiotics include amoxicillin/clavulanate (500 mg PO q8h) or clindamycin (300 mg PO q6h) plus ciprofloxacin (250 to 500 mg PO q12h).

When exploration of the wound reveals joint space penetration, the patient should be hospitalized for surgical exploration, irrigation, débridement, and possible soft tissue closure by a hand specialist. Antibiotics should be started as soon as possible, ideally in the emergency department. Appropriate choices are cefazolin (1 g IV q8h) plus penicillin (2

Figure 18-7.

Mechanism of clenched fist injury.

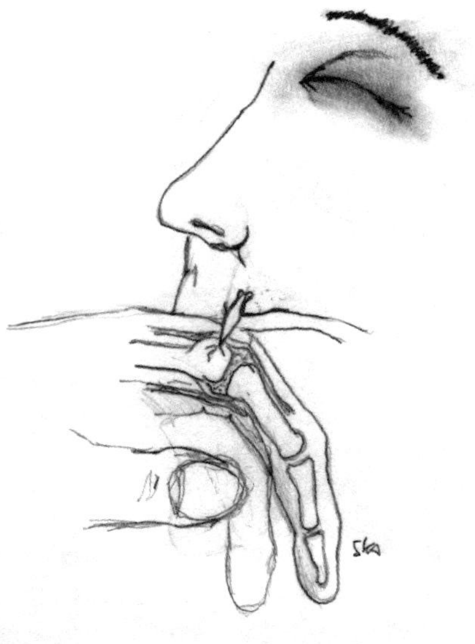

to 4 million U IV q4-6h), nafcillin (1 to 2 g IV q4-6h) plus penicillin (2 to 4 million U IV q4-6h), or ampicillin/sulbactam (1.5 g IV q6h).

Open hand bite. As opposed to the clenched fist injury, the open hand bite generally involves less force and, thus, less underlying tissue damage. These wounds still require thorough examination, exploration, and copious irrigation to remove foreign matter and reduce bacterial contaminants. Depending on the extent of injuries, patients may be managed as inpatients or as outpatients with close followup care.

One prospective randomized study examined the impact of empiric antibiotic coverage for human hand bites less than 24 hours old with no sign of infection on initial presentation.[16] In patients who received antibiotics, there were no infections. Of the patients who did not receive antibiotics, 47% developed infections. The authors concluded that empiric prophylactic antibiotic coverage is indicated for all patients with human hand bites.

Current recommendations for uninfected wounds suggest a β-lactam antibiotic with a β-lactamase inhibitor such as amoxicillin/clavulanate (500 mg PO TID for 5 to 7 days) or clindamycin (300 mg PO q6h) plus ciprofloxacin (250 to 500 mg PO q12h). Infected wounds require parenteral antibiotics; appropriate choices are cefazolin (1 g IV q8h) plus penicillin (2 to 4 million U IV q4-6h), nafcillin (1 to 2 g IV q4-6h) plus penicillin (2 to 4 million U IV q4-6h), or ampicillin/sulbactam (1.5 g IV q6h).

Animal

Animal bites lead to approximately 300,000 emergency department visits, 10,000 hospitalizations, and 20 deaths annually. Approximately 80% of animal bites are inflicted by dogs, 10% by cats, and 10% by other animals. Dog bites become infected in 3% to 18% of patients, and 30% to 80% of cat bites become infected.[20]

Dogs and cats carry a large number of organisms in their mouths that are pathogenic to humans if bitten. In a multicenter prospective study, the Emergency Medicine Animal Bite Infection Study Group showed that 50% of the people who had infected dog bites and 63% of those who had infected cat bites had sustained their bite injuries to their hands.[20] The average time from the bite to the onset of symptoms of infection was 24 hours for dogs and 12 hours for cats. *Pasteurella* sp grew in 50% of infected dog bites and 75% of infected cat bites, making this species the most commonly isolated organism in both types of infected animal bites. A combination of aerobic and anaerobic organisms grew from a total of 56% of all wounds (48% from dogs and 63% from cats). Other aerobes frequently cultured were *Streptococcus*, *Staphylococcus*, and *Moraxella*. Anaerobic infections usually were mixed and more often were found in cat bites and abscesses than were other types of infections.

Based on the culture results and patient outcomes of this study, the authors recommended antibiotic treatment for all animal bites of the hand.[20] Empiric antibiotic treatment begins with a β-lactam and a β-lactamase inhibitor, a second-generation cephalosporin, or a combination of penicillin and a first-generation cephalosporin or clindamycin and a fluoroquinolone. For minor wounds in otherwise healthy individuals with good followup care, treatment is with an antibiotic such as amoxicillin/clavulanate (250 to 500 mg PO q8h). In patients with large wounds or with other medical conditions, hospitalization for parenteral antibiotic administration may be warranted, using cefazolin (1 g IV q8h) plus penicillin (2 to 4 million U IV q4-6h) or ampicillin/sulbactam (1.5 g IV q6h).

Table 18-2 lists infectious organisms and treatment recommendations for several animal bites.[21]

Diabetes

Patients with diabetes are thought to be at greater risk for hand infections due to both systemic and local factors.[22] Diabetes is associated with alterations in cell-mediated defense and wound healing, plus the ischemia associated with angiopathy of small and large vessels. Diabetic neuropathy alters the perception of pain and may result in the patient not recognizing an infection until later in its course.

It is a common belief that diabetes complicates the course of a hand infection. One retrospective study considered the course of hand infections in diabetic patients at a Veterans Administration hospital and in a nationwide database of all Veterans Administration hospitals.[23] The results of the study showed that, in persons with diabetes, hand infections required amputations less often than did foot infections. Hand infections in diabetic patients appear to be best managed with parenteral antibiotics, and although they frequently require local débridement, amputation of a digit or hand is rarely necessary.

Because infections in diabetic patients often involve Gram-negative organisms, they must be covered in any treatment regimen. Although antibiotic choice ultimately depends on the culture results, empiric selection is cefazolin (1 g IV q8h) plus gentamicin, or cefoxitin (2 g IV q6h), or ampicillin/sulbactam (1.5 g IV q6h) (see Table 18-1).

Human Immunodeficiency Virus and Intravenous Drug Abuse

It is well known that the human immunodeficiency virus (HIV) alters the host response to infection. In a study of hand infections in patients who had AIDS or were seropositive for HIV, the most common pathogen was *S. aureus*.[24] A number of cases involved polymicrobial infections, and several were Gram-negative infections. Of 11 patients who underwent amputation, seven were infected with Gram-negative organisms. It appears that Gram-negative infections produce worse outcomes in this patient population.

In this study,[24] the type of injury was more important in determining outcome than was the degree of immunocompromise. It is important to note that *E. corrodens*, an anaerobic Gram-negative rod associated with 15% to 20% of human bite infections, is thought to be especially virulent in HIV-positive patients. The study recommends the

Table 18-2.

Antibiotic treatment by infecting animal.[21]

Animal	Infectious Organism	Comments	Treatment
Bat	Unknown	Prophylaxis within 12 hours or treat established infection	Amoxicillin/clavulanate or doxycycline
Cat	*Bartonella henselae*	Cat scratch fever	Azithromycin or erythromycin
Cat	*Pasteurella*	Soft tissue infection	Amoxicillin/clavulanate; with penicillin allergy: clindamycin plus trimethoprim-sulfamethoxazole
Catfish	Toxins	Usually toxins but may become infected secondarily	Amoxicillin/clavulanate
Dog	*Capnocytophaga canimorsus*	Systemic spread/sepsis	Penicillin, clindamycin, or ciprofloxacin
Dog	*Pasteurella, Staphylococcus, Streptococcus,* anaerobes	Cellulitis, deep-seated infections	Amoxicillin/clavulanate; with penicillin allergy: clindamycin plus trimethoprim-sulfamethoxazole
Fish	*Mycobacterium marinum* (aquarium)	Chronic skin ulcers and pustules	Clarithromycin 500 mg BID or doxycycline 100 mg QD or rifampin and ethambutol (each course for 3 months)
Hamster	*Acinetobacter*	Soft tissue infection	Imipenem or antipseudomonal penicillin
Hamster	*Leptospira* sp	Leptospirosis	Penicillin G IV or doxycycline PO or IV
Mouse	*Leptospira* sp	Leptospirosis	Penicillin G IV or doxycycline PO or IV
Opossum	*Pasteurella multocida*	Soft tissue infection	Amoxicillin/clavulanate; with penicillin allergy: clindamycin plus trimethoprim-sulfamethoxazole
Pig	Polymicrobial	Soft tissue infection	Amoxicillin/clavulanate
Poultry	*Streptococcus, Clostridium*	Soft tissue infection	Amoxicillin/clavulanate or clindamycin
Rabbit	*Francisella tularensis*	Tularemia	Gentamicin

Animal	Infectious Organism	Comments	Treatment
Raccoon	Unknown	Prophylaxis within 12 hours or treat established infection	Amoxicillin/clavulanate or doxycycline
Rat	*Leptospira* sp	Leptospirosis	Penicillin G IV or doxycycline
Rat	*Streptobacillus moniliformis*	Rat bite fever or systemic infection	Penicillin or doxycycline
Rat	*Pasteurella multocida*	Soft tissue infection	Amoxicillin/clavulanate; with penicillin allergy: clindamycin plus trimethoprim-sulfamethoxazole
Skunk	Unknown	Prophylaxis within 12 hours or treat established infection	Amoxicillin/clavulanate or doxycycline
Snake	*Acinetobacter, Hafnia, Klebsiella, Pseudomonas, Salmonella, Shigella, Staphylococcus*	Soft tissue infection	Ceftriaxone
Spider (black widow, brown recluse)	None	Not infectious	None
Squirrel	*Francisella tularensis*	Tularemia	Gentamicin
Waterfowl	*Pseudomonas aeruginosa*	Soft tissue infection	Ceftazidime or ciprofloxacin

use of a first-generation cephalosporin such as cefazolin (1 g IV q8h). In the event of a bite infection or in intravenous drug abusers, an aminoglycoside such as gentamicin was added to the cephalosporin.

Environmental Factors

Wounds exposed to marine environments can become infected with *Aeromonas hydrophila*, *Vibrio vulnificus*, or *Mycobacterium marinum*.

Wounds contaminated by soil may become infected by the fungus *Sporothrix schenckii*, which causes sporotrichosis. This presents as a painless ulcerating nodule, often associated with a regional lymphadenopathy.[25] Treatment consists of oral potassium iodide; amphotericin B is the drug of choice for refractory or deep-seated infections. *Enterobacter agglomerans* infection also occurs in soil-related injuries.

Special Considerations

Rabies

There were five reported cases of rabies in humans in the United States in 2000, all of which were fatal.[26] These were the first cases to be reported since December 1998, which means that all individuals bitten by animals now must be evaluated for rabies treatment.

Several animals serve as reservoirs for rabies. Among domestic animals, dogs, cats, and ferrets are common sources of rabies transmission to humans. Worldwide, dogs are the most common reservoir for human exposure to rabies, but because of vaccination programs, dogs are rarely responsible for human rabies in the United States. There are now more cases of rabid cats than rabid dogs in the United States. Among wild animals, raccoons, coyotes, foxes, skunks, and bats are common sources of rabies. Between 1980 and 1999, there were 21 cases of bat-associated human rabies, with no bite detected in 17 of the 22 cases. Therefore, simple exposure to bats places humans at high risk for rabies. Members of the rodent family (hamsters, guinea pigs, gerbils, chipmunks, rats, mice, and squirrels) and lagomorphs (hares and rabbits) rarely cause rabies.

Rabies is caused by *Lyssavirus*, an RNA-containing rhabdovirus found in the saliva of infected animals. Transmission occurs when infected saliva comes into contact with a break in the skin (bite or scratch) or mucous membranes. The virus then spreads to the central nervous system, causing encephalomyelitis. Although only 20% of untreated individuals bitten by a known rabid animal develop rabies, human rabies is almost always fatal. Therefore, it is incumbent on the physician to identify individuals at high risk for contracting rabies and to initiate treatment.

Treatment is designed to prevent an individual from becoming clinically infected by the rabies virus and consists of two components: passive immunization by inoculation of rabies antibodies and active immunization through a series of rabies vaccinations. The 1999 human rabies prevention recommendations of the Advisory Committee on Immunization Practices, Centers for Disease Control and Prevention,[27] are summarized as follows:

- Determine whether the individual has been bitten by an animal that poses a high risk for rabies transmission (Table 18-3). Captured animals can be observed to see if rabies develops, or, if the animal is to be killed, a brain sample can be examined for the rabies virus.
- Clean the wound thoroughly with soap and water, then use a virucidal agent such as povidone-iodine to kill any surface rabies virus.
- Determine the patient's rabies vaccination status (see also "Tetanus").
- If the patient is **unvaccinated**, administer rabies postexposure prophylaxis as follows:

Table 18-3.

Rabies postexposure prophylaxis guide, United States, 1999.[27]

Animal Type	Evaluation and Disposition of Animal	Postexposure Prophylaxis Recommendations
Dogs, cats, and ferrets	Healthy and available for 10 days observation	Should not begin prophylaxis unless animal develops clinical signs of rabies*
	Rabid or suspected rabid	Immediately vaccinate
	Unknown (escaped)	Consult public health officials
Skunks, raccoons, foxes, and most other carnivores; bats	Regarded as rabid unless animal proven negative by laboratory tests†	Consider immediate vaccination
Livestock, small rodents, lagomorphs (rabbits and hares), large rodents (woodchucks and beavers), and other mammals	Consider individually	Consult public health officials. Bites of squirrels, hamsters, guinea pigs, gerbils, chipmunks, rats, mice, other small rodents, rabbits, and hares almost never require antirabies postexposure prophylaxis

*During the 10-day observation period, begin postexposure prophylaxis at first sign of rabies in a dog, cat, or ferret that has bitten someone. If the animal exhibits clinical signs of rabies, it should be euthanized immediately and tested.
†The animal should be euthanized and tested as soon as possible. Holding for observation is not recommended. Discontinue vaccine if immunofluorescence test results of the animal are negative.

- Passive immunization with **rabies immune globulin** (RIG) human, a hyperimmune globulin. It provides protection almost immediately and lasts more than 21 days. Rabies immune globulin is administered only once; it can be administered through ***but not beyond*** the seventh day of the five-vaccination antirabies series described below. The current recommendation calls for 20 IU of RIG/kg in all patients, including children. (More than 20 IU/kg should not be administered due to enhanced suppression of active immunization.) If possible, inject the entire dose directly into and around the site of injury. Otherwise, administer the RIG at a site distant to and separate from the rabies vaccination site.
- Active immunization with a series of five **antirabies vaccinations.** Using one of the three approved vaccines, administer the first vaccination as soon as possible after exposure, followed by vaccinations at 3, 7, 14, and 28 days after the first one. Because RIG suppresses host response to the vaccine, all five vaccinations are required for full protection. Antibody response occurs in 7 to 10 days and lasts at least 2 years. Again, because it takes time for the immune system to produce its own antibodies, the recommendation is to administer RIG up until the third vaccination on day 7 to confer protection until the body is fully immunized.

• In 1997, a human rabies vaccine was approved for **preexposure prophylaxis** for individuals who are at high risk for rabies exposure (veterinarians, wildlife and fish and game personnel). The vaccine is good for 2 years after completion of a series of three vaccinations. Individuals exposed to rabies in the past who have undergone full postexposure prophylaxis also are considered fully immunized. A fully immunized individual who is bitten by a rabid animal (or one at high risk for rabies) needs only two antirabies vaccinations, one administered on the day of exposure and one 3 days later, and ***not*** RIG.

The rabies virus may lie dormant in the human body for 4 months to more than 1 year. A patient with a delayed presentation still requires and benefits from treatment. Both RIG and the antirabies vaccinations are safe to use in pregnant patients.

Tetanus

Tetanus immunization status should be determined for all patients with hand injuries. Tetanus is a neurologic syndrome caused by the ubiquitous bacterium *Clostridium tetani*, which produces an exotoxin, tetanospasmin, that is responsible for the clinical manifestations of tetanus. Treatment is aimed at neutralizing this exotoxin with antibodies. Passive immunization is achieved with the administration of hyperimmune immune globulin; active immunization is achieved with a toxoid that increases the body's production of antibodies.

Approximately 70% of persons who develop tetanus in the United States are older than 50 years and are inadequately immunized. In recent years, cases of tetanus in the United States have had a mortality rate of 24%.[28]

Treatment recommendations are based on the date of the patient's last immunization and the risk of contracting tetanus (the dirtier the wound, the higher the risk) (see Table 5-1, page 52). A wound is considered dirty if it is more than 6 hours old; is contaminated with soil, saliva, feces, or dirt; contains avulsions or puncture or crush wounds; or was caused by a missile, burn, or frostbite. No additional treatment is needed for patients who have had the complete series of three vaccinations, with the last one being within 10 years if the wound is clean, or within 5 years if the wound is dirty.

A patient who is at least 7 years old who is uncertain of the date of his or her last immunization or has an incomplete (less than three) immunization series must receive an adult tetanus and diphtheria toxoid (Td) booster. A dirty wound also requires immunization with tetanus immune globulin.

For a patient who is at least 7 years old who has never been immunized, the primary immunization series may be started in the emergency department with one Td inoculation, followed by the remaining two injections 6 weeks and 6 months later.

Pregnant patients may receive either the tetanus immune globulin or the tetanus toxoid; neither has been shown to be teratogenic.

References

1. Robson MC, Duke WF, Krizek TJ. Rapid bacterial screening in the treatment of civilian wounds. *J Surg Res.* 1973;14:426-430.
2. Robson MC, Heggers JP. Delayed wound closures based on bacterial counts. *J Surg Oncol.* 1970;2:379-383.
3. Jebson PJL. Infections of the fingertip. *Hand Clin.* 1998;14:547-555.
4. Abrams RA, Botte MJ. Hand infections: treatment recommendations for specific types. *J Am Acad Orthop Surg.* 1996;4:219-230.
5. Hook EW, Hooton TM, Horton CA, et al. Microbiologic evaluation of cutaneous cellulitis in adults. *Arch Intern Med.* 1986;146:295-297.
6. Gonzalez MH, Kay T, Weinzweig N, et al. Necrotizing fasciitis of the upper extremity. *J Hand Surg (Am).* 1996;21:689-692.
7. Bisno AL, Stevens DL. Streptococcal infections of skin and soft tissues. *N Engl J Med.* 1996;334:240-245.
8. Bilton BD, Zibari GB, McMillan RW, et al. Aggressive surgical management of necrotizing fasciitis serves to decrease mortality: a retrospective study. *Am Surg.* 1998;6:397-400.
9. Kaul R, McGeer A, Low DE, et al. Population-based surveillance for group A streptococcal necrotizing fasciitis. A*m J Med.* 1997;103:18-24.
10. Rahmouni A, Chosidow O, Mathieu D, et al. MR imaging in acute infectious cellulitis. *Radiology.* 1994;192:493-496.
11. Stamenkovic I, Lew PD. Early recognition of potentially fatal necrotizing fasciitis. *N Engl J Med.* 1984;310:1689-1693.
12. Stone DR, Gorbach SL. Infectious diseases in dermatology. *Dermatol Clin.* 1997;15:213-220.

13. Brown DR, Davis NL, Lepawsky M, et al. A multicenter review of the treatment of major truncal necrotizing fasciitis with and without hyperbaric oxygen therapy. *Am J Surg.* 1994;167:485-489.
14. Fontes RA, Ogilive CM, Miclau T. Necrotizing soft infections. *J Am Acad Orthop Surg.* 2000;8:151-158.
15. Boles SD, Schmidt CC. Pyogenic flexor tenosynovitis. *Hand Clin.* 1998;14:567-578.
16. Zubowicz VN, Gravier M. Management of early human bites of the hand: a prospective randomized study. *Plast Reconstr Surg.* 1991;88:111-114.
17. Jebson PJL. Deep subfascial space infections. *Hand Clin.* 1998;14:557-566.
18. Murray PM. Septic arthritis of the hand and wrist. *Hand Clin.* 1998;14:579-588.
19. Barberi RA, Freeland AE. Osteomyelitis of the hand. *Hand Clin.* 1998;14:589-604.
20. Talan DA, Citron DM, Abrahamian FM, et al. Bacteriologic analysis of infected dog and cat bites. *N Engl J Med.* 1999;340:85-92.
21. Glaser C, Lewis P, Wong S. Pet-, animal-, and vector-borne infections. *Pediatr Rev.* 2000;21(7):219-232.
22. Gunther SF, Gunther SB. Diabetic hand infections. *Hand Clin.* 1998;14:647-656.
23. Pinzur MS, Bednar M, Weaver F, et al. Hand infections in the diabetic patient. *J Hand Surg (Br Eur).* 1997;22B:133-134.
24. McAuliffe JA, Seltzer DA, Hornicek FJ. Upper-extremity infections in patients seropositive for human immunodeficiency virus. *J Hand Surg.* 1997;22A:1084-1090.
25. Moran GJ, Talan DA. Hand infections. *Emerg Med Clin North Am.* 1993;11:601-619.
26. Human rabies—California, Georgia, Minnesota, New York, and Wisconsin, 2000. *MMWR Morb Mortal Wkly Rep.* 2000;49:1111-1115.
27. Human rabies prevention—United States, 1999. Recommendations of the Advisory Committee on Immunization Practices (ACIP). *MMWR Morb Mortal Wkly Rep.* 1999;48(RR-1):1-21.
28. Diphtheria, tetanus, and pertussis: recommendations for vaccine use and other preventive measures. Recommendations of the Immunization Practices Advisory Committee (ACIP). *MMWR Morb Mortal Wkly Rep.* 1991;40(RR10):1-28.

CHAPTER 19

Burns and Cold Injuries

Robert C. Satonik, MD, FACEP

The upper extremity, especially the hand, is the most commonly burned area of the body, being involved in up to 80% of all burns.[1,2] The hand is of immense functional importance, and the goal of treatment is to provide the patient with the best possible functional and cosmetic outcomes.

This chapter addresses injuries caused by thermal, chemical, and electrical burns and by cold exposure. Regardless of the mechanism of injury, the key to management is assessing the extent of injury in terms of both area involved and depth. These key points determine the care required and the need for and timing of specialty referral.

Anatomy

A detailed discussion of hand anatomy is provided in Chapter 1. Some specific anatomic considerations of burns and cold injuries to the hand are as follows:

- The entire hand represents 2.5% of total body surface area, with 1% each accounting for palmar and dorsal aspects of the hand proper and 0.5% accounting for the fingers.[3]
- The skin on the dorsal aspect of the hand is thinner and more flexible. The thinness predisposes it to a greater incidence of severe injury and the need to maintain flexibility for optimal outcome.
- The palmar aspect of the hand is afforded some protection by thicker skin and a reflexive response to close the hand into a fist when injury occurs.

Burns

Mechanism of Injury

It is helpful to have an understanding of the pathophysiology of a burn injury as it relates to the potential sources.

Thermal Injuries

In thermal injuries, the heat exposure may be direct or indirect. Direct exposure results from contact with flames, scalding, hot surfaces or objects, and hot tar. Indirect sources include steam and heated vapors.[3]

Direct heat exposure. Flames account for up to 50% of all thermal injuries. The central area of direct contact with the flames produces the deepest injury, with a surrounding zone of lesser injury. Scald injuries occur most commonly in children. The initial contact point typically has the most severe injury, with a larger surrounding injury secondary to the runoff or splattering of the hot liquid. The presence of an immersion line should raise the consideration of a nonaccidental injury.

Hot object burns typically occur on the hand and fingers as the victim reaches for or grasps a hot object. The injury usually is localized, and the outline of the object often is evident. Hot tar burns typically are occupation related. The thermal contact and heat transfer often are prolonged as the adherent tar mass continues to transfer heat until it is cooled. Most tar that is used for roofing applications is heated to 500°F.

Indirect heat exposure. Injuries from steam and vapors cause a diffuse burn pattern, but they can be just as severe as direct heat injuries. The evaluation and treatment of these injuries remain the same as for all burns.

Chemical Injuries

Acids cause coagulation necrosis, which results from the desiccating action of the acid on tissue proteins. This stimulates the development of an eschar, which helps prevent further injury. Some acids produce an exothermic reaction, with the skin releasing heat, which causes a secondary thermal injury.

Alkalis produce damage from liquefaction necrosis and generally are more severe than burns caused by acids. The liquefaction allows deeper penetration of the chemical agent. The alkalis combine with proteins and lipids in the tissue, forming soluble protein complexes and soaps, which then allow the hydroxyl ions to penetrate deep into the tissue.[4] Alkali injuries often appear superficial on initial presentation, but they may continue to evolve over the next several days.

Electrical Burns

Electrical burns are classified based on source voltage. High-voltage current traditionally has been defined as 1000 V or greater. High-voltage sources generally are located outside the home and in the workplace. Typical residential power lines in the United States are 7620 V. Common household current is 110 V, and large home appliances require 220 V. Clinically, contact with 600 V or greater produces injury patterns typical of high-voltage injury.[5] High current produces direct tissue heating, which results in neural injury, vasospasm, thrombosis, and myonecrosis. Current flow through body areas with a smaller cross-sectional area such as the hand is potentially more destructive.

Airbag Injuries

These injuries represent a unique mix of frictional, chemical, and thermal burns. Airbag injuries typically occur on the dorsum of the hand. The frictional component results from the rapid deployment of the airbag. The average velocity of deployment is 144 mph, which inflates the standard 60-L driver's side airbag in 10 milliseconds.[6] The chemical injury results from the ignition of the airbag canister. The major byproduct is sodium hydroxide, an alkali, which is spread as an aerosol during deployment and as a heated gas during deflation venting of the airbag.[6]

Airbag deflation occurs within several seconds after deployment via ports located at the 3 and 9 o'clock positions on the steering wheel. This deflation venting process typically accounts for the thermal injury. A second, far less common source of thermal injury from airbags occurs when the chemicals used to ignite the charge canister self-ignite, which may occur on exposure to temperatures above 300°F or to live electrical wires.[6]

History

A definitive discussion of burn management is beyond the scope of this chapter; the key is to treat the entire patient, not just the burned extremity.

Some key points to consider in the patient's history are the following:

- Mechanism of injury
- Whether the dominant or nondominant hand is injured
- Previous injury to or disability of the burned hand
- Occupation and recreational activities
- Tetanus immunization status
- Comorbid conditions, such as advanced age, smoking, vascular disease, diabetes, steroid use, and immune compromised state.

Physical Examination

When examining a burned hand, it is important to note the motor function, sensation, and vascular status and to determine the extent (percentage of body surface area) and depth of injury. To evaluate motor function, the physician should observe the position of the hand, assess the passive and active motion at the joints, and test the strength. Sensation of the named nerves of the hand should be documented, as should two-point discrimination testing of the digits. The quality of the radial and ulnar pulses should be noted, and the capillary refill time should be documented. It may be necessary to assess the palmar arch vessels with Doppler.

The size of the burn is estimated by using the patient's palm as a marker for 1% body surface area. The digits and hand should be evaluated for circumferential injury because circumferential burns are at high risk for the development of elevated compartment pressures.

Depth of injury is pivotal to proper care (Figure 19-1). It is helpful to modify the traditional first-degree through third-degree burn depth assessment. Second-degree burns should be further classified as superficial or deep. A fourth-degree injury class is added to describe hand burns with burn injury to the underlying bone, muscle, and tendon.

First-degree (superficial) burns are limited to the epidermis. Patients present with erythema and pain and heal well in a short period of time.

Second-degree (partial-thickness) burns involve the epidermis and varying amounts of the dermis. In general, the dermal appendages (hair follicles and sweat glands) are intact and provide the source for healing. Patients present with painful blisters. Some scarring and pigment change may occur. With superficial partial-thickness burns, healing typically occurs within 3 weeks. Burns that do not heal within 3 weeks are considered to be deep partial-thickness burns and have a course similar to that of full-thickness burns. **Deep partial-thickness burns** require skin grafting.

Third-degree (full-thickness) burns involve the epidermis, dermis, and dermal appendages. Patients present with a painless, charred wound. These injuries require skin grafting.

Fourth-degree burns involve the underlying muscle, tendon, and bone and require extensive reconstruction.

Special Considerations

In patients with electrical burns, it is critical to look for contact burns. **Contact burns** have central charring with a zone of gray-white necrosis and only minimal peripheral injury. The benign appearance of the contact burn masks the potential for significant underlying injury. The patient with an electrical burn requires additional evaluation of the cardiovascular, nervous, and musculoskeletal systems, with particular attention to signs of the development of rhabdomyolysis.

Chemical burns, especially alkali injuries, often appear superficial and minor when the patient first presents to the emergency department. It is important not to be lulled into a false sense of security and to

Figure 19-1.

Depths of burns.

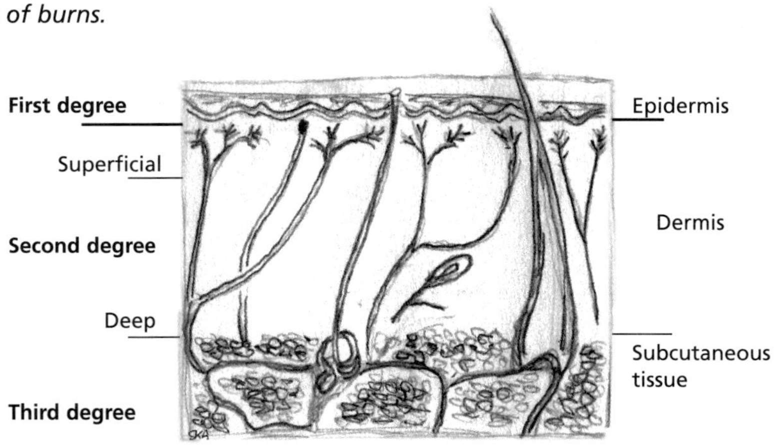

undertreat this burn. Neglected, this burn allows liquefactive necrosis to continue and the injury pattern to progress.

Treatment

The primary consideration in the initial care of the burned hand is to establish the extent and depth of injury because these parameters determine all further care. Superficial and superficial partial-thickness burns can be managed with simple care at home and should heal well in 7 to 10 days without significant scarring or residual disability.[3] All other burns require urgent referral to a specialist. The second-degree burn should be approached with caution because it often is difficult to determine whether it is a superficial or deep partial-thickness injury on initial examination in the emergency department. The more severe burns require excision and early split-thickness skin grafting.

General Care

Analgesic agents should be provided for pain relief; NSAIDs often provide pain relief for the more superficial burns, whereas parenteral agents may be required for more severe injuries. The burn area should be cleansed with a mild soap. Loose, floppy blisters and skin should be débrided, but intact blisters should be left as a biological dressing. The patient's tetanus immunization status should be checked and updated as needed.

Dressings and Splints

The optimal dressing has been described as easy to apply and remove, requiring few dressing changes, painless, promoting healing, and not encouraging infection.[1] At this time, no dressing meets all of these requirements. In general, the dressings should be fashioned with sterile gauze, and the digits should be wrapped individually. Luce[2] recommends wrapping the digits in Xeroform (Sherwood Medical, St Louis, Mo), a bacteriostatic petrolatum gauze dressing.[2] For a minor burn, when immediate mobilization is desired, a dressing can be made by placing a surgical glove, with the fingertips cut off, on the patient's hand over an antibiotic cream.[1] When splinting is required in more severe burns, most recommend that the burned hand be splinted in the following fashion[7]:

- The wrist in dorsiflexion
- The MCP joints in 90 degrees of flexion
- The IP joints in full extension or 20 degrees of flexion

Antibiotics

Systemic antibiotics should not be administered prophylactically in the emergency department. Patients who present with burn wound cellulitis should be treated with antistaphylococcal agents. Such patients typically present several days after the injury with redness, increased warmth, increasing pain, lymphangitis, and fever.

Antibiotic creams generally are used on all burns; several of the more commonly used products are as follows[3]:

- Silver sulfadiazine (Silvadene) is a bacteriostatic agent that has good broad-spectrum coverage. It is painless on application and helps protect the healing epithelium. Silver sulfadiazine is expensive; it also can cause neutropenia and is contraindicated in pregnant patients and patients with a sulfa allergy.

- Bacitracin (neomycin, polymyxin B, and bacitracin zinc) is an inexpensive bacteriostatic agent with good Gram-positive coverage. It is used most commonly on the face and lips, as well as in more superficial hand burns.
- Mafenide (Sulfamylon) is a bacteriostatic agent that penetrates the burn eschar well, with good Gram-negative coverage. It is, however, painful on application and is a carbonic anhydrase inhibitor, which may create a metabolic acidosis.
- Biobrane (Bertek [Dow Hickam] Pharmaceuticals, Morgantown, West Virginia) and 3M Tegaderm (3M Health Care, St Paul, Minn) are two commonly used synthetic occlusive membranes. They are useful for burn coverage in areas that are clean and flat. They act as an artificial skin, sealing and protecting the wound, and can be left in place for 7 to 10 days.

Hospitalization

Some of the criteria for the admission of patients with hand burns are as follows[3,8]:

- Circumferential hand and finger burns
- Burns that involve more than 2% to 3% body surface area that are full thickness
- Significant burns of the hands, face, genitalia, perineum, feet, or major joints
- High-voltage electrical injuries
- Patients with other significant injuries and comorbid conditions

Home Care

Patients with burns who are discharged from the emergency department should be given the following instructions:

- Change the dressing once or twice a day. Rinse the burn with a mild soap and water, apply the antibiotic cream, and redress the wound.
- Elevate the hand to prevent swelling.
- Watch for signs of infection, such as redness, increased pain, fever, and red streaking up the arm.
- Drainage from the wound is normal, especially if Silvadene is used. It typically leaves a watery green-gray discharge on the dressing and a protein coagulum in the wound.

Followup Care

All except the most superficial burns should be rechecked in 24 hours to reassess burn depth and extent. Any patient with a deep partial-thickness, mixed-thickness, or full-thickness burn who is not hospitalized should see a burn specialist in 2 to 4 days.

Referral

After the initial assessment and treatment of a burn to the hand, most patients can be treated as outpatients and managed by a primary care physician. However, in general, patients with the following injuries or situations should be referred to a specialist in burn management:

- Circumferential injuries
- Depth of injury greater than superficial partial thickness
- Significant comorbid conditions
- Occupations or life interests that require a great deal of manual dexterity
- Vascular, motor, or neurologic compromise
- Alkali injuries (because the full extent of injury is not evident on initial examination)

Complications

Early complications include infection, which is characterized by wound cellulitis, increased pain, fever, and lymphangitis, and the development of compartment syndromes.

Escharotomy is indicated for compartment syndromes when there is evidence of decreased perfusion in the burned hand. Escharotomy generally should be performed by a specialist in burn management. The first step is to decompress the forearm, which is accomplished with medial and lateral incisions down the forearm, ending at the MCP joints of the thumb and fifth digit. Once the forearm is decompressed, perfusion in the hand is reassessed. If perfusion is still compromised, a digital escharotomy is indicated. Digital escharotomy is typically performed on the radial aspect of the thumb and the ulnar aspect of the digits between the digital neurovascular bundle and the extensor tendons. This escharotomy location provides the patient with the best possible functional outcome if the digital nerve is injured through exposure or edema.

Late complications usually are the result of scarring and resulting contracture. The four most commonly seen late complications are as follows[8]:

- **Web space syndactyly**, which results from contracture of the dorsal web space margins
- **Digital flexion contractures**, which may involve only the skin or may involve the underlying joint capsule
- **Boutonnière deformity**, which results from deep injury to the dorsal PIP region
- Dorsal skin deficiency secondary to skin loss

Special Considerations in Treatment

Removal of Hot Tar

Tar adheres quickly to the underlying skin, and attempts at manual removal result in greater tissue injury as the skin is pulled off with the adherent tar. Most petroleum distillates readily dissolve tar, but their harsh nature adds injury to already burned tissue. Neosporin ointment (polymyxin B, neomycin, and bacitracin zinc) is the most widely recommended agent; it acts as an emulsifying agent and should be used four times daily. Over time, some tar is removed at each dressing change. The use of mayonnaise or petroleum jelly also has been described.[3]

Chemical Burns

These burns can appear deceptively superficial. Few specific antidotes exist. Most dry powders can be brushed off, whereas copious water irrigation is the mainstay of treatment for most chemical burns. During irrigation of an alkali injury, it is helpful to measure pH as a guide to treatment. pH should be measured 10 to 15 minutes after the irrigation is stopped; this allows for back diffusion of the offending agent. If pH is measured immediately after the completion of irrigation, the results may reflect pH of the irrigant.

Several chemical agents require unique management and are discussed separately.

Hydrofluoric acid is a destructive chemical that causes severe injury by releasing fluoride ions. It is used in the semiconductor industry, in glass etching, and in household products such as rust removers, metal and brick cleaners, and wheel brighteners. Contact with concentrations of greater than 50% result in immediate pain, blanching, and blistering. Contact with lower concentrations may result in delayed onset of symptoms of up to 24 hours; this often is seen with concentrations of less than 20%.[4]

Systemic effects can be seen with a contact surface as small as 2.5% body surface area (the size of the hand). Resultant hypocalcemia, hypomagnesemia, and hyperkalemia cause cardiac and neurologic systemic toxicity. Treatment begins with immediate irrigation with water for 20 to 30 minutes. For brief exposures to concentrations of less than 20%, copious irrigation may be the only treatment required. Persistent pain is a marker of more severe injury that requires further treatment.

The next stage of treatment is aimed at neutralization of the fluoride ions. Both calcium and magnesium bind with fluoride and limit its toxicity. The greatest experience has been with calcium gluconate, and it remains the recommended agent. The first step is to apply calcium gluconate gel, which is made by mixing an ampule of calcium gluconate with two or three packages of Surgilube (E. Fougera & Co, a division of Altana, Inc, Melville, NY).[9] The gel is applied topically to the burned skin. Persistent pain is an indicator for further treatment. A major limitation of the gel is its inability to penetrate the depth of the wound.

If the patient's pain persists, the second step is local infiltration of the wound with calcium gluconate. A 10% calcium gluconate solution is used, and 0.5 mL/cm^2 burned tissue is infiltrated with a 30-gauge needle.[4] Pain relief usually is quick, and persistent pain is an indicator for additional treatment. A major drawback to the local infiltration technique is the need to remove the fingernails if they are involved in the injury. The final option is an intra-arterial infusion, which is indicated when other stepwise treatments have failed or in the case of severe injury. An arterial catheter is placed in the appropriate vascular supply (typically the brachial artery for hand infusion). A three-way stopcock is attached. The stopcock is connected to a pressure-monitoring device and the infusion syringe. The infusion syringe is set up in a 50-mL syringe that contains 10 mL of 10% calcium gluconate and 40 mL of

5% dextrose. This infusion is administered over 2 to 4 hours and may be repeated in 4 hours if symptoms persist.[4] The pressure-monitoring device helps ensure that the infusion catheter remains in the artery. The intra-arterial infusion is time and resource consuming, and in general, these patients should be hospitalized. Other indications for admission include the following:

- More than 1% total body surface area exposure to a solution with a concentration of more than 50%
- More than 5% total body surface area exposure to a hydrofluoric acid solution of any concentration
- Inhalational exposure to a solution of more than 60% concentration

Phenol (carbolic acid) is a corrosive organic acid that is commonly used in industry and medicine. It rapidly denaturates proteins, forming a painless brown or white coagulum. The coagulum forms a nearly instantaneous barrier to simple water irrigation. Lavaging or soaking with polyethylene glycol (PEG 300 or 400) is helpful. If polyethylene glycol is not available, glycerol or isopropyl alcohol is useful.[4]

White phosphorus is used in munitions, insecticides, rodenticides, and fertilizers. Its unique property is that it ignites on contact with air. The patient presents with flaming droplets of inorganic phosphorus imbedded beneath the skin. Initial care includes débridement of visible particles and large-volume water irrigation. A Wood's lamp may be helpful in identifying the particles. Rinsing with 1% copper sulfate solution has been described.[4] The copper sulfate combines with the phosphorus to form a dark coating on the particles. This dark coating aids in location to facilitate débridement and helps limit further oxidation. The copper sulfate rinse must be copiously irrigated because copper sulfate can cause hemolysis and renal failure.

Elemental sodium and potassium explode on contact with water. The particles should be covered with mineral oil or cooking oil; then, they can be irrigated. Burning particles should be smothered or extinguished with a class D fire extinguisher.[4]

Cold Injuries

Cold injuries are most common on the exposed areas of the hands, face, nose, ears, and feet. As with burn injuries, the management of cold injuries to the hands is determined by the extent of injury and the area involved. Cold injuries can be categorized as nonfreezing or freezing injuries on the basis of the presence or absence of ice crystal formation in the involved tissue.[10]

Mechanism of Injury

Nonfreezing injuries are the milder form of cold injuries. Although these cold injuries can be painful, no specific treatment except rewarming is required. **Chilblain** results from long-term exposure to cold and damp conditions and is characterized by burning, itching, and erythema. On rewarming, tender blue nodules appear; they may last for several days and then resolve spontaneously. **Frostnip** is on a continuum with frostbite. Frostnip is a superficial freeze injury without ice crystal formation in the tissue. The involved skin is pale due to the intense vasoconstriction. The symptoms resolve on rewarming, and no tissue loss occurs.

Frostbite, a freezing injury, is the most severe form of cold injury. It is characterized by ice crystal formation in the involved tissue and commonly results in permanent tissue injury and loss.

Physical Examination

Frostbite is described in two phases with three zones of injury and clinically classified similar to thermal injuries. **Phase 1** of frostbite is the actual freezing process of the involved tissue, with the formation of extracellular and then intracellular ice crystals. This results in dehydration and cellular damage. **Phase 2** occurs as the area is rewarmed. This primarily is a reperfusion injury, with the development of interstitial edema and the release of chemical mediators that cause further injury.

The three zones of frostbite injury are described by their anatomic location.[10] The **hyperemia zone** is the most proximal and superficial area of injury and typically heals well. The **stasis zone** is an area of severe but potentially reversible damage; this is the injury zone at which treatment is directed. The **coagulation zone** occurs in the most distal aspects of the involved area and has irreversible tissue injury.

The clinical classification of frostbite severity parallels that of thermal burns. First-degree and second-degree injuries are considered superficial and generally have a good prognosis; third-degree and fourth-degree injuries are considered to be deep and generally have a poor prognosis.[10]

First-degree frostbite is a partial-freeze injury with erythema, edema, and hyperemia. There is no tissue loss or blister formation, and the skin often desquamates several days after rewarming.

Second-degree frostbite is a full-thickness injury with edema, erythema, and clear blister formation. During the week after the injury, hard black eschars develop. These eventually fall off to reveal healed tissue.

Third-degree frostbite involves damage that extends into the subcutaneous tissue, with skin necrosis, hemorrhagic blister formation, and blue-gray discoloration of the skin. The involved skin has no sensation and classically has been described as feeling like a block of wood.

Fourth-degree frostbite has damage that extends into the underlying muscle, bone, and tendon, with dry black mummification.

Treatment

The cornerstone of frostbite treatment is removal of the patient from further cold exposure and rewarming. Any cold, wet, or constrictive clothing should be removed. It is important to treat the entire patient; frostbite victims often are hypothermic and dehydrated and may have associated traumatic injuries.

Rewarming should take place in a warm water bath of 40° to 42°C (104° to 107.6°F) for 10 to 30 minutes with active motion of the hand in the bath. Rewarming often is painful, and analgesia usually is required. Rewarming should continue until the skin is pliable and erythematous.[10] It is important to measure the temperature of the water because tap water may be as hot as 50° to 60°C (122° to 140°F), which can cause a scald injury. Likewise, dry heat should be avoided because it can desiccate already damaged tissue. Most recommend débriding or aspirating clear blisters and leaving hemorrhagic blisters intact.[10] The use of aloe vera cream and ibuprofen is thought to limit further injury caused by the release of prostaglandins and thromboxane contained in the blisters. The digits should be kept separated and wrapped in dry sterile dressings. Elevation is recommended to help control edema. Tetanus immunization status is important because frostbite wounds are considered to be tetanus prone. In general, prophylactic antibiotics are not recommended.

Hospitalization

Patients with all except the most superficial cases of frostbite should be hospitalized. Full demarcation of the injury may not occur for 3 to 4 weeks. The dry black eschars that develop are protective of the healing tissue beneath. Early surgical intervention is not indicated and may contribute to increased tissue loss through the accidental débridement of healing tissue. However, surgical intervention is indicated if wet gangrene develops.

Home Care

Patients who can be discharged to home should be given the following instructions:

- Change the dressings twice a day after applying topical aloe vera cream.
- Take ibuprofen for pain and to reduce further injury. Other pain medications might also be used.
- Watch for signs of infection, such as redness, increased pain, fever, or red streaking up the arm.

Followup Care

All except the most superficial frostbite injuries should be rechecked in 24 hours to reassess their depth and extent. Any patient with second-degree or third-degree frostbite injuries who is hospitalized should see a hand specialist in 2 to 4 days.

Complications

Patients who develop infection typically present with **wet gangrene** (ischemic necrosis with surrounding cellulitis) and require hospitalization with surgical consultation. Antibiotics are given, and even amputation may be necessary.

Long-term complications associated with frostbite injuries include the following[10]:

- Permanent cold sensitivity
- Chronic pain
- Hyperhidrosis (excessive sweating)

- Growth plate arrest in pediatric patients, typically occurring in the distal phalanges with resultant shortening and radial deviation
- Posttraumatic arthritis in fourth-degree injuries

Conclusion

Treatment is guided by a careful evaluation of hot and cold injuries to the hand, with a knowledge of anatomy and the stages of possible injury. Most patients require close followup with a hand specialist for these types of injuries. Adherence to the basic tenets of management on the basis of the depth and size of injury ensure the best possible outcome.

References

1. Belliappa PP, McCabe SJ. The burned hand. *Hand Clin.* 1993;9:313-324.
2. Luce EA. The acute and subacute management of the burned hand. *Clin Plast Surg.* 2000;27:49-63.
3. Drueck C. Emergency department treatment of hand burns. *Emerg Med Clin North Am.* 1993;11:797-809.
4. Harchelroad FP, Ballister JM. Chemical burns. In: Tintinalli JE, Kelen GD, Stapczynski JS, eds. *Emergency Medicine: A Comprehensive Study Guide.* 5th ed. New York, NY: McGraw-Hill; 2000:1286-1292.
5. Rabbon J, Alder J, Rosen C, et al. Electrical injury from subway third rails: serious injury associated with intermediate voltage contact. *Burns.* 1997;23:515.
6. Vitello W, Kim M, Johnson RM, et al. Full thickness burn to the hand from an automobile airbag. *J Burn Care Rehabil.* 1999;20:212-215.
7. Lister G. *The Hand: Diagnosis and Indications.* 3rd ed. New York, NY: Churchill Livingstone; 1993.
8. Sundine MJ, Kao SD. Burns of the hand and upper extremity. In: Jebson PJL, Kasdan ML, eds. *Hand Secrets.* Philadelphia, Pa: Hanley & Belfus; 1998:43-44.
9. Borkhart KK, Brent J, Kirk MA, et al. Comparison of topical magnesium and calcium treatment for dermal hydrofluoric acid burns. *Ann Emerg Med.* 1994;24:9.
10. Rabold MB. Frostbite and other localized cold-related injuries. In: Tintinalli JE, Kelen GD, Stapczynski JS, eds. *Emergency Medicine: A Comprehensive Study Guide.* 5th ed. New York, NY: McGraw-Hill; 2000:1227-1231.

CHAPTER 20

Pediatric Injuries

Jonathan I. Singer, MD, FACEP

The management of hand injuries in children, in general, is similar to that for adults. An emergency physician who is accustomed to managing adult hand injuries can comfortably render care to children who have comparable injuries. However, there are subtleties that, if recognized, can lead to improved healing for the child (and the parent) as well as reduced anxiety for the physician.

Presenting Complaints

An estimated 5% of pediatric visits to a community emergency department and 10% to 20% of visits to a pediatric emergency department follow traumatic events. The most frequently injured anatomic areas are the face and scalp. Injuries to the forearm, especially the area about the distal volar wrist crease, and digital injuries are the next most common.

In a pediatric emergency department, the most commonly reported categories of hand and digit injuries are lacerations (38%), soft tissue events (29%), fractures (19%), and ligament disruption (8%).[1] Younger children disproportionately present with lacerations, burns, bites, and stings. Older children tend to sustain more fractures and sprains, the majority of which occur as a result of participating in sports or fist fights.[2]

Physiology

Hand-Digit Unit

A variety of congenital defects may involve the hand-digit unit, including syndactyly, dysplasias, and part deficiencies.[3] In the absence of a congenital defect, an infant's hand and digits at birth resemble those of an adult. However, for the child's hand-digit unit to become fully functional, a neurologic maturation process must occur. This physiologic advancement progresses at an accelerated rate during the first 18 months of life.

Developmental Stages

Although there are minor variations, the physiologic development of the hand-digit unit progresses through defined stages.

Three Months

By 12 weeks of age, infants are capable of grasping with either hand and briefly retaining offered objects.

Three to Six Months

Between 3 and 6 months of age, infants can bring their hands together spontaneously in the midline. A 6-month-old can change the orientation of the arms and reach either hand toward a desired moderate-sized object, bring the object to the midline, and achieve oral contact. At 5 to 6 months old, infants first digitally pursue, without success, smaller objects. By 6 months of age, infants make raking motions of the digits toward smaller objects. Digital movements toward a smaller object are likely to occur first with the ulnar aspect of the hand.

Six to Twelve Months

By 6 to 7 months of age, the radial functions of the hand-digit unit improve. The thumb is first used in conjunction with the palm, followed by other digits. Between 6 and 9 months, the radial-palmar grasp mechanism becomes more refined. Infants master accurate apposition of the thumb and digits during this time and are capable of picking up pea-sized objects with a reasonable pincer motion.

Twelve to Eighteen Months

By 12 months of age, neurologically normal children can execute a pure pincer motion with small objects without ulnar support. At 15 to 18 months, all healthy infants are capable of inserting their fingers into small openings.

Fine motor hand and digit skills continue to develop beyond the first 1.5 years of life. By 18 months, most children have developed motor and sensory skills comparable to those of adults but lack the proportionate sense to protect their hand-digit units from injury.

Patterns of Injury

Contributing Factors

The state of motor refinement, potential for exposure to environmental hazards (household appliances, playground equipment), and lapses in parental supervision are among the physiologic and behavioral factors that most commonly contribute to pediatric bodily injury.[2] With hand and digit injuries, the age of the child greatly influences the pattern of injury.[1,4]

Impact of Age

Familiarity with the spectrum of age-related injuries allows the clinician to interpret the likelihood for unintentional versus intentional (abuse) injury (Figure 20-1).

Infant (Younger Than 1 Year)

It is unlikely that an infant will be brought to an emergency department for a newly discovered scenario such as conjoined digits or superfluous digits. A child younger than 1 year may sustain a **hair tourniquet syndrome**, in which a human hair or a thread from clothing entwines a digit or digits; autoamputation can result from the tissue entrapment.

Toddler (1 to 2 Years Old)

The rate of developmental change between the first and second years of life is enormous. Inquisitive toddlers typically use their hands (which have developed beyond their cerebral powers) to explore their home environments. Highly mobile toddlers incur a wide variety of contact injuries. For example, a common injury is a partial-thickness dry contact burn of the digits with or without thenar or hypothenar injury from touching a kerosene heater. The tops of these heaters range from 300° to 550°F, and an inadvertent contact of less than 1 second can cause severe burns. Gas fire floor furnaces and steam vaporizers placed in proximity to curious toddlers are a major source of partial-thickness scald injuries. Toddlers freely insert digits or hand-held implements into electrical outlets and sustain localized, low-voltage electrical injuries. They also will insert digits into objects and then be unable to extract them.

Preschooler (2 to 5 Years Old)

Between 2 and 3 years old, children maximize self-injury due to minimal lapses in parental supervision. Preschool-aged children are at risk for hand contact thermal injuries. Implements likely to cause injuries at this age are hot barbecue grills (and charcoal briquettes), hair dryers, curling irons, and motorcycle tailpipes. Boiled water, pooled grease, and hot food sludges may cause scald injuries to the hand but rarely in exclusion of other body parts. At 3 to 4 years old, children sustain digit injuries as a consequence of unnatural reaches. Lacerations occur from grasping broken glass or sharp knives. Bites inflicted by other children are common. By age 5, most children possess near-adult levels of motor dexterity, but residual degrees of incoordination may predispose to digital crush injuries. Subungual hematoma, nail bed

Figure 20-1.

Impact of age on type of injury.

Infant (<1 year)
- Congenital amputation
- Traumatic amputation (hair tourniquet)
- Physical abuse

Toddler (1-2 years)
- Contact injury
- Entrapment
- Physical abuse

Preschooler (2-5 years)
- Contact injury
- Abrasion, contusion
- Human bite
- Laceration
- Crush injury
- Physical abuse

Early Schooler (5-13 years)
- Bite, envenomation
- Laceration
- Foreign body
- Blast injury
- Amputation
- Fracture
- Physical abuse

Adolescent (>13 years)
- Fracture
- Dislocation
- Laceration
- Crush injury
- Blast injury
- Ring degloving
- Physical abuse

injury, partial pulp avulsion, and distal digit amputation are prevalent unintentional injuries in 5-year-olds.

Early Schooler (5 to 13 Years Old)

The incidence of bites, envenomations, soft tissue injuries such as abrasions, superficial avulsions, and retained foreign bodies peaks in early school-aged children. Digital fractures are most prevalent. Physeal, phalangeal shaft, and intra-articular fractures increase in frequency with advancing age[5] in direct correlation with participation in sports. Sports that require catching an object have the most profound effect on digits. Partial amputations from ignition of fireworks also are seen in this age group.

Adolescent (Older Than 13 Years)

Sports-induced digital injuries in this age group include impacted fractures of the proximal portions of the PIP or DIP joint, Salter type I epiphyseal fractures of the distal phalanges, crushing fractures of the distal tuft, and avulsion fractures of the MCP joint. A fall on an outstretched arm typically results in a distal radial or ulnar fracture in a child younger than 12 years, but in an adolescent, the identical fall results instead in a scaphoid fracture.

Adolescents who engage in sports, particularly those that require handling balls or tackling, are subject to dislocations. Proximal interphalangeal joint dislocations are most common, followed in order of frequency by CMC joint dislocations at the base of the thumb and MCP joint dislocations. Overuse injuries that involve the hand or wrist may occur.

Adolescents who enter the workforce may sustain ring degloving injuries when a finger ring becomes caught on a stationary object as the individual is jumping or falling. Fingertip amputations and tendon lacerations may result from contact with blades. Mutilation may occur on contact with rotary blades when using a lawnmower, and industrial machinery can cause avulsions or amputations. Devastating injuries may be seen in older individuals who explode ammunitions.

Contemplating Abuse

One of the universal rules when evaluating traumatic injuries is to be vigilant about identifying physical abuse. Estimates vary, but it is possible that 10% to 20% of pediatric trauma victims assessed in emergency departments have sustained intentional injuries. Recognition and reporting by emergency department staff members are necessary to prevent escalation and permanent injuries.[2]

Any body surface or organ system, including the hand or digits, can be the primary target of child abuse. The hand alone may be intentionally injured without another anatomic area sustaining injury. Alternatively, a hand injury may be incidental to another primary target. Children who are physically disciplined may use their hands to lessen the impact on other body parts and sustain injuries to their hands in the process. In a study from a children's hospital of child abuse team referrals, more than 8% of physically abused children sustained injuries to the hand-digit unit.[4]

There is no reliable profile for predicting which children with hand injuries have been abused. Abuse should be considered anytime there is an unusual history or clinical scenario.

History

There should be heightened concern in the presence of a dysfunctional family unit, an aberrant past medical history, and an unusual explanation by the historian (Figure 20-2). When the mechanism of injury exceeds the child's expected capabilities according to his or her developmental stage, abuse should be considered. For example, a 6-month-old does not possess the capability to pincer grasp a fork and insert the prongs into an electrical outlet to sustain a burn.

Physical Examination

The shape, pattern of distribution, and extent of a hand injury may differentiate an accidental injury from one that was inflicted intentionally. For example, accidental dry thermal contact results in a partial-thickness burn to the palmar aspect of the hand and spares the dorsum. An exploratory injury typically is unilateral. The injury to a hand burned by steam is not circumferential. Accidental hot water immersion produces a deeper burn at the points of initial contact and secondary splash marks. But circumferential hand injury with a clear-cut immersion line (a stocking-glove pattern) suggests that the hand was immersed forcibly. If the contralateral hand has a mirror image burn, forcible restraint was used. Also, human bites leave a characteristic double arch. An adult's bite to a child's hand leaves heavier bruising and a wider (≥3 cm) canine-to-canine mark than a child's bite.

Figure 20-2.

Indicators of possible child abuse.

Parent Profile
- Social isolation
- Stressed, disorganized
- Admits to violence
- Poor self-image

Child Profile
- Lacks primary care
- Delayed immunizations
- Previous injuries
- Abused sibling

Historical Alarms
- Delay in coming to emergency department
- Disclaims abuse
- Story changes
- Self- or sibling-induced

Physical Alarms
- Child passivity
- Beyond child's development
- Incompatible mechanism
- Mirror image injury

Common Challenges of the Pediatric Encounter

Challenges Imposed by Patients

Eliciting the history of an injury can be difficult. Infants are expressive but preverbal in terms of intelligible speech. Toddlers are verbal, but their speech may be understood only by their parents. Preschool-aged children have cognition and, when willing, can clearly relate the symptoms of illness. For an injury, however, they may not be able to interpret circumstances or answer the straightforward "when, where, and how" questions. Early school-aged children, who typically fear abandonment in the emergency department, may be overwhelmed by their injuries and be verbally hesitant. Through previous experiences, older children may have grown to distrust physicians and nurses; they may fear getting in trouble as a result of the situation and may communicate poorly. Adolescents exhibit less paranoia. With only slight reticence, they are fully expressive regarding mechanism of injury, location of pain, and perception of their current disabilities. However, fears of mutilation or retribution may alter their expressivity.[6]

All children, regardless of age, recognize physical pain, but younger children may not be able to localize the source of pain when asked. Early in life, children learn that health care workers provide painful shots; they distrust the uniform denial: "This won't hurt." Children are reluctant to have injured hands examined because they do not want to renew or create more pain. Depending on the child's developmental stage, this reluctance may manifest as protective withdrawal or regressive behaviors such as crying, flailing, or kicking. Even the calmest child may rock, sweat, demonstrate rapid speech, and alter vital signs when he or she submits an injury to scrutiny.

Challenges Imposed by Parents

Some parents are unable to recount histories, even if they observed the events. And some parents, upon witnessing unexpected, painful injuries to their children, may recall other traumatic experiences and become unable to cope. In emergency departments, parents are counted on to placate their children, but many do so with anxiolytic speech in proximity to their children. Unfortunately, some parents exhibit aversions to the examination room setting; they are quick to retreat to the waiting room to supervise their other children or plead separation from the injured child when there is a protest. Parents of older children sometimes elicit confrontational behaviors by stressing a child's own responsibility for the injury. They may quarrel with their children, or even with each other. Some parents openly resent hospitals and express undue concerns about the physicians' skills. And in rare situations, parents may be openly hostile to the point of threatening harm to health care workers.

Challenges Imposed by Professional Staff

Most people who work in emergency departments are tolerant of pediatric emergencies and urgencies and display concern and empathy for ill and injured children. However, an unfortunate few show no overt expression of affection for the pediatric population, and their displeasures may be easily transmitted to parents and children. The common clues include lack of eye contact, circumspect voluntary distancing from the family, and banning of a parent or parents from the treatment area. Reduced verbalizations, terse responses to inquiries, and judgmental affect compound mistrust and jeopardize the family's opportunity to cope. Intolerant health care workers tend to overemphasize the importance of physical restraint devices. Equally as awkward, some physicians and nurses request that a parent "corral" an injured body part without assessing the physiologic or psychologic impact of restraint.

Overcoming Barriers

As daunting as these challenges may seem, they are not insurmountable. Figure 20-3 lists recommendations for making the evaluation and management process less traumatic for everyone involved.

Noteworthy Differences in the History and Physical Examination

History

A pediatric encounter involving an injured hand or digit should begin with a discussion between the physician and the child. First, the physician should establish that he or she will only speak and plans no immediate physical harm. A little creativity is required; nonthreatening topics of interest can be addressed before the medical interrogation begins. The physician should sit on a stool or chair at face-to-face level with the child. Patience is required in attempts to coerce a child into responding. Questions should be open-ended and asked one at a time, noting the child's emotional tenor and nonverbal clues in addition to verbal responses. If a particular line of questioning is met with reluctance, the medical sleuthing can stop temporarily. One solution is to change to a neutral topic, return to an introductory ice-breaker, and reinitiate the pursuit for historical details. Badgering is not an effective approach to a child who refuses to answer. Rather, it is best to indicate respect for the child's refusal to disclose. After speaking with the child, the physician should interview the parent to clarify issues, confirm the parent's observations, and fill in important gaps such as allergies and immunization status. The physician also should seek information about the family and siblings, looking for the potential of abuse.

Before the Physical

While still at a distance, the physician should inform the child how the examination will be performed, using age-appropriate language, then ask for the child's cooperation. Full disclosure of the elements and order of the examination should decrease the child's fears, as will an assurance that inspecting, not touching, will happen first. Two-point discrimination can be demonstrated on the physician's own hand using paper clips, not needles, emphasizing that the clip creates a painless sensation. Active range of motion will modestly renew the child's pain, so the physician should tell the child that they will stop if there is too much pain. After previewing each aspect of the examination, the child should be

Figure 20-3.

Overcoming barriers in the pediatric encounter.

Physician-Child
- Keep distance during history-taking
- Acknowledge child's autonomy
- Reduce child's situational anxiety
- Use age-appropriate calming speech
- Reassure, explain, bargain
- Delay painful manipulation until the end
- Acknowledge when you create pain

Parent-Child-Physician
- Encourage proximity of parent and child
- Keep unit together for history and physical examination
- Involve parents in all decision-making
- Support parents' desire to reduce pain
- Seek assistance from a calming parent
- Promote coping (humor, nonprocedural talk)
- Praise parents who participate in care

permitted to ask questions. Answers to questions on degree of pain should defer specific quantification. If pressed, the physician can suggest depictions such as "pressure," "squeezing sensation," or "poking sensation." The "bee sting" comparison will lead to immediate decompensation and should be avoided. Most young children, even those with no personal experience, fear stitches. If the child asks, "Will I need stitches?" a useful response is, "No, but we might have to put the skin together with thread."

The next step is to confirm that the parent is willing and capable of providing physical and psychologic support. For example, the physician could ask the parent to remove the child's bandages and see if this challenge is met with hesitancy before progressing. At this point the physician should approach the child and reestablish a seat at the child's eye level, touching nothing, seeking trust, willing to stay calm even in the face of frank withdrawal. A claim of, "I gotta go potty!" (from the child) can be answered with, "OK, sure. We'll wait 'til you're done." If another stall is attempted, the parent can be asked to help reduce the child's stress. If all these efforts fail, the physician must focus on the task at hand and go forward.

The Physical

The anatomy and function of the hand and digits in a child are identical to those in an adult,[3] so in a compliant child, the order and detail of the examination should resemble those of the adult examination.[5] If the child is only marginally compliant, noninvasive evaluation may be necessary, including observation of the hand's resting stance, rotary malalignment, and other deformities. If the child is totally noncompliant, the physician can only attempt to evaluate vascular and neurologic integrity before providing anesthesia. An Allen test should be performed at the wrist or at the base of the injured digit, and capillary refilling time should be established. If the child is uncooperative for two-point discrimination, the physician should look for a dry volar fingertip of denervation injury; facial changes may indicate sensation. Provision of systemic analgesics, sedatives, or local or regional anesthesia may then permit direct wound inspection, palpation, and assessment of tendon and motor function.[3]

Local Anesthesia

Topical

Vasoconstrictors such as epinephrine, norepinephrine, phenylephrine, and cocaine are not routinely recommended for use in tissues with blood supplied by an end artery such as a digit. A topical emulsion of prilocaine and lidocaine, EMLA cream, has been shown to be effective on extremities. The limiting factor to its routine use is the slow rate to develop sufficient anesthesia. It may require up to 1 hour to modify perceived pain from deep tissue manipulation.[8]

Infiltrative

Digital blocks are performed in children as they are in adults (see Chapter 4).[3] The preferred technique is to enter the dorsal web space, advancing toward the bony cortex with a small (27- to 30-gauge) needle. The anesthetic agent is placed along the dorsal and volar surface of the digit, aspirating to avoid intravascular infusion prior to injection. The volume and concentration of the subcutaneous wheal should not exceed the maximal recommended dose (Table 20-1). Typically, for the average child, this translates to a maximum of 1 mL to either side of the digit in an infant and 2 mL to either side in an older child.[9]

Most pediatric emergency physicians use lidocaine in the stock 1% solution or a 1% buffered solution (0.1 mEq of sodium bicarbonate/mL of stock lidocaine). Both produce pain relief in several minutes. Because the duration of analgesia with lidocaine is brief, some hand surgeons substitute longer-acting agents such as bupivacaine or mepivacaine.

Imaging

To Film or Not To Film

Routine radiographic examination of all pediatric upper extremity injuries is not the standard practice in any community. The emergency physician must therefore rely on the patient's history and physical examination findings to assess the need for x-rays. The presence of both gross deformity and point tenderness is the best discriminator of pediatric fracture. These findings are noted in more than 80% of children with fractures. Ecchymosis is a fairly powerful discriminator of fracture in upper extremity injuries in adults but not in children.[10]

Technical Issues

Plain films should be confined to the area where the trauma is localized. Comparison films of the unaffected extremity should not be obtained routinely. They should be obtained, however, if there is a question of an abnormal trabecular pattern or bone density. Comparison films may also be of value in uncovering epiphyseal widening or a secondary ossification center. As with interpretation of radiographs in adults, the emergency physician should not try to interpret poor-quality films. Films should be repeated if there is motion, poor positioning, or inadequate penetration.

Table 20-1.

Anesthetic agents for pediatric digital block.

Agent	Concentration	Maximum Dose	Onset	Duration
Lidocaine	1-2%	5 mg/kg	2-5 min	1-2 h
Bupivacaine	0.25-0.5%	2 mg/kg	2-10 min	4-8 h
Mepivacaine	1-2%	6 mg/kg	3-5 min	2-3 h

Misreads

The rate of discordance between emergency physicians' and radiologists' interpretations of all pediatric plain films ranges from 1% to 11%. Of all misinterpretations, pediatric upper extremity misreads form the largest group.[11] The epiphyseal plates appear different at different ages and can be mistaken for a fracture, or an occult fracture may erroneously be read as a normal epiphyseal region. Figure 20-4 illustrates the **Salter-Harris classification system** for fractures involving the growth plate. These classifications have both prognostic and therapeutic implications.

Treatment

The general principles for treating injured hands and digits in adults hold true for pediatric patients with most mild to moderate injuries, including open and closed fractures, dislocations, tendon injuries, abrasions, contusions, soft tissue injuries including burns, lacerations, subungual hematomas, nail bed injuries, and bite wounds. Treatment directed at retaining functional capacity and cosmetic appearance usually results in healing. With devastating injury such as complete digit amputation, a hand specialist should direct the ultimate repair.

Infants, toddlers, and early school-aged children have the capacity to regrow tissue with an incomplete distal fingertip amputation. In young patients, partial amputations with moderately large defects of bone and

Figure 20-4.

Salter-Harris fracture classification.

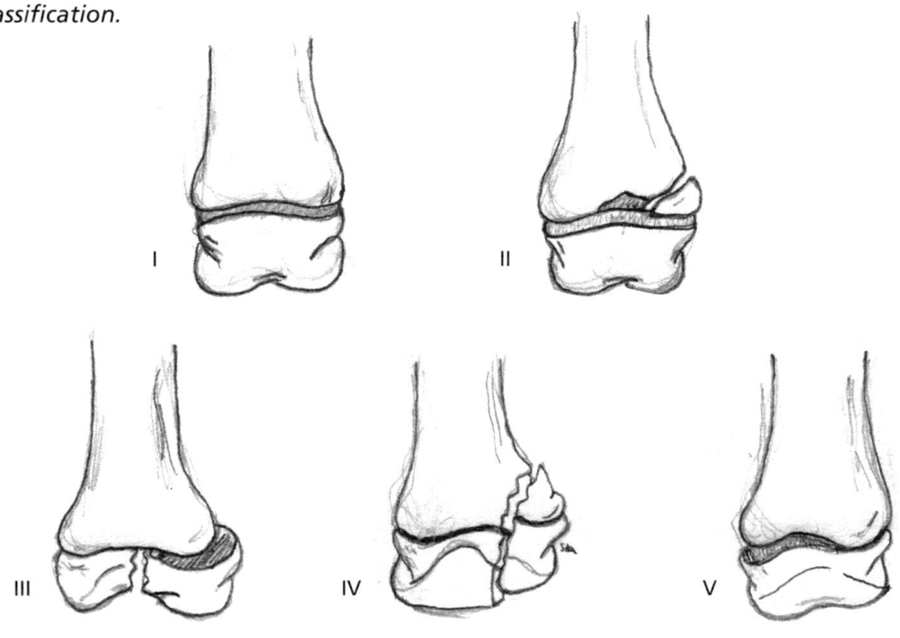

soft tissues, distal to the DIP joint, can be left to heal by secondary intention.[12] After consultation, it may be appropriate not to sacrifice exposed bone to obtain direct closure of an amputation. The injury may be cleaned, dressed, and splinted and the patient treated with antibiotics and analgesics while followed as an outpatient.

As a general rule, a child's physical injury heals faster with fewer complications than a similar injury in an adult. For example, a toddler who closes a door on his finger may sustain a tuft fracture with or without nail bed injury, and if an open fracture is created, there will be no infection. The child will slough the fingernail in 1 week and develop a new, almost normal nail in 3 to 4 months. An adult with a comparable injury, even with meticulous surgical repair, may incur retarded healing time with infection. A permanently deformed nail and a finger that is predisposed to recurrent paronychia are more likely sequelae in an adult.

The principles of analgesia, rest, elevation, and splinting hold true for managing pediatric hand injuries. The injured hand should be splinted in the safe position with the wrist neutral or in slight extension, the MCP joints flexed 90 degrees, the IP joints in full extension, and the thumb in abduction. For children younger than 5 years, it may be difficult to keep the hand settled in any splint device. For this reason, successfully retained splints require multiple layers. The functional dressing (tube gauze, Adaptic, Kling, and splint) must be covered with a redundant network of tape, burn netting, or both. This permits the child to slip out of nonfunctional materials. Occasionally, a long arm cast may be needed simply to keep the dressing in place.

To monitor the emotional impact of the injury and the emergency department visit, assess physical healing, and ensure recovery of normal function, pediatric patients require early followup care (within 1 week). This helps prevent the prolonged disability that can result from mistreated or misdiagnosed conditions such as fracture, dislocation, or tendon injury.

References

1. Bhende MS, Dandrea LA, Davis HW. Hand injuries in children presenting to a pediatric emergency department. *Ann Emerg Med.* 1993;22:1519-1523.
2. Chadwick DL. The diagnosis of inflicted injury in infants and young children. *Pediatr Ann.* 1992;21:477-483.
3. Ablove RH, Moy OJ, Peimer CA. Pediatric hand disease: diagnosis and treatment. *Pediatr Clin North Am.* 1998;45:1507-1524.
4. Johnson CF, Kaufman KL, Callendar C. The hand as a target organ in child abuse. *Clin Pediatr.* 1990;29:66-72.
5. Overton DT, Uehara DT. Evaluation of the injured hand. *Emerg Med Clin North Am.* 1993;11:585-600.
6. Gratz RR. Children's responses to emergency department care. *Ann Emerg Med.* 1984;13:322-333.
7. Algranati PS. Effect of developmental status on the approach to physical examination. *Pediatr Clin North Am.* 1998;45:1-23.
8. Kennedy RM, Luhmann JD. The "ouchless emergency department." Getting closer: advances in decreasing distress during painful procedures in the emergency department. *Pediatr Clin North Am.* 1999;46:1215-1247.

9. Emslander HC. Local and topical anesthetic for pediatric wound repair: a review of selected aspects. *Pediatr Emerg Care.* 1998;14:123-129.
10. Rivara FP, Parish RA, Mueller BA. Extremity injuries in children: predictive value of clinical findings. *Pediatrics.* 1986;78:803-807.
11. Brunswick JE, Elkhanipour K, Fuchs S, et al. Emergency medicine resident interpretation of pediatric radiographs. *Acad Emerg Med.* 1996;3:790-793.
12. Almquist EA. Hand injuries in children. *Pediatr Clin North Am.* 1986;33:1511-1522.

CHAPTER 21

Sports Injuries

Paul J. Donovan, DO, FACEP

Hand injuries are common during sports participation. An estimated 5% to 10% of all sports-related injuries involve the hand and wrist.[1] Although the initial assessment, physical examination, and emergency treatment are in general similar for athletes and nonathletes, optimal care of the injured athlete often is directed at protected mobilization and aggressive orthopedic followup care to return the athlete to play in an expeditious yet safe manner. The nature of the injury could be traumatic or overuse (inflammatory), with the traumatic variety predominating in emergency department patients. Football, hockey, and basketball players are commonly at risk. Falls on an outstretched wrist (hyperextension) are common in sports and can result in carpal fractures (of which the most common is a scaphoid fracture), lunate and perilunate dislocations, and other significant ligament injuries, such as scapholunate dissociation. The spectrum of sports-related injuries also includes tendon injuries and similar injuries via other mechanisms.

Ligament Injuries

Ulnar Collateral Ligament Injury

Ulnar collateral ligament injuries are most common in skiers (hence the common name **skier thumb** or **ski pole thumb**), although they frequently occur in hockey and football players. Campbell originally described this injury in 1955 as an overuse injury. Although both the ulnar and radial collateral ligaments stabilize the thumb at the MCP joint, injuries to the ulnar collateral ligament are most common.

Physical Examination

The patient often gives a history of a fall with valgus stress applied to the thumb at the MCP joint. Pain and swelling typically are noted over the ulnar aspect of the MCP joint of the thumb. Gentle stress should be applied to the MCP joints in extension and with 10 to 20 degrees of flexion, with slight valgus stress to the accessory and ulnar collateral ligament proper, respectively. Stress also should be applied to the MCP joint of the asymptomatic thumb for comparison. Laxity is present with grade II and grade III injuries, but only pain is present with a grade I injury.

Radiography

Radiographs may show an avulsed fragment, but they typically are normal. If the film shows an intra-articular avulsed fragment that is more than 25% of the articular surface, this has treatment implications and may mandate open reduction and internal fixation or percutaneous fixation.

Treatment

Emergency treatment includes thumb spica immobilization, ice, and NSAIDs. The length of immobilization depends on the extent of the injury and may be as short as 2 weeks for grade I injuries and 4 to 6 weeks for grade II injuries. Metacarpophalangeal joint instability and large intra-articular fragments often require surgical repair for a more stable outcome.

Complications

Complete (grade III) ulnar collateral ligament tears can be complicated if the adductor aponeurosis is interposed between the torn ligament ends, which is called a **Stener lesion**. This requires surgical repair and can result in chronic instability if the injury is not recognized.

Scapholunate Dissociation

A scapholunate dissociation is a ligament injury to the scapholunate joint of the carpal bones of the wrist that usually results from a fall on an outstretched hand during sporting activity. The force generated across the scapholunate joint can result in a spectrum of ligament injury from a simple sprain (grade I) to complete disruption.

Physical Examination

Typically the patient presents with pain over the dorsum of the wrist just distal to the radial styloid with or without associated swelling and ecchymosis. There may be tenderness in the anatomic snuffbox area as well.

Radiography

Because the differential diagnosis of any wrist injury should include a scaphoid fracture, proper wrist films, including scaphoid views, should be obtained. If these are negative and scapholunate dissociation is suspected, then a bilateral clenched fist view with ulnar deviation should be obtained. Radiographically, evidence of this injury consists of diastasis of the intercarpal space between the scapholunate joint of more than 3 mm (**Terry Thomas sign**). A **signet ring sign** may be present, which results from volar rotation of the scaphoid and appears as a cortical ring-like opacity overlying the scaphoid. The scaphoid also appears shortened as a result of volar rotation. On lateral radiography, an increased scapholunate angle of more than 80 degrees is considered evidence of instability, but this is a difficult radiographic sign to elicit.

Treatment

A short arm thumb spica, ice, NSAIDs, and close orthopedic followup care are recommended. Sprains are treated definitively with 4 to 6 weeks of immobilization. For obvious diastasis, surgical repair or reconstruction is necessary.

Complications

This injury is often overlooked and misdiagnosed as a wrist sprain. Missed injuries can result in significant long-term disability, pain, and limitation of motion.

Tendon Injuries

Extensor Tendon Injury

This common injury often is referred to as **baseball finger** or **mallet finger**. It occurs in baseball, football, basketball, and volleyball when a player's attempt to catch a ball causes sudden forced flexion at the distal phalanx. The spectrum of injury ranges from tendon avulsion to the break of a small or large intra-articular fragment off of the dorsal proximal aspect of the distal phalanx.

Physical Examination

Typically the patient presents with obvious flexion deformity at the DIP joint with swelling and is unable to extend the DIP joint.

Radiography

Films can be normal if the injury is caused by tendon avulsion. More commonly they demonstrate a small dorsal avulsion at the proximal aspect of the distal phalanx.

Treatment

Emergency treatment consists of splinting the DIP joint in slight hyperextension for a minimum of 6 to 8 weeks. Ice, NSAIDs, and early orthopedic followup care are recommended. A large intra-articular fragment may necessitate surgical repair.

Complications

Incorrect diagnosis or an inadequate period of immobilization can result in permanent inability to extend at the DIP joint. A swan-neck deformity can result.

Flexor Digitorum Profundus Avulsion

A sudden forced hyperextension at the DIP joint is the usual mechanism of injury with an FDP avulsion, or **jersey finger**. It occurs almost exclusively when a football player attempts to tackle an opposing player (Figure 21-1 and Figure 21-2). This can occur in any digit, including the thumb, but about 75% of these injuries affect the ring finger.

Physical Examination

The patient is unable to flex the distal phalanx at the DIP joint. Although the patient may notice a palpable pop and minimal pain initially, swelling and pain are common on examination.

Radiography

Radiographs usually are normal, although they may show an intra-articular avulsion off the volar proximal aspect of the distal phalanx.

Treatment

Emergency treatment consists of splinting in approximately 45 degrees and 30 degrees of flexion at the PIP and DIP joints, respectively. The use of ice and NSAIDs may be helpful. Early orthopedic followup care is recommended. Definitive treatment typically includes surgical repair.

Complications

Failure to recognize this injury results in permanent inability to flex at the DIP joint, as does improper treatment.

Trigger Finger or Trigger Thumb

This condition usually results from repetitive trauma or overuse of the thumb or fingers. A tendon nodule usually forms in response to chronic or intermittent inflammation. As a result, the patient experiences pain and difficulty with use, with a snapping sensation when flexing the affected digit.

Physical Examination

Often, a palpable tendon nodule is present. Active and passive range of motion testing may be accompanied by a palpable snapping sensation.

Radiography

Radiographs are needed to rule out associated avulsion fracture after traumatic events; otherwise, films typically are normal.

Figure 21-1.

Flexor digitorum profundus tendon avulsion, or jersey finger.

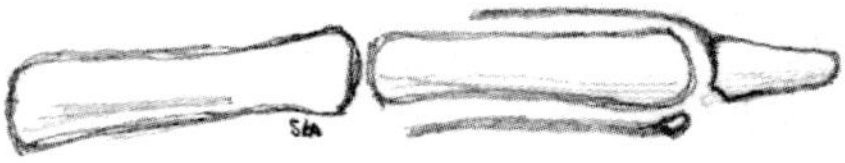

Figure 21-2.

Mechanism of injury, jersey finger.

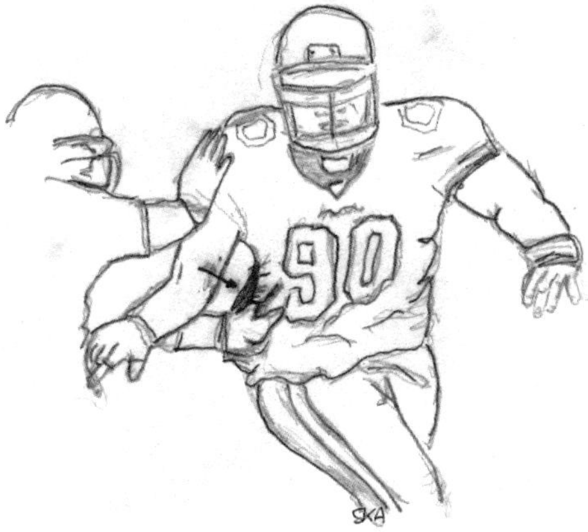

Treatment

Splinting in flexion to comfort, ice, NSAIDs, and early orthopedic followup care are recommended. If symptoms persist, a steroid injection often is helpful. Surgical release of the tendon sheath may be indicated for chronic symptoms.

Complications

Occasionally, tendon rupture occurs around the site of the tendon nodule.

de Quervain Disease (Tenosynovitis)

This condition involves the first dorsal extensor compartment of the wrist and the base of the thumb. The abductor pollicis longus and extensor pollicis brevis tendons occupy this compartment as they traverse over the radial styloid. Typically this is an overuse condition that is common in golfers, racquet sports players, and fly fishermen, although it can result from direct or repetitive trauma.

Physical Examination

Pain and tenderness usually are present over the snuffbox tendons. Occasionally, crepitus is noted on either active or passive range of motion of the tendon. The **Finkelstein test** is considered positive when pain is reproduced through passive stretching of the thumb tendons as the patient holds the thumb in the palm of the hand while the wrist is ulnar-deviated by the examiner.

Radiography

Radiographs typically are normal.

Treatment

The use of ice, NSAIDs, and immobilization with a thumb spica splint for a brief period (1 to 2 weeks) are recommended. A steroid injection into the tendon sheath may also be helpful.

Complications

For recurrent or persistent symptoms, surgical release of the tendon sheath is an option.

Carpal Fractures

Scaphoid Fracture

The scaphoid is the most commonly fractured carpal bone of the wrist; approximately 70% of carpal fractures involve the scaphoid.[1]

Physical Examination

Typically the patient presents with a history of mechanism consistent with scaphoid injury. Pain and tenderness are present over the snuffbox, especially with slight ulnar deviation. There may also be associated swelling and ecchymosis.

Radiography

Appropriate views include PA, lateral, and scaphoid, which is an ulnar-deviated view that elongates the scaphoid and may help uncover some nondisplaced fractures.

Treatment

A thumb spica splint in mild wrist flexion and slight radial deviation along with ice, NSAIDs, and orthopedic followup care within 1 week are recommended. Whether the splint should be carried up above the humeral epicondyle to prevent pronation and supination of the forearm is an area of controversy related to the location of the fracture. Because distal third scaphoid fractures generally have a better outcome than proximal two-thirds fractures due to a better blood supply distally, a short arm thumb spica splint is adequate for any distal third scaphoid fracture. If the fracture involves the proximal two thirds of the scaphoid or is displaced (by more than 2 mm), a sugar tong splint that incorporates a thumb spica component is necessary to prevent forearm pronation and supination.

Complications

Any patient with a clinically positive examination (snuffbox tenderness) but a negative radiograph should have a thumb spica splint applied and obtain followup care within 1 week. Magnetic resonance imaging is the modality of choice for occult scaphoid fractures. Long-term complications include malunion, nonunion, and missed fractures with subsequent avascular necrosis of the scaphoid.

Hook of the Hamate Fracture

Most fractures of the hamate involve the hook of the hamate, which serves as the attachment of several ligaments and digital tendons. Typically, the mechanism of injury is the impact of the handle of a bat or racket against the hypothenar eminence or the direct impact of a fall on this area.

Physical Examination

The hook of the hamate is located approximately 2 cm distal and radial to the pisiform in the distal carpal row. If a fracture is present, palpation usually reveals pain, tenderness, and swelling.

Radiography

Posteroanterior, lateral, and carpal tunnel views allow visualization of this fracture.

Treatment

A short arm volar splint along with ice and NSAIDs are necessary, with orthopedic followup in 1 to 2 weeks. Generally, undisplaced fractures can be treated with casting for 8 to 12 weeks. If the hook is displaced and nonunion occurs, excision usually is necessary to minimize complications.

Complications

Inadequate radiographs or physical examination may result in failure to properly diagnose this injury. Because of the tenuous blood supply, nonunion is common with displaced or improperly immobilized fractures.

Triquetrum Fracture

This typically is an avulsion fracture of the dorsal aspect of the triquetrum that results from soft tissue avulsion or bony impingement.

Physical Examination

Pain and tenderness occur over the dorsal radial aspect of the wrist.

Radiography

A lateral view of the wrist usually demonstrates this fracture.

Treatment

A short arm splint is recommended until the patient is asymptomatic (usually 3 to 4 weeks), along with ice and NSAIDs. Orthopedic followup care is recommended in 1 to 2 weeks.

Complications

Rarely, symptomatic nonunion occurs; this usually is treated with excision.

Reference

1. Rettig A. *Clinics in Sports Medicine: Hand and Wrist Injuries.* 3rd ed. Philadelphia, Pa: WB Saunders Co; 1998.

Additional Reading

Hart R, Rittenberry T, Uehara D. *Handbook of Orthopedic Emergencies.* Philadelphia, Pa: Lippincott-Raven; 1999.

Reid DC. *Sports Injury and Assessment.* New York, NY: Churchill Livingstone; 1992.

CHAPTER 22

Occupational Injuries

Thomas Harter, MD, Russell Shatford, MD, and Stephen McCabe, MD

This chapter addresses some aspects of occupational hand injuries that are relevant to emergency care and presents some views and suggestions that generally are not covered in the medical literature. Some of this information is based on the authors' experiences and subjective opinions and does not necessarily represent the views of most hand surgeons. Topics include theories on restricted or modified work restrictions, acute care recommendations, and cumulative trauma disorders such as carpal tunnel syndrome, tendonitis, and lateral epicondylitis.

The Emergency Physician's Perspective

The most important responsibility bestowed on all physicians is to provide the best possible care for all patients. The care of occupational hand injuries places an extra burden on emergency physicians. Competition and rising health care costs have forced employers to actively participate in the management of health care delivery. As a result, they seek high-quality care at the lowest cost. Today physicians and employers both must be mindful that health care is a business as well as a profession.

Emergency physicians should consider the evaluation and treatment of occupational hand injuries from the same perspective as the hand surgeon. They also must be able to see the injured employee from the positions of the employer and the insurance carrier. Emergency physicians must be familiar with state Workers' Compensation laws and with the specific rules, regulations, and responsibilities of the health care provider, employer, and employee. Also mandatory is immediate, clear, and concise communication with the injured employee and employer regarding a plan for future expectations and needs. Although it may not be possible to provide an exact diagnosis and a definitive plan before the emergency department workup is completed, a differential diagnosis and possible outcomes should be explained.

The prevailing attitude among employers seems to be that, because of their expense, specialists are to be avoided unless absolutely necessary, and that emergency department treatment is inefficient, time consuming, and not cost effective. Employers understand that the choice of provider can have widespread financial repercussions and affect overall workplace morale. Employers also want to make sure that their injured workers receive the best possible medical care at cost-effective prices, although most would likely pay the maximum rate for satisfactory outcomes. Why? Because an injured employee will then be loyal and strive to be productive. For the employer, it's just good business. This point of view, while not universal, still represents the best approach.

Most medium-sized to large-sized cities in the United States have at least one large company that fits the following profile: thousands of employees, present in the location for at least two generations, workers who are relatively healthy, long-term employees. Such a company is able to compile good data and knowledge about outcomes; it also has preferences for certain providers. Even a very safe company has injured employees and, over time, gains experience with the health care system and the quality of the local providers. As a result, this company believes that it knows which emergency physicians provide cost-effective, high-quality care. Any emergency physician should want to be known as the first choice for such a company, as well as smaller companies, insurance carriers, and anyone else looking for physicians and hospitals that provide high-quality care.

How, then, does a physician get referrals from these companies? What is required to meet their needs? Why should an occupational injury be viewed differently than any other injury?

The Workers' Compensation system evolved during the 1800s and 1900s and is a factor in the success of the industrialized world. The concept of a no-fault system is an incentive for businesses to be productive without the risk of financial loss from litigation, and for workers to be employed without the risk of financial loss from injury. Employers and their insurance carriers are responsible not only for medical bills but also for lost wages and compensation for permanent medical impairment. Obviously, the choice of provider can result in a wide range of possible outcomes for the employer and employee depending on medical decisions, so it is crucial for the emergency physician to understand the system.

What are the requisites for good care and good decision-making? How can the emergency physician deliver high-quality care at cost-effective prices? How can he or she satisfy both the injured employee and the company and continue to get good referrals? One of the first lessons a provider learns when dealing with an occupational injury is that decisions can significantly affect cost. The emergency physician might be asked to give an opinion as to whether a medical problem is truly caused or aggravated by work. The importance of taking the best possible history and performing the best possible physical examination cannot be overemphasized. In work-related injuries, the history can be more complicated than in non–work-related injuries. Decisions often must be made with limited information. To be successful, the physician must always be objective and never take sides, even though the injured patient is not paying the bill. Both the employer and the employee must trust the decisions made by the physician. Some niche "workers' comp" physicians find themselves out of business after a brief interval of siding with management; they serve no purpose if they are not trusted by injured workers. This is easy to discuss in theory, but it can be difficult to tell an injured, sore, tired worker that he or she must return to work or that the injury was not job related. Sometimes, it may not be possible to make an informed decision based on limited information. If that's the case, the emergency physician should simply say so. Even if the emergency physician is not responsible for the decision of causation, the history documented at the time of evaluation is a major factor in the ultimate decision. What may seem inconsequential at the time of the initial evaluation can result in an unfair financial burden for whoever is determined to be responsible.

All physicians have been accused of ordering unnecessary tests to protect themselves from malpractice litigation. Pressure from employers to save costs makes decisions even more difficult, and emergency physicians face this conflict often. Ultimately, the physician must always do what is best for the patient and order whatever tests are necessary. Unfortunately, sometimes the appropriate response to an employer who is not satisfied with the physician's medical recommendations is that the company use another provider. "Yes, I want to care for occupationally injured patients, but no, I am not going to compromise patient care."

Work Restrictions

Most physicians believe that the sooner a patient returns to work after an injury, the more quickly he or she recovers, both mentally and physically. Some employers allow injured employees to return to work as soon as possible after injury in a restricted capacity, but others do not allow return to work until recovery is complete. The emergency physician should be knowledgeable about a company's specific policies, and if in doubt, should ask about them at the time of the evaluation. Most patients are honest but may not be familiar with company policy. And human nature being what it is in this situation, time off work for a work-related injury would be agreeable to most. Of course, after a certain period of time (which varies from state to state), the employer must pay the injured worker for being off work. This amount of money varies; in some situations, depending on the company, the employee might be paid more for ***not*** working than for working, and this income usually is tax free. On the other hand, the employer may provide incentives for employees who limit lost time from work-related injuries and reward them for good attendance records.

When an employee is not able to work because modified or light work is not available, the medical decision as to when the injured worker is 100% recovered can be difficult, particularly when symptoms are subjective and cannot be quantified. This problem is made more difficult when an employee is not motivated to return to work. If restricted work is available, there is no problem. So why wouldn't every employer have restricted work? In theory, an injured employee would get paid his or her regular rate or salary while working in a restricted capacity. Most other workers would go along with this, particularly if the injury were acute. However, when the injury is a repetitive strain-type disorder with subjective symptoms, fairness becomes the issue, particularly if the injured employee is perceived by fellow employees as not being motivated to recover. Why should someone be paid the same for doing less work than fellow employees? (New Testament gospels are not readily adopted in today's workplace.) For some companies, the hassles that go along with having restricted work do not justify the savings. The company has insurance to pay injured employees while they are off, so it's the insurance company's problem to get them back to work, right? Even though emergency physicians do not usually get involved with long-term problems, they still should understand the pros and cons of restricted or modified work. The emergency physician who is pressured by a patient to be "taken off work" can explain to that patient that he or she (if not totally disabled) can work if modified work is available, and that the company must make the decision about working in a restricted capacity. The emergency physician may be faced with the dilemma of giving narcotics for pain while simultaneously allowing a patient to return to work in a restricted capacity. Some patients even threaten a physician indirectly by implying the possibility of further injury to self or other employees if forced to return to work. Emergency physicians also frequently hear: "They don't have light work! They ***say*** they do, but they really don't." For all these reasons, communication and cooperation among physician, patient, and employer are mandatory. What may seem to be a relatively simple and straightforward problem can become complicated, and the emergency physician should respond accordingly.

Common sense descriptions of what an injured employee can and cannot do are best left general and flexible. The physician is not in a position to see the job being done and should not be pressured for exactness. Instead, the physician should encourage the employer and employee to work together and compromise if necessary to succeed in keeping the injured patient in the workplace.

Care of Acute Injuries

Obviously, the emergency medical care of occupational hand injuries should not be any different from that of nonoccupational injuries. The specific care of lacerations and soft tissue injuries is covered in other chapters, but a brief discussion here of some specific recommendations concerning the emergency care process is relevant.

Sometimes emergency department personnel such as nurses or assistants, when called to a room to render treatment for a hand laceration, see their role simply as helping the physician set up and obtaining the necessary equipment and supplies. Then, when the procedure begins, they leave. Considering that all care for lacerations, even simple ones, is ***surgery*** and should be respected as such, the more help the better. Particularly for hand trauma, in which the extent of the injury is unknown, atraumatic bloodless exploration is mandatory. To obtain the best result, as with all surgical procedures, appropriate exposure is necessary. Four (or six) hands are better than two.

For example, when treating an asymptomatic partially divided tendon, depending on the position of the finger or hand at the time of injury, the tendon may not be visible in the wound unless the position at the time of the injury is duplicated. To obtain an adequate view, it is necessary for an assistant to retract the skin using two hands while the physician does the exploration. During exploration, the physician must be confident that the deepest, least easily accessible part of the wound has been visualized.

Plain lidocaine or **bupivacaine** is recommended for finger metacarpal blocks using a 3-mL syringe with a 30-gauge needle for injection. Except for simple lacerations, a **metacarpal block** is preferable to a local block injected directly into the edges of a laceration, resulting in less edema in the wound itself and less pain when performed properly. Hemostasis can be maintained with a finger tourniquet (Tourni-cot, Mar-Med Co, Grand Rapids, Mich), a commercially available device that is inexpensive and comes in enough sizes to be used safely on all fingers (and toes).

Excision is recommended for all but the simplest, cleanest wounds by removing 0.5 to 1 mm of skin circumferentially, or more if necessary depending on the severity of injury. Crushed or contaminated soft tissue and fat also should be sharply débrided. Unlike for other areas of the body, the need to eliminate "dead space" by using deep sutures in fat or fascia generally is not necessary in the hand or fingers. **Monofilament nylon** (5-0, PC-3 or 6-0, PC-1) is best for skin closure. **Fast-absorbing cat gut suture** (6-0 or 5-0) is the ideal suture for nail bed lacerations. The nail plate should be removed before nail bed repair and should not be sewn through either for repair or to attempt to hold the nail plate on the nail bed for protection. After nail plate removal, cleaning and débridement of areolar tissue with a No. 15 blade is all that is necessary before replacing the nail plate beneath the eponychium.

Also, all physicians repairing hand or finger lacerations should use at least **2.5× magnification** for optimal results.

Cumulative Trauma Disorders

Carpal Tunnel Syndrome

Carpal tunnel syndrome is a symptom complex that is associated with many diseases, but it usually is idiopathic, particularly in the occupational setting. The patient presents with complaints of sensory change in the fingers that are innervated by the median nerve associated with nocturnal paresthesias, burning pain, and diminished dexterity. Physical examination may reveal sensory changes in the median nerve distribution, and in advanced cases, weakness or atrophy of the abductor pollicis brevis tendon. Hypertrophy of the synovial tissue surrounding the median nerve in the proximal palm, resulting in diminished blood flow to the nerve, may be the cause of nerve irritation. The synovial tissue presumably increases in volume in response to the increased demands of repetitive work. The carpal tunnel is a fixed-volume structure of bone and ligament that cannot expand with increased pressure. The resulting increase in pressure is transferred to the relatively soft median nerve, compromising blood supply and resulting in an ischemic nerve. The diagnosis is made when a nerve conduction study shows slowing of nerve conduction velocity across the carpal tunnel with elevated median nerve sensory and/or motor latency. In the occupational setting, it is best to stay with a diagnosis of numbness until a nerve conduction test is positive with objective findings. Initial treatment includes cessation of the job activity that precipitated the problem, wrist splinting, elevation if edema or swelling is present, and anti-inflammatory medication. Carpal tunnel syndrome that results from repetitive strain or overuse is rarely a surgical emergency, as might be the case after a single traumatic event such as a severe contusion.

A key to solving the problem is educating the patient about carpal tunnel syndrome and the difficulty in predicting a long-term outlook, while communicating this dilemma to the company. There is no definitive test, including nerve conduction studies, that can predict which individuals will be able to perform repetitive work without problems. Likewise, there is no guarantee that surgical intervention will allow a patient to return to repetitive work without a recurrence of symptoms. Undoubtedly, one of the major reasons for the large expense companies bear for the treatment of carpal tunnel syndrome is the failure of surgical intervention to cure the problem and allow patients to return to work symptom free. Emergency physicians probably should refer patients suspected of having carpal tunnel syndrome to physicians who are interested in and have experience managing the problem in the occupational setting, not necessarily hand surgeons. As suggested earlier, employers and insurance companies view surgical specialists not only as expensive but also as essentially capable of converting a straightforward claim into a problem that never ends. There is no satisfactory test to determine a patient's motivation to recover after elective surgery; a patient with objective pathology who undergoes a perfectly executed operation by an experienced hand surgeon will not recover unless he or she is motivated to do so.

Tendonitis

de Quervain Disease (Tenosynovitis)

Patients with de Quervain disease (tenosynovitis), or **first compartment tendonitis**, present with pain, swelling, and tenderness on the radial side of the wrist aggravated by movement of the thumb and wrist, especially in an ulnar-directed motion (Figure 22-1). Chronic overuse usually is the cause, but the problem can occur after an acute traumatic event such as a contusion or laceration. Physical examination demonstrates tenderness to palpation over the radial styloid, sometimes associated with swelling and crepitus. The **Finkelstein test** (Figure 22-2) is performed by having the patient flex the thumb and then wrap the fingers around the thumb. The examiner then holds the hand and moves it in an ulnar direction while keeping the forearm immobile. Pain over the first compartment is considered diagnostic. Initial treatment should include rest, a soft thumb spica splint, NSAIDs, and avoidance of the precipitating activity. If symptoms have been present for several weeks, a local steroid injection should be considered. The recommended dose is 1 mL betamethasone with 1 mL plain lidocaine in a 3-mL syringe with a 27-gauge needle.

First compartment tendonitis must be differentiated from degenerative arthritis at the thumb CMC joint. This condition is not caused by work but can be aggravated by work; it is a common condition among workers. The initial emergency treatment is the same.

Intersection Syndrome

Pain and swelling on the radial side of the wrist approximately 4 cm proximal to the radial styloid associated with erythema and crepitus should alert the emergency physician to this condition. Formerly thought to be caused by friction between the muscle bellies of the first and second compartments, intersection syndrome is now thought to be the result of inflammation of the synovium in the second extensor compartment containing the radial wrist extensors. Treatment consists of wrist splinting with the wrist extended to 15 degrees, NSAIDs, and rest. Tendonitis in the other four extensor compartments or flexor surface is much less common than first or second compartment tendonitis, but when suspected, it should be treated in a similar manner.

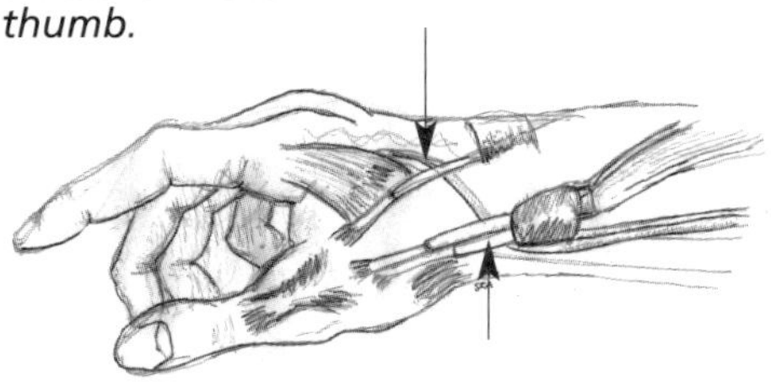

Figure 22-1.

de Quervain disease (tenosynovitis) involves the sheaths of the long abductor and short extensor tendons of the thumb.

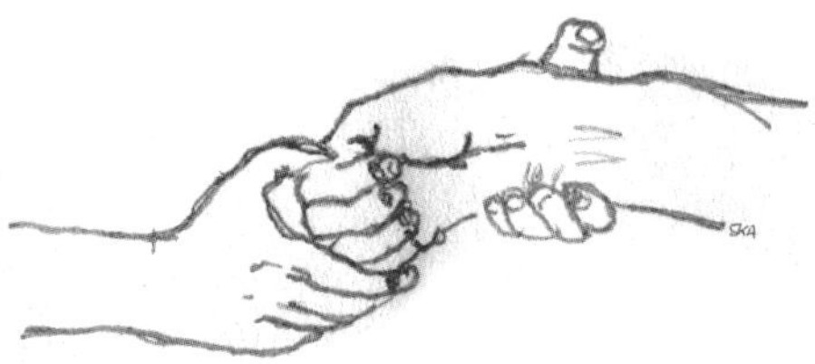

Figure 22-2.

Finkelstein test for de Quervain disease.

Trigger Finger and Trigger Thumb

This condition is characterized by a catching or snapping sensation that is relieved when the digit moves from a fixed flexed position to an extended posture. It is associated with pain in the palm over the A1 pulley caused by inflammation of the tenosynovium in the tendon sheath. Occasionally, the finger or thumb gets caught in an extended position that is relieved by flexion. Most cases are caused by a discrepancy in the diameter of the tendon, which normally is smaller than the diameter of the surrounding sheath, allowing the tendon to glide through freely. Occasionally, the patient and physician assume the problem is in the PIP joint because the sensation of catching seems to localize there. Physical examination usually reveals no tenderness to pressure at the PIP joint or proximal phalanx but marked tenderness in the palm over the A1 pulley. Treatment consists of rest, NSAIDs, and steroid injection. Often, the patient can be helped temporarily by wearing a finger splint over the dorsum of the finger with the PIP and DIP joints extended.

Lateral Epicondylitis

Lateral epicondylitis, or **tennis elbow**, actually is much more common in nonathletes than in tennis players. It usually is seen in the fourth and fifth decades of life and presents as pain over the lateral epicondyle associated with wrist extension. Physical examination reveals tenderness over the lateral epicondyle, exacerbation of pain with wrist extension against resistance, and pain with passive wrist flexion. The pathology is thought to be inflammation of the extensor muscles and supinator at their origin from the lateral epicondyle, possibly from tears. The exact nature and cause of the pathology remain unknown. Treatment consists of rest, a localized pressure splint applied directly over the epicondyle, NSAIDs, and steroid injection. Lateral epicondylitis usually is a self-limiting condition; attempts to avoid activities that precipitate the pain plus patience are often rewarded with resolution of the problem. Many surgical procedures have been described to correct the problem, but none have been uniformly successful. Excellent results have been achieved with the **Wolff procedure**, which consists of an exploration of the extensor muscles and a transverse division of the fasciae that surround them. However, as with any elective operation in an occupational setting, the patient will not recover unless motivated.

Medial epicondylitis is much less common than lateral epicondylitis and is treated in a similar manner.

Summary

The intrusion of multiple variables from a complex economy have made the practice of medicine more challenging than ever. The emergency physician must be knowledgeable not only of his or her specialty but also of the constantly changing rules and factors that influence decision-making. Understanding the needs of occupationally injured patients and their companies is vital for emergency physicians.

Additional Reading

Green DP. *Operative Hand Surgery*. Philadelphia, Pa: Churchill Livingstone; 1999:1404-1417, 2022-2042.

McCabe SJ. *Hand, Wrist, and Arm Sourcebook*. Lincolnwood, Ill: Lowell House; 2000:259-269.

CHAPTER 23

Common, Nonurgent, and Chronic Complaints

Gregory C. Hoskins, MD

Emergency and primary care physicians see patients who have a multitude of chronic hand conditions. Structures in the hand lie in close proximity to each other, and symptoms often overlap, making hand pathology a difficult diagnostic challenge. The most common hand conditions are discussed here. Many conditions are minor, but some can be debilitating without successful treatment. Seemingly trivial complaints may involve conditions that are progressive and irreversible. A solid understanding of hand pathology is necessary to recognize and treat serious conditions reliably.

Nerve Compression Syndromes

Patients with nerve compression syndromes present with sensory or motor complaints in the hand. These syndromes result from mechanical compression of the nerves proximal to or within the hand. Knowledge of the anatomy of the upper extremity is necessary to correctly determine the most likely point of compression.

Compression may result from direct external forces or from overuse of the hand or arm. Abnormal structures near a nerve such as ganglion cysts, thickened tendon sheaths, bone fragments, tumors, or aneurysms also have been implicated as causes. In addition, pregnancy and systemic diseases such as diabetes mellitus, myxedema, rheumatoid arthritis, gout, and alcoholism may contribute through various mechanisms.

Pressure on a nerve results in intraneural edema, which leads to microvessel obliteration and causes axonal ischemia and demyelination. The nerve may eventually degenerate and undergo fibrosis. Depending on the severity of degeneration, nerves may or may not be able to recover when the compression is relieved.

It is important to localize the point of compression to treat these syndromes effectively. History, physical examination, and knowledge of the neuroanatomy of the hand and arm usually indicate the most likely point of compression. In some cases, electromyography is necessary.

History-taking should focus on occupational or other activities that may be causing compression through overuse or repetitive trauma. Through the physical examination, the physician must carefully map out the distribution of sensory and motor deficits. Nerve innervation within the hand generally is predictable, but variations do occur and may make the diagnosis difficult. Nerves are especially susceptible to compression at certain anatomic sites where they travel through narrow spaces or take a superficial course; compression at these sites accounts for most of the syndromes encountered. Conditions that can mimic nerve compression syndromes include cervical radiculopathy, thoracic outlet syndrome, peripheral neuropathy, and peripheral vascular disease.

The cornerstone of treatment is the release of compression on the involved nerve. In mild cases, this might be accomplished by modifying or ceasing the inciting activity. Splinting joints in a neutral position to relieve pressure on the involved nerve often is helpful. Nonsteroidal anti-inflammatory drugs are recommended. Injections of steroids and local anesthetic agents temporarily decrease or alleviate symptoms in most patients and have been shown to decrease the need for surgical decompression in some patients. ***Due to the risk of intraneural injection, which may cause permanent nerve damage, only experienced physicians or those being directly supervised by an experienced physician should perform steroid injections.*** A short course of oral steroids has been suggested as an alternative, but the evidence is inconclusive as to the effectiveness of this approach. Pyridoxine (vitamin B-6) has been used for the treatment of carpal tunnel syndrome and may provide some benefit; severe cases usually require surgical decompression.

Patients should be informed that prolonged or progressing symptoms require aggressive care, and they should seek followup care with a primary physician or be directly referred to a hand specialist.

Carpal Tunnel Syndrome

Carpal tunnel syndrome is the most commonly encountered nerve compression syndrome. It results from compression of the median nerve as it travels through the carpal tunnel, which is created by the concave alignment of carpal bones with the anterior coverage of the transverse carpal ligament. The carpal tunnel houses the median nerve and all of the flexor tendons and their sheaths.

Diagnosis

This syndrome tends to occur in two patient populations: middle-aged women, who often experience worsening symptoms at night, and workers who repetitively flex and extend their wrists, use a strong gripping action, or are exposed to excessive vibration or repetitive trauma. Early symptoms typically include pain, tingling, and numbness in the distribution of the median nerve, which includes the palmar surface of the thumb, the radial two thirds of the palm, the index and middle fingers, and the radial aspect of the ring finger. Pain may be referred to the elbow and shoulder, and symptoms may progress to include motor weakness and loss of fine motor coordination, affecting the opponens pollicis, abductor pollicis brevis, and first and second lumbricals. Muscles innervated by the radial and ulnar nerves closely mimic the function of these muscles, so no motor test can precisely determine which muscles are impaired. Overall weakness may be detected in the affected hand. Late findings may include atrophy of the involved muscles.

The **Phalen test** is performed by holding the wrist in a fully flexed position for several minutes; this reproduces or worsens symptoms if carpal tunnel syndrome is present. This is a useful and reliable test. The **Tinel sign** is elicited by gently tapping or holding pressure over the median nerve at the wrist; tingling along the median nerve dermatome should occur in patients with carpal tunnel syndrome. This is a less reliable test because it can create false-positive results. Electromyography may be used to confirm the diagnosis.

Treatment

Treatment can be started in the emergency department. Emphasis should be placed on the need to modify or cease activity identified as a possible cause. Nonsteroidal anti-inflammatory drugs are recommended. Splinting the wrist in a neutral position during the day and night for several weeks is warranted if symptoms are severe. Eventually, surgical decompression may be warranted, although carpal tunnel syndrome has a high rate of recurrence even after surgery.

Pronator Teres Median Nerve Compression Syndrome

This syndrome, also affectionately called **honeymoon paralysis**, occurs secondary to compression of the median nerve as it passes between the two heads of the pronator teres muscle just distal to the cubital fossa. Causes include fibrous bands, direct trauma, and prolonged external pressure.

Diagnosis

Symptoms may be the same as those of carpal tunnel syndrome and may involve weakness of the muscles that flex the wrist and fingers. The most important distinguishing symptom is a sensory deficit in the palm, which indicates compression of the palmaris branch of the median nerve arising proximal to the carpal tunnel.

Treatment

Symptoms usually are mild and self-limited. Splinting of the forearm in a position between pronation and supination may be helpful in more severe cases.

Anterior Interosseous Syndrome

This syndrome results from compression of the anterior interosseous branch of the median nerve that arises in the cubital region just distal to the heads of the pronator teres.

Diagnosis

Typically the patient presents with a decreased ability to flex the distal phalanx of the thumb and index finger, causing impairment of writing and decreased grip strength. The patient is unable to pinch a sheet of paper between the pads of the thumb and index finger. The anterior interosseous muscle is purely a motor nerve, innervating the flexor pollicis longus and flexor digitorum profundus muscles. This syndrome often coexists with pronator teres median nerve compression syndrome.

Treatment

Treatment follows the general principles of other nerve compression syndromes.

Cubital Tunnel Syndrome

This is a common compression syndrome that involves the ulnar nerve as it passes through the cubital groove, which is located at the elbow along the posterior aspect of the medial epicondyle of the humerus. An aponeurotic band holds the ulnar nerve tightly against the groove in flexion and more loosely in extension. Flexion of the elbow increases pressure exerted on the nerve at this location, as do wrist extension, shoulder abduction, and forward flexion. The ulnar nerve is superficial at this location and vulnerable to external compression. A sudden inadvertent strike of the elbow at this location is referred to as a hit to the **funny bone**.

Diagnosis

Sensory symptoms generally are the first to develop, corresponding to the superficial position of these fibers, followed by motor deficits of the intrinsic muscles of the hand. More severe compression begins to affect the deeper nerve fibers that innervate the flexor carpi ulnaris and flexor digitorum profundus muscles.

Patients often report shooting pains, tingling, or numbness in the ulnar aspect of the palm and little finger. Flexing the elbow and extending the wrist for 3 minutes likely worsens symptoms. Patients may demonstrate weak abduction and adduction of the little finger. Weakness on flexion of the wrist in an ulnar direction may be noted, as may weakness on flexion of the DIP joints. Atrophy of the hypothenar region and first web space and clawing of the ring and little fingers may be noted in long-term cases.

Treatment

Treatment is similar to that for other nerve compression syndromes, including activity modification and NSAIDs. Patients should be encouraged to avoid prolonged flexion of the elbow and may benefit from the use of a pillow or an Ace wrap to keep the elbow extended during sleep. The elbow should be padded to protect against external compression, which typically occurs when resting the elbows on a desk while working at a computer. Surgery may be necessary if other therapy fails.

Guyon Syndrome

A less common site of ulnar nerve compression is Guyon's canal, through which the palmar branches of the ulnar nerve enter the hand. This canal runs between the pisiform and the hook of the hamate and is covered by the volar carpal ligament and palmaris longus muscle. The canal is a narrow passageway that contains the superficial and deep palmar branches of the ulnar nerve, the flexor carpi ulnaris tendon, and the ulnar vein and artery.

A ganglion cyst, an aneurysm or thrombosis of the ulnar artery, or any object that intrudes into this narrow space is likely to cause nerve compression. This may occur traumatically with anterior dislocation of the ulnar head, with carpal fracture, or with repetitive compression of the hypothenar region, as occurs with bicycle riding or the operation of a pneumatic drill.

Diagnosis

Compression at Guyon's canal causes a pattern of symptoms similar to that of cubital tunnel syndrome, but there is no involvement of the dorsal branch of the ulnar nerve, which branches proximally to Guyon's canal. Therefore, sensation at the dorsal little finger and the dorsal ulnar aspect of the ring finger and hand is spared in this syndrome. Patients with Guyon syndrome may have difficulty grasping and performing fine movements and may have paresthesias across the volar aspect of the little finger and the volar ulnar aspect of the ring finger.

If compression occurs slightly distal to Guyon's canal and affects the deep but not the superficial palmar branch of the ulnar nerve, a purely motor syndrome known as **pisohamate hiatus syndrome** results. It occurs in a space formed between the hamate and the pisiform carpal bones and covered by the pisohamate ligament and the tendinous arch of the palm. Symptoms include weakness of the interosseous and hypothenar muscles. The presence of sensory symptoms suggests a more proximal site of nerve compression.

Treatment

Treatment considerations are similar to those for other nerve compression syndromes.

Radial Nerve Compression Syndrome

The radial nerve is most often compressed at the midhumeral level, where it travels in a groove along the posterior aspect of the humerus. Causes include midshaft humeral fractures, prolonged compression, and very heavy use of the triceps muscles, as occurs with weight lifting.

Diagnosis

Patients may present with wrist drop and a decreased ability to extend the fingers or abduct the thumb. The wrist is likely held in a pronated position. The patient may note sensory deficits on the dorsal aspect of the hand, excluding the ulnar aspect and the fingertips. In the case of **Saturday night palsy**, symptoms might occur on wakening after a night of heavy drinking led to the patient sleeping on top of the affected arm. Symptoms may last several weeks but typically resolve spontaneously.

Treatment

Treatment is similar to that for other nerve compression syndromes. Splinting the wrist in an extended position improves the function of the hand by causing the patient to use the intrinsic muscles.

Painful Joints or Tendons

Rheumatoid Arthritis

Rheumatoid arthritis is an idiopathic systemic disease that causes hyperplasia of the synovial tissue of the joints and tendons. This disease causes an inflammatory arthritis that may lead to the destruction of cartilage and bone. It is common, affecting about 1% of the US population, and women two to three times more often than men.[1] The course of the disease ranges from a mild, nondestructive arthritis in a few joints to a profoundly destructive and even fatal process. Rheumatoid arthritis has no known cure.

Diagnosis

Rheumatoid arthritis typically affects multiple joints in a symmetric manner. Patients note morning stiffness in the involved joints, most often the PIP and MCP joints. As the disease progresses, patients may note enlargement of the PIP (**Bouchard nodes**) and MCP joints secondary to a pannus formed by proliferating synovial tissue. Radiographs may reveal soft tissue swelling, joint space narrowing, marginal erosions, and periarticular osteoporosis. Arthrocentesis should be performed if there is concern of infection or crystal-induced arthritis. Findings of sterile synovial fluid without crystals and an elevated white blood cell count to 50,000 cells/mm^3 support the diagnosis.

The classic **Z deformity** develops as the metacarpals drift in a radial direction and the fingers and carpal bones drift in an ulnar direction (Figure 23-1 and Figure 23-2). A swan-neck or boutonnière deformity

Figure 23-1.

Classic Z deformity of rheumatoid arthritis.

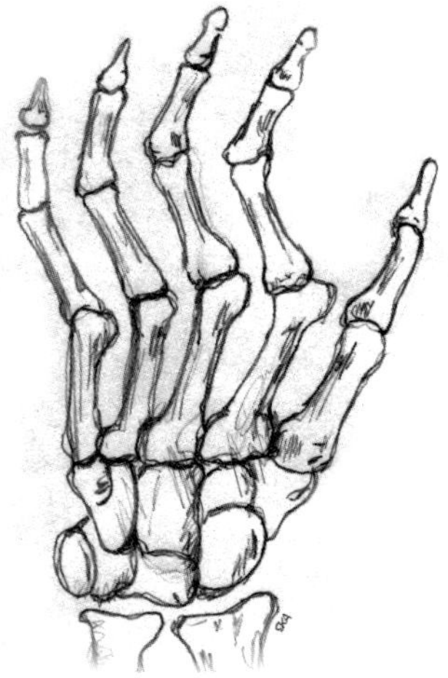

Figure 23-2.

Rheumatoid arthritis.

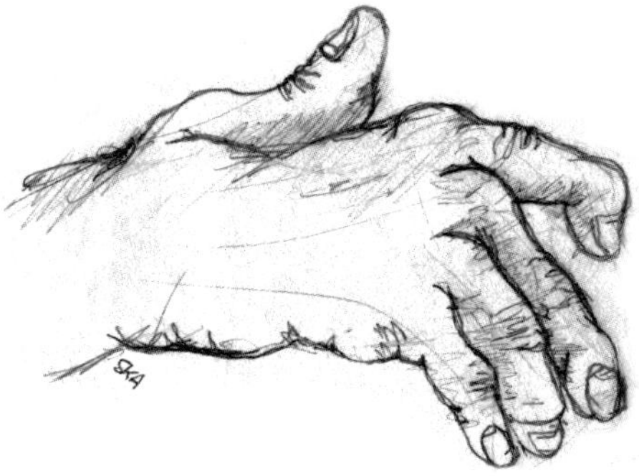

may develop as joint destruction progresses. Rheumatoid nodules may be noted, most commonly over the olecranon, extensor surface of the forearm, and dorsum of the fingers. They are composed of a collagenous matrix that may undergo central necrosis and drainage. Tenosynovitis is common, and tendons may develop adhesions to thickened tendon sheaths and eventually rupture. Trigger finger is another complication. Patients with rheumatoid arthritis may have involvement of the cervical spine and are at risk for atlantoaxial instability. ***Caution should be used during intubation or any other procedure that involves manipulation of the cervical spine in patients suspected of having rheumatoid arthritis.***

Treatment

Measures should be taken to alleviate symptoms as well as to slow the progression of the disease. Patients should be encouraged to perform exercises to maintain range of motion and to strengthen the musculature that surrounds the involved joints. Tenosynovitis, tendon rupture, and various deformities are treated aggressively. Nonsteroidal anti-inflammatory drugs are beneficial because rheumatoid arthritis is an inflammatory disease. Corticosteroids, administered orally or via direct injection, may be effective in slowing the progression of the disease, but long-term use may lead to osteoporosis and a worsened outcome. Treatment is most effective if started early, before cartilage damage takes place, and there are many options for medical therapy. Referral to a hand specialist and a rheumatologist is warranted for any patient who has not been previously diagnosed or treated.

Osteoarthritis

Osteoarthritis is far more common than rheumatoid arthritis and affects nearly every individual to some extent by middle age. It is caused by the progressive loss of articular cartilage. This process may be idiopathic, related to chronic repetitive trauma, or related to a previous destructive process in the joint. Inflammatory mediators have a role in osteoarthritis but not to the extent that they do in rheumatoid arthritis. Risk factors include obesity, diabetes mellitus, and a genetic predisposition.

Diagnosis

Patients have pain with use, decreased range of motion, and crepitus of the involved joints. The DIP joints and the CMC joints of the thumb are most commonly involved, although the PIP and MCP joints may also be involved. Enlargement of the DIP joints (**Heberden nodes**) results from osteophytes that develop on the dorsal aspect of the joint. Proximal interphalangeal joint enlargement (Bouchard node) may occur as in rheumatoid arthritis but is caused by osteophyte formation, not synovium proliferation. Carpometacarpal joint involvement, specifically the trapeziometacarpal joint, can cause significant disability. Patients have difficulty with any task that requires movement of this joint, such as turning a key or opening a jar. The **grind test** (axial loading with rotation of the thumb) and the **crank test** (axial loading with passive flexion and extension of the thumb) both elicit pain and crepitus. This may indicate basal joint osteoarthritis and possible instability, and surgery may be necessary. Mallet finger, ganglion cyst formation, tenosynovitis, and nerve compression syndromes are common complications of osteoarthritis. Radiographs reveal subchondral sclerosis, cysts, joint space narrowing, and marginal osteophytes. Soft tissue swelling is less pronounced than in rheumatoid arthritis.

Treatment

Treatment focuses on pain relief and the prevention of further disability. Activity that might contribute to this condition should be modified or stopped. The patient should be encouraged to perform low-impact exercises to strengthen muscles and to maintain range of motion. Nonsteroidal anti-inflammatory drugs may be helpful but have a limited role because this is not primarily an inflammatory process. Acetaminophen is an effective pain reliever that lacks the adverse effects on renal function and gastric mucosa caused by NSAIDs. Steroids are not useful in osteoarthritis. Patients with basal joint degeneration and instability should receive a short arm thumb spica splint and be referred to a hand specialist.

Kienböck Disease

This disease presents as arthritis of the wrist secondary to avascular necrosis of the lunate. The cause is not completely understood, although previous trauma has been implicated.

Diagnosis

Kienböck disease most often affects men between the ages of 20 and 40. Patients present with pain, stiffness, and swelling over the dorsal aspect of the wrist and may have difficulty holding heavy objects. Initially, isolated tenderness may be noted on palpation of the lunate (on the dorsal aspect of the wrist just distal to the radius and near the midline). Symptoms worsen as degeneration of the lunate progresses. Gradually, the other carpal bones and the distal radius may be affected. Eventually, the entire wrist joint may be destroyed, causing severe disability and deformity. Radiographs of the wrist reveal increased density of the lunate in comparison with the other carpal bones. The lunate may fragment, and adjacent bones may show signs of degeneration.

If the scaphoid and lunate bones appear separated (**Terry Thomas sign**), the patient may instead have scapholunate dissociation secondary to a ligament tear. The patient may note a slipping or snapping sensation when moving the wrist.

Treatment

If there is radiographic evidence of Kienböck disease, the wrist should be splinted in the neutral position with a short arm splint. Nonsteroidal anti-inflammatory drugs may be helpful. If no radiographic evidence exists but the disease is suspected, the wrist should be splinted for 3 weeks. If pain exists without radiographic evidence, a bone scan should be considered. Surgery may be needed if the disease progresses, and referral to a hand specialist is recommended.

Avascular Necrosis of the Scaphoid

This disease usually results from a traumatic fracture of the scaphoid that heals improperly. Due to the tenuous blood supply of the scaphoid that flows in a distal-to-proximal direction, proximal fractures are more at risk for this complication than are distal fractures. In **Preiser disease**, this condition occurs spontaneously with no history of trauma.

Diagnosis

The patient initially has pain and tenderness along the area of the scaphoid, most reliably in the anatomic snuffbox. Decreased strength and range of motion may be noted. Radiographs of the wrist should be obtained; an oblique and a PA view with the wrist in ulnar deviation may be helpful if routine films are negative. A fracture or lucency may be noted in the scaphoid, or the scaphoid may appear to have increased density (as with Kienböck disease). Patients with recent or remote trauma who have snuffbox tenderness should be assumed to have a scaphoid fracture until proved otherwise. Bone scans should be obtained if pain continues despite splinting.

Treatment

Patients with snuffbox tenderness but no radiographic abnormalities should be splinted for 1 to 2 weeks and then reevaluated. A radiographically visible fracture should be treated with a long arm thumb spica splint for at least 6 weeks, and the patient should be referred to a hand specialist. Avascular necrosis requires prompt referral. If nonunion of the scaphoid persists or significant degeneration has occurred, surgery is indicated.

de Quervain Disease (Tenosynovitis)

Tenosynovitis results from inflammation and thickening of the tendon sheath. This may be caused by overuse or secondary to another condition, such as rheumatoid arthritis, osteoarthritis, or gout. Movement of the involved tendon produces pain and may create an audible or palpable crepitus as it rubs against the inflamed tendon sheath. de Quervain disease involves the abductor pollicis longus and extensor pollicis brevis tendons and is the most common tenosynovitis of the hand and wrist. Treatment of this condition is a guideline for the treatment of other forms of tenosynovitis.

Diagnosis

Patients with de Quervain disease present with pain over the radial styloid that is exacerbated by movement of the thumb. They may note a creaking noise or sensation as the tendon moves. A history of overuse or a new activity supports the diagnosis. Radiographs should be obtained to rule out bony involvement if trauma has occurred. Calcification of the tendon may be seen in chronic cases. Consider alternative diagnoses, such as infectious tenosynovitis, avascular necrosis of the scaphoid or lunate, arthritis of the wrist, ganglion cyst, or a nerve compression syndrome.

Treatment

The involved tendon should be immobilized to facilitate healing. A short arm thumb spica splint is used to immobilize the thumb and wrist. Nonsteroidal anti-inflammatory drugs are helpful. Steroid injection into the involved tendon may be helpful. Chronic tendonitis with significant impairment may require surgical synovectomy to release the tendon from the thickened tendon sheath.

Trigger Finger

Trigger finger results from a nodule that develops on the flexor tendon of the finger. The nodule has difficulty sliding past the proximal pulley, which holds the tendon sheath to the finger (Figure 23-3). The nodule may result from repetitive trauma or be related to rheumatoid arthritis or diabetes mellitus. The thumb and the ring and middle fingers are most often affected.

Diagnosis

The patient may report pain or a catching sensation on flexion or extension of the involved finger. Symptoms may be referred to the PIP joint or the IP joint of the thumb, although the point of friction is the pulley located at the MCP joint. Diffuse swelling may be noted, or a nodule may be palpated in the distal palm near the base of the finger. Occasionally, the nodule becomes trapped on one side of the pulley, causing the finger to be locked in flexion or extension (**locked finger**). The patient may wake up with this condition, and the finger may gradually unlock during the day. Radiographs are not helpful. **Dupuytren disease** should be considered as an alternative diagnosis in a patient who has a distal palmar nodule. Flexor tendon ganglion cysts also may be mistaken for trigger finger.

Figure 23-3.

Trigger finger. **A)** *Nodule distal to pulley with finger in extension.* **B)** *Tendon nodule locked proximal to pulley.*

A

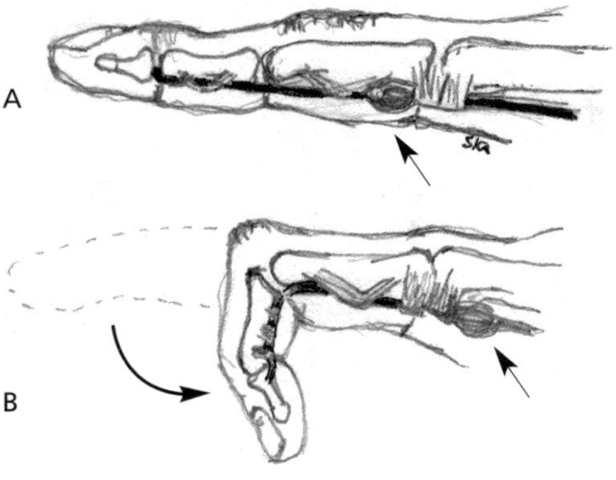

B

Treatment

Initial treatment is similar to the treatment for tenosynovitis. The finger should be immobilized in extension for 2 weeks, and NSAIDs are recommended. Steroid injection into the tendon sheath may be helpful and should be considered before surgical release. Failure of initial therapy warrants referral to a hand specialist.

Deformities

The following deformities typically are chronic and progressive and often are not the primary reason a patient seeks medical care (Figure 23-4). Patients may have accepted their debilitating conditions as untreatable results of aging or chronic disease, but treatment may prevent progression of the deformity or even reverse it.

Boutonnière Deformity

This deformity results from a disruption of the central portion of the extensor tendon as it connects to the dorsal base of the middle phalanx. The extensor mechanism, or central slip, can be damaged by direct trauma to the PIP joint, forceful flexion of the PIP joint against resistance, or joint dislocation.

Diagnosis

With boutonnière deformity, the PIP joint is flexed due to the unopposed action of the flexor tendons against a damaged extensor mechanism. The DIP joint is extended because the portion of the extensor tendon that runs lateral to the central slip remains intact. As the lateral bands (traveling on each side of the central slip) sublux around the PIP joint, the degree of flexion deformity of the PIP joint and extension deformity of the DIP joint increases.

Injury to the central slip may not be apparent on initial presentation. A patient may present with this deformity weeks later as subluxation of the lateral bands begins to exert a proximal pull on the distal phalanx.

Figure 23-4.

A) *Normal balance of digit.* **B)** *Mallet finger deformity.* **C)** *Swan-neck deformity.* **D)** *Boutonnière deformity.* **E)** *Claw deformity.*

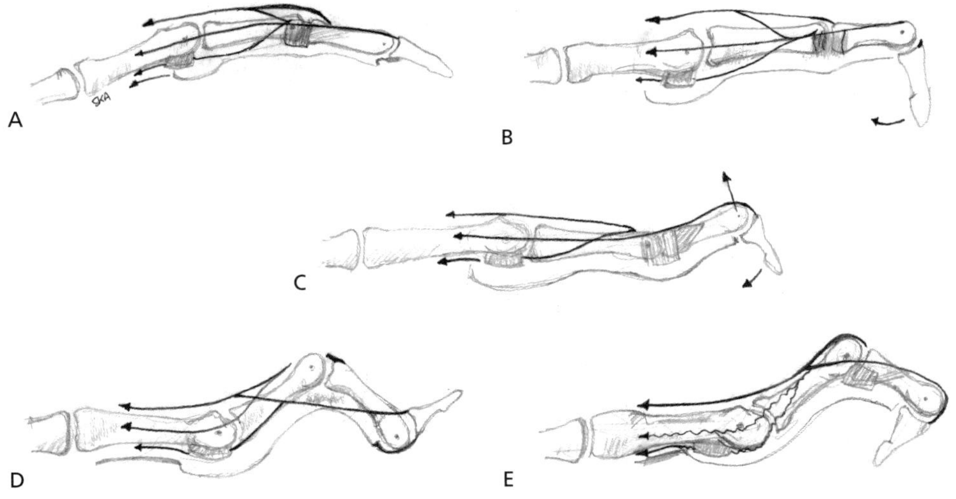

Treatment

Therapy involves splinting the PIP joint in an extended position regardless of whether the deformity is acute or chronic. The DIP joint should remain unencumbered. Acute injuries should be left splinted for at least 4 weeks. Chronic deformity makes full extension of the PIP joint more difficult to achieve, and gradually increased extension through repeated splinting may be necessary. Referral to a hand specialist is indicated in both cases.

Swan-Neck Deformity

This deformity occurs when the volar support of the PIP joint is weakened due to either trauma or a systemic disease such as rheumatoid arthritis. Contraction of the intrinsic muscles or chronic mallet finger also may cause progression to the swan-neck deformity.

Diagnosis

As the volar support weakens, the PIP joint becomes hyperextended. This creates tension on the flexor tendons and causes flexion of the DIP and MCP joints. The swan neck shape is essentially the opposite of the boutonnière deformity.

Treatment

Swan-neck deformity is a chronic condition and difficult to correct. Splinting of the entire digit in a neutral position and referral to a hand specialist are recommended.

Mallet Finger

Mallet finger results from traumatic rupture of the extensor tendon at the DIP joint.

Diagnosis

The patient may present acutely with a painful and swollen fingertip that cannot be actively extended or may present days to weeks after the injury when the pain and swelling have resolved and the dysfunctional joint becomes noticeable. Radiography of the digit may reveal a small avulsion fracture of the dorsal base of the distal phalanx. In chronic cases, the distal phalanx may sublux volarly due to the unopposed flexor force. Chronic mallet finger may progress to a swan-neck deformity.

Treatment

Treatment of acute or chronic mallet finger involves splinting the DIP joint in 15 degrees of hyperextension. No other joints should be immobilized. Splinting should be continued for 6 weeks for acute conditions and 8 weeks or longer for chronic conditions. The patient should be informed that flexing the DIP joint during this rehabilitation period may cause the extensor insertion to be damaged again.

These patients should be referred to a hand specialist. Cases refractory to splinting and those with avulsion fractures that involve more than one third of the DIP joint surface require surgical pinning.

Claw Hand

This is a chronic condition that results from denervation of the intrinsic muscles of the hand due to injury to the ulnar or median nerve, or to both.

Diagnosis

The deformity develops only if the flexors remain functional, so complete loss of ulnar and median nerve function does not result in claw hand. Loss of function of the intrinsic muscles (the lumbricals and interossei) allows hyperextension of the MCP joints. Intact deep and superficial flexors cause profound flexion of the DIP and PIP joints, which are ineffectively extended due to the abnormal position of the MCP joints.

Treatment

Early intervention through splinting of the MCP joints in a neutral position can prevent further degeneration and allow the extensor tendons to oppose flexion of the PIP and DIP joints. Surgery may eventually be needed to prevent this devastating deformity and to maintain some hand function.

Dupuytren Contracture

This is a disease of the palmar and digital fasciae that results in debilitating deformity of the hand (Figure 23-5). The cause of this disease is poorly understood, but there may be a dominant genetic component. Men are affected 7 to 10 times more frequently than women. The disease is most common in persons of northern European descent; it also is called **Viking disease**. Apart from a genetic predisposition for the disease, risk factors include diabetes mellitus, epilepsy, pulmonary disease, alcoholism, smoking, HIV infection, and age older than 40.

Diagnosis

Early in the course of the disease, painless nodules may be noted near the distal palmar creases. The involved fascia becomes increasingly thick and causes the fingers to flex at the MCP joint. The ring finger typically is affected first; then, the little, middle, and index fingers and thumb are progressively involved. Patients may note an increasing difficulty with certain tasks, such as putting on gloves or putting their hands in their pockets.

Treatment

Splinting the hand does not change the course of the disease, nor do other conservative therapies. Surgical fasciotomy is necessary and generally is considered when the MCP joint is contracted greater than 30 degrees, the PIP joint has any degree of contraction, or the condition is disabling to the patient. Early referral to a hand specialist is recommended.

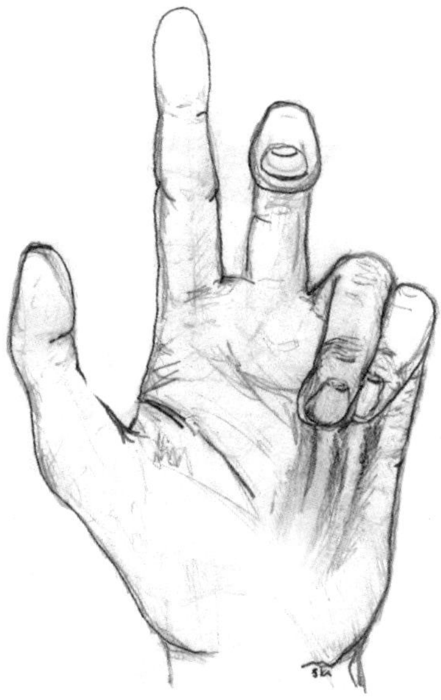

Figure 23-5.

Dupuytren contracture.

Masses

A mass in the hand may be a primary complaint that causes pain or impairment, displeasing cosmesis, or concern of significant disease. Masses are not uncommon. An emergency physician also may be asked to examine a mass as a secondary complaint. Generally, masses are nonemergent, but as many as 10% of soft tissue masses are malignant.

Ganglion Cysts

This is the most common tumor of the hand. It develops spontaneously from an adjacent tendon sheath. The cyst communicates with the tendon sheath through a valve that allows synovial fluid to escape the sheath and become trapped in the cyst. This may result from a traumatic tear to the ligaments that support the tendon, allowing it to herniate out of the normal position.

Diagnosis

Ganglion cysts often are asymptomatic but can cause significant impairment. The patient may note pain or decreased range of motion with movement of the involved tendon or may develop a nerve compression syndrome. Occasionally, a cyst ruptures and causes diffuse swelling and pain. Infection should be considered if warmth, erythema, and increased pain develop.

The synovial fluid may periodically escape back into the tendon sheath, causing the pathognomonic history of a mass that waxes and wanes. Palpation of a soft fluid-filled cyst makes the diagnosis easy, but ganglion cysts may feel hard and therefore can be difficult to distinguish from a solid tumor. A cystic mass will transilluminate. Ganglion cysts most commonly occur in one of four locations: the dorsal radial aspect of the wrist, the volar radial aspect of the wrist, the proximal finger flexor crease, or the dorsal aspect of the DIP joint (**mucous cyst**) (Figure 23-6).

Figure 23-6. *Ganglion cysts.*

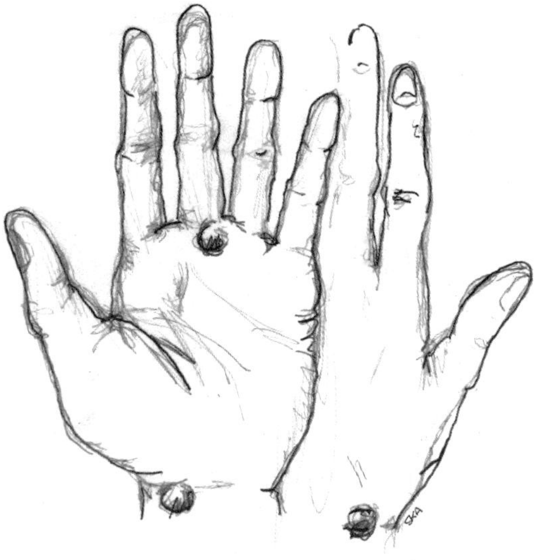

Treatment

Ganglion cysts are benign and may resolve spontaneously with conservative therapy. Restricted motor movement, avoidance of localized trauma, and NSAIDs are first-line therapy.

Drainage is the treatment of choice when a cyst becomes symptomatic. Most cysts can be drained with very little risk of complications, but the patient should be informed that there is a high recurrence rate. The skin overlying the cyst should be anesthetized with 1% lidocaine without epinephrine, and then an 18-gauge needle should be inserted. The cyst may be easier to locate if the needle is inserted just proximal to it and angled along the tendon over which it lies. The contents of a ganglion cyst are clear and colorless, with a viscosity that resembles jelly, and often are too thick to be aspirated by the negative pressure of the syringe alone. Gentle pressure on the cyst during aspiration helps propel the fluid through the needle and into the syringe. Ganglion cysts that continue to recur despite drainage may require surgical excision, but there still is a 5% to 10% recurrence rate.

If the aspirate is not clear and thick, an infection or some other diagnosis should be considered. Aspirating ganglion cysts along the volar radial aspect of the wrist requires caution. The cyst may lie beneath the radial artery or might be an aneurysm, and drainage may cause damage to the radial artery. Also, ganglion cysts in the wrist located near the radial, median, or ulnar nerve may be damaged by the insertion of a large-bore needle.

Other Masses

Fortunately, the presence of a primary malignant tumor or metastasis below the elbow is rare, but any mass that is not clearly identifiable warrants referral to a specialist. The following are examples of common masses.

Giant Cell Tumor

This is a common soft tissue tumor in the hand that is often referred to as **localized nodular synovitis**. It occurs as a gradually enlarging firm nodular mass along the palmar aspect of the finger near the tendon sheath. It is typically asymptomatic and causes only cosmetic complaints. Similar lesions located near the flexor creases at the base of the digits may be fibromas related to Dupuytren disease. Occasionally, radiographic evidence of cortical erosion may be noted. This mass is treated with local excision by a hand specialist, and recurrence is common.

Epidermal Inclusion Cyst

This mass may develop at any site of previous penetrating injury, commonly on the fingertip or the volar aspect of the palm or fingers. It is a painless, slow-growing soft tissue mass. Unlike a ganglion cyst, an epidermal inclusion cyst does not transilluminate. A foreign body granuloma is another mass that is often associated with previous trauma.

Enchondroma

An enchondroma is the most common neoplasm of the bones in the hand, and it is benign. It is normally painless, but it may lead to a pathologic fracture, which typically is how it is discovered. These neoplasms are most often located in the proximal phalanx, but they can be found in any bone. Radiography reveals a central intramedullary lucency with a thin cortex. All suspicious lesions require referral to a hand specialist for treatment and to rule out malignant bone tumors. Osteomyelitis also should be considered.

Lipoma

This is the most common soft tissue neoplasm of the hand. Lipomas occur most frequently in the thenar area of the palm or in the first web space. They are typically painless but can cause nerve compression syndromes or functional impairment. As with all soft tissue masses in the hand, referral to a hand specialist for further evaluation is prudent.

Glomus Tumor

This is a benign tumor that usually occurs under a fingernail. It typically is very painful and may create a blue discoloration under the nail and cause cold intolerance of the involved area. There is increased pain with submersion in cold water.

Carpal Boss

This is a painless bony mass located at the base of the second and third metacarpals. It is created by one or more bony projections off the proximal aspect of these metacarpals, the trapezium, or the trapezoid. Radiography assists in the diagnosis. Occasionally a ganglion cyst is associated with a carpal boss.

Malignant Lesions

Squamous cell carcinoma is the most common malignancy of the hand and generally is found on the dorsal aspect where exposure to ultraviolet radiation from the sun is most likely. **Basal cell carcinoma** and **melanoma** also may occur, most frequently on the palms. **Subungual melanoma** should be considered when evaluating a painless discolored lesion under the nail. Although rare, malignant soft tissue tumors can occur in the hand, and any soft tissue mass should be considered malignant until proved otherwise. The most common soft tissue sarcomas in the hand are **synovial sarcoma**, **malignant fibrous histiocytoma**, **epithelioid sarcoma**, and **liposarcoma**. These lesions often metastasize, usually to the lungs or lymph nodes. As mentioned, malignant tumors also can occur in the bones of the hand and should be considered whenever an unexplained radiolucent or radiodense lesion is noted on radiography.

Raynaud Phenomenon or Disease

Raynaud phenomenon or disease is a paroxysmal vasospastic disorder that usually affects the fingers but can affect the toes, earlobes, and tip of the nose. Women are affected five times more frequently than are men, usually during childbearing age. Symptoms initially may occur in only one or two digits but can progress to involve both hands symmetrically. Involved digits become pale to extremely white or cyanotic during episodes. Areas of discoloration are often sharply demarcated from normal-appearing skin. The patient may note pain, tingling, numbness, or decreased fine motor movements. Paroxysms may last minutes to hours and often are triggered by cold exposure, fatigue, or emotional stress.

The spectrum of this disorder is broad, ranging from mild and nonprogressing symptoms to a progressive and highly destructive process that causes gangrene and amputation. The term **Raynaud phenomenon** is used if the syndrome is related to another disease, whereas the term **Raynaud disease** is reserved for the syndrome when there is no underlying cause. Typically, this term is not used until a thorough search for an underlying cause is performed and 24 months have elapsed since the initial presentation. This terminology is problematic in that many causes are not discovered for years after the onset of symptoms. Furthermore, many diseases associated with Raynaud phenomenon are serious and potentially treatable, and the possibility of an underlying cause should not be dismissed. In nearly half of all patients with this syndrome, an underlying cause is ultimately discovered.

The diseases most commonly associated with Raynaud phenomenon are the collagen vascular diseases (scleroderma, systemic lupus erythematosus, rheumatoid arthritis, dermatomyositis, polymyositis). Other causes include arterial occlusive disorders (atherosclerosis, thoracic outlet syndrome), neurologic disorders (nerve compression disorders, spinal cord tumors), pulmonary hypertension, blood dyscrasias, trauma (excessive vibration, electric shock, cold injury), reflex sympathetic dystrophy, and various drugs (β-blockers, cisplatin).

Diagnosis

The initial diagnosis is made clinically based on the symptoms. A bone scan may be helpful in some cases and demonstrates decreased perfusion into the involved digits during episodes. Pulses should be equal in patients with Raynaud phenomenon. Blood pressures should be measured in both arms to rule out subtle differences caused by arterial occlusion. Eventually, studies to look for collagen vascular disease and other underlying causes must be performed, but a rigorous workup is not necessary on the initial presentation.

Treatment

Patients who smoke should be encouraged to stop because smoking may be a contributing factor. Calcium channel blockers have been used with varying success rates. Underlying disease should be treated. Exposure to factors that trigger episodes such as cold and stress should be reduced.

Reflex Sympathetic Dystrophy

Also referred to as **complex regional pain syndrome** or **sympathetically maintained pain**, this syndrome is thought to be due to an abnormal hyperactive sympathetic reflex that causes signs and symptoms in the involved extremity. The syndrome usually is triggered by an injury that occurred days to weeks earlier. There is much debate over how to define this syndrome, and reflex sympathetic dystrophy has undoubtedly been overdiagnosed. The syndrome does exist, however, and objective evidence can be used to make the diagnosis.

Diagnosis

Reflex sympathetic dystrophy is most often diagnosed in the hand. Patients with this syndrome may complain of one or more of a multitude of symptoms that include pain, stiffness, edema, skin discoloration, vasomotor instability, variations in hand temperature, and hyperhidrosis. Pain usually is described as severe burning. Skin discoloration ranges from erythema to cyanosis. Raynaud phenomenon (vasoconstriction and cold intolerance) may be noted. Abnormal posturing is not a symptom. Atrophy of the skin and subcutaneous tissue may occur, creating a shiny appearance with the loss of skin creases, and the palmar fascia may thicken. Osteoporosis may develop, causing the characteristic "punch-out" lesions on radiographs.

Many specialists believe that the diagnosis of reflex sympathetic dystrophy should not be made without trophic changes, edema with stiffness, radiographic evidence of bone demineralization that is asymmetric compared with the opposite extremity, and a positive three-phase radionuclide bone scan. Malingering, conversion disorder, diabetic neuropathy, nerve compression syndromes, and peripheral vascular disease should be considered as alternative diagnoses.

Treatment

The physician must demonstrate respect for the patient's pain and confidence that therapy will be successful. Initial treatment involves exercise and therapy focused on decreasing the response to painful stimuli. The patient should be advised to stop smoking because this can contribute to the increased sympathetic tone and can exacerbate symptoms. Sympatholytic drugs such as phentolamine and local and stellate ganglion nerve blocks have been used with varying success rates. Sympathectomy is sometimes performed in severe cases. Psychiatric referral may be helpful. Referral to a hand specialist is warranted if the patient has severe disability or requires diagnostic confirmation.

Reference

1. Harrison TR, Fauci AS, eds. *Harrison's Principles of Internal Medicine.* 14th ed. New York, NY: McGraw-Hill: 1997:1402.

Additional Reading

Agur A, ed. *Grant's Atlas of Anatomy.* 9th ed. Baltimore, Md: Williams & Wilkins; 1991.

American Society for Surgery of the Hand. *The Hand: Primary Care of Common Problems.* 2nd ed. New York, NY: Churchill Livingstone; 1990.

Berry T, ed. *The Hand as a Mirror of Systemic Disease.* Philadelphia, Pa: FA Davis; 1963.

Blackburn W. *Approach to the Patient With a Musculoskeletal Disorder.* Birmingham, Ala: Professional Communications; 1999.

Cailliet R. *Hand Pain and Impairment.* 4th ed. Philadelphia, Pa: FA Davis; 1994.

Chang M, Chiang H, Lee S, et al. Oral drug of choice in carpal tunnel syndrome. *Neurology.* 1998;51:390-393.

Dammers J, Veering M, Vermeulen M. Injection with methylprednisolone proximal to the carpal tunnel: randomized double blind trial. *BMJ.* 1999;319:884-886.

Jebson P, Kasdan M, eds. *Hand Secrets.* Philadelphia, Pa: Hanley & Belfus; 1998.

Kasdan M, Janes C. Carpal tunnel syndrome and vitamin B6. *Plast Reconstr Surg.* 1987;79:456-462.

Knoop K, Stack L, Storrow A, eds. *Atlas of Emergency Medicine.* New York, NY: McGraw-Hill; 1997.

Lister G, ed. *The Hand: Diagnosis and Indications.* 3rd ed. New York, NY: Churchill Livingstone; 1993.

Snider R, ed. *Essentials of Musculoskeletal Care.* Rosemont, Ill: American Academy of Orthopedic Surgeons; 1997.

Stutts J, Kasdan M, Hickey S, et al. Reflex sympathetic dystrophy: misdiagnosis in patients with dysfunctional postures of the upper extremity. *J Hand Surg [Am].* 2000;25:1152-1156.

Tubiana R, Thomine J, Mackin E, eds. *Examination of the Hand and Wrist.* St Louis, Mo: Mosby; 1996.

CHAPTER 24

Unique Injuries

Arthur F. Proust, MD, FACEP, and Brian T. Stubitsch, MD

Hand trauma that results from wringers, cornpickers, snowblowers, high-pressure injection devices, and nail guns is uncommon and offers a clinically challenging spectrum of injuries. These injuries often require surgical intervention, so prompt recognition and treatment can greatly influence outcomes. The epidemiology, pathophysiology, clinical presentation, and management of each type of injury are reviewed.

Wringer Injuries

Many of the terms that describe entities in medicine are derived from Latin or Greek words. Occasionally, however, a particular illness or injury becomes associated with its causative agent. **Wringer arm**, which was coined by MacCollum[1] in 1938 in a description of 26 cases, falls into this category. This injury occurs when an extremity becomes entrapped in the roller mechanism of a wringer washer, which came into widespread use in the 1920s.

MacCollum concluded that the severity of injury is determined by the speed of the rollers and the length of time the extremity is subjected to the crushing force.[1] In 1941, Allen[2] reported on the importance of compression in reducing limb edema and subsequent ischemia in his review of 107 patients. In 1950, while comparing the available treatment modalities, Hausmann and Everett[3] recommended early skin grafting. And in 1954, Posch and Weller[4] advocated the need for hospitalization and early split-thickness skin grafts to minimize scar formation and prevent secondary infection.

More recently, degloving injuries of the hand associated with industrial roller injuries have been treated with full-thickness skin grafts from avulsed skin flaps.[5] Devascularized digits have been revascularized with the use of microsurgical techniques. Also, palmar avulsion flaps have been revascularized with primary arteriovenous anastomosis.[6]

Epidemiology

The introduction of automatic washing machines in the 1940s reduced the incidence of wringer arm as a type of crushing injury. However, in 1970, wringer washers accounted for 5.5% of all washing machine shipments; 124,000 were shipped in 1980. These washers have long life expectancies; they are most likely to be found in homes within low socioeconomic areas, in homes headed by older individuals, and in locales that lack adequate plumbing and sewer facilities.[7]

Industrial roller injuries are high-energy variants of wringer injuries. Although the number of injuries seems to be increasing, the true incidence is unknown. Rollers are found in a variety of industries, including printing, baking, and farming.

Mechanism of Injury

Wringer injuries result from compressive, thermal, and shearing forces that are applied to a limb while it is trapped between the rotating rollers.[7] Injury severity is affected by the speed of rotation of the rollers, the narrow space between rollers, the duration of entrapment, the extent of struggle, and the method of release.[8]

Compressive Force

The compressive force is a direct consequence of the extremity being forced into a narrow gap between the rollers and is principally responsible for edema, contusion, and neuropraxia. Edema and other tissue responses lead to further limb ischemia.[8-10]

Thermal Force

Thermal forces are the result of friction that develops between the rollers and the extremity. Subsequent burns are of varying degrees and severity.

Shearing Forces

Shearing forces are created by the rollers as they move superficial soft tissue over deeper fixed structures, which results in lacerations, avulsions, fractures, and the formation of subcutaneous hematomas. Countertraction of the extremity opposite the direction of the roller rotation exacerbates the shearing injury.[8]

Clinical Presentation

Wringer injuries occur most commonly in the pediatric population, with the highest incidence between the ages of 3 and 5 years[11] and a 2:1 ratio of boys to girls. The average age of patients decreases as injuries become more proximal.[7,11,12]

In industrial roller injuries, victims are primarily men, with an average age of 36 years.[13]

Injury Location

Injuries are grouped as hand and wrist, forearm and elbow, and arm and axilla. The forearm and elbow group is the most commonly involved location because the progress of the rollers often arrests in the antecubital fossa.[14] The right extremity is entrapped in 59% of cases, and the left in 41%; bilateral injuries are rare.[11]

Injury Type

The most common type of wringer injury is a **friction burn**. The severity varies from mild erythema to badly burned, nonviable skin. Ten percent to 12% of associated injuries include minor lacerations, with most occurring in the first web space and thenar eminence. Fractures or dislocations occur in 2% to 5% of patients, and the incidence of hematomas ranges from 2% to 10%.[7,11,14]

Complex injuries that involve nerves and tendons, amputations, and wounds that require flap reconstruction with wringer injuries are rare; only 43 instances were discovered in a retrospective review dating back to 1938. Only five cases of Volkmann ischemic contracture and three cases of vascular occlusion that required fasciotomy were found.[14]

Modern industrial rollers exert pressures in excess of 800 psi as compared to wringer washers, which do not exceed 15 psi.[13] As a result, in the workplace, there is an increased incidence of fracture-dislocations, nerve and tendon injuries, amputations, and degloving injuries that require flap reconstruction and skin grafting.[5,6,13]

Management

Initial management must begin with a comprehensive history and a thorough sensory, motor, musculoskeletal, and soft tissue examination. Radiographs of the involved areas, including proximal and distal joints, are needed to rule out adjacent fractures and dislocations.

Initial emergency department management must focus on pain management and wound care, as well as on an assessment of complex injuries that mandate emergency orthopedic referral and subsequent surgical care.

Wound Care

Wound care consists of gentle cleansing and débridement. Lacerations that can be closed primarily should be repaired at this time. Blisters and hematomas should undergo prompt incision and drainage. Prompt fasciotomy should be performed if there is an increase in compartment pressure. Fractures should be reduced and splinted as indicated. The extremity should be wrapped lightly with a nonadherent dressing and elevated.

Compressive Dressings

The use of compressive dressings is controversial. Comparisons of elastic and nonelastic compressive dressings from previous reports are inconclusive because of differences in the time of presentation, the use of steroids, and associated injuries.[2,3,9,11] Chamberlain and Soltes[12] noted that studies with and without compressive dressings had similar outcomes. Nonelastic compressive dressings reduce the likelihood of constriction being applied to the extremity and therefore are preferred.[3]

Skin Grafts

The incidence of skin grafts ranges from 11% to 70%. Factors that may account for this wide range include early versus delayed treatment, the use of compressive dressings, and changes in safety features of wringer washers. Skin grafts, if needed, should be performed early to reduce associated infection and wound contraction. The likelihood of split-thickness skin grafts is increased for those who delay treatment.[8,11] Complex degloving injuries have been repaired with full-thickness skin grafts from revascularized avulsed skin flaps.[5,6]

Antibiotics

The prophylactic use of antibiotics is reserved for contaminated industrial wounds with open fractures, degloving injuries, or amputations; parenteral first-generation cephalosporins are used.[13] Good wound care is a more dependable method of minimizing the risk of infection with noncomplex wringer injuries.[7] In this situation, antibiotic prophylaxis does not prevent the conversion of burns from partial to full thickness. Hyaluronidase injected locally into the wound has been shown experimentally to reduce wound edema associated with wringer injuries. However, there are insufficient data to advocate this clinical approach.[15]

Pain

Significant pain is associated with wringer injuries. The liberal use of parenteral narcotics is advocated. Stellate ganglion block to prevent vasospasm is reserved for more chronic problems following upper extremity compression.[14]

Hospitalization

Hospitalization is considered routine for wringer and industrial roller injuries and may be prolonged for those who delay treatment.[11] Complications from industrial roller injuries must be anticipated and include compartment syndrome that requires fasciotomy, wound infection, skin graft rejection, and limited functional recovery.[5,6,13] Outpatient management of wringer injuries has been recommended for patients who have no evidence of complex injury or areas of full-thickness skin loss, patients who will be in close proximity to the health care facility, and those who have reliable caregivers. This approach should be taken with caution.[14]

Cornpicker Injuries

Agriculture is one of the most hazardous industries, accounting for an injury/death rate of 46 per 100,000 workers. In contrast, all other occupations combined account for an injury/death rate of 13 per 100,000 workers. Farm machinery is associated with an extensive number of hand injuries, with the cornpicker implicated in particular.[16] Farm soil, corn husk, grease, and oil contamination compound these severe mechanical injuries.

Epidemiology

Victims usually are male, with a wide age range. The dominant hand usually is injured. Injuries occur seasonally, from September through December with peak incidence in October and November. Because farmers often work alone in the field, they may be trapped for extended periods of time before being discovered.[17]

Mechanism of Injury

The cornpicker machinery consists of pointed shoes, snapping rollers, chain, and auger, and the combine, which strips the corn from its husk. The pointed shoes, or snouts, guide rolls of corn into gathering chains and pull the stalks into snapping rollers. These rollers, which are located side by side and rotate in opposite directions, strip the ears of corn off the stalks. The gathering chain and auger then carry the ears of corn and feed them to the combine, where they are husked and shelled.[18]

Cornpicker injuries most often occur when the gathering chains or snapping rollers become occluded (usually as a result of damp corn stalks, weedy field conditions, or harvesting too quickly) and the farmer tries to disengage the obstruction by using a tool or pulling the stalks. When cleared, the machine immediately engages and pulls the stalks or tool, along with the farmer's hand, into the snapping rollers. All of these injuries could be prevented by simply turning the machine off before releasing the obstruction.[19]

The hand usually sustains both a severe friction burn and a crush injury with an avulsion force.[16,17,19-22] Amputation or devascularization of three or more digits, defined as **mutilation**, is quite common[19,23] (Figure 24-1). The width of the hand or prominence of the metacarpal head usually prevents further advancement into the rollers. The wrist and forearm may be crushed or avulsed if the hand passes through the rollers. There is marked soft tissue and skeletal injury. Fractures of the digits, hand, and forearm usually are displaced and comminuted. More proximally, the elbow and shoulder may dislocate; ligaments and tendon attachments often are disrupted.[23]

Clinical Presentation

Severe mutilation with amputation or digit devascularization, degloving, crushing, and friction burns are common.[16,17,20-22]

Maxim et al[24] characterized three classic patterns of injury in 1954. **Type I**

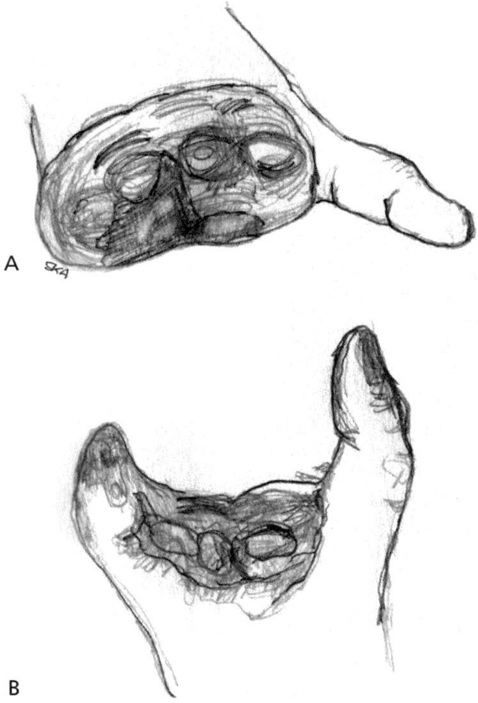

Figure 24-1.

Cornpicker injuries. **A)** *Amputation of all fingers, with the thumb spared.* **B)** *Devascularization of the little finger and amputation of the ring, middle, and index fingers, with the thumb spared.*

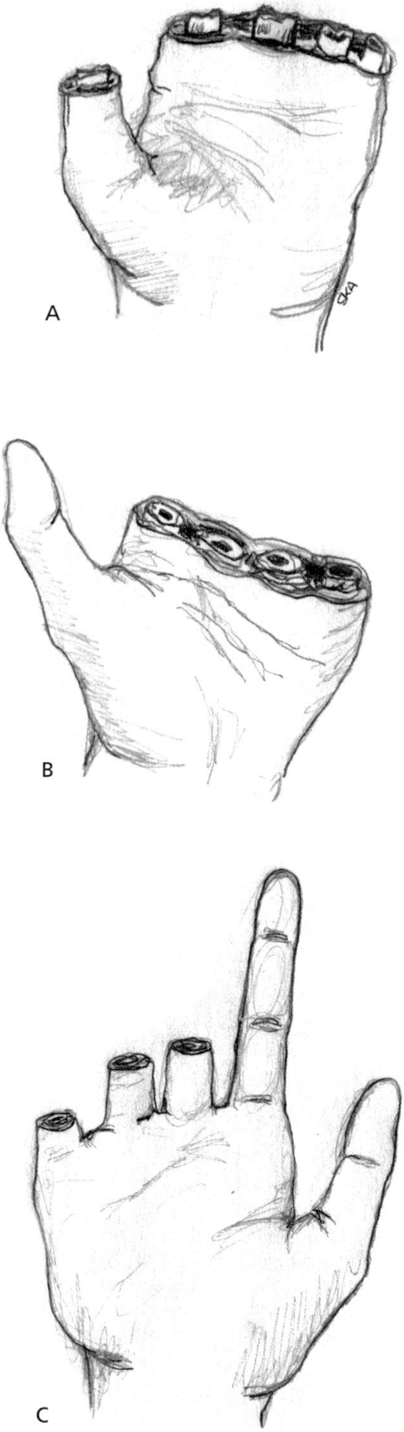

Figure 24-2.

Classifications of mutilating cornpicker injuries. **A)** *Type I injury, amputation or devascularization of all digits.* **B)** *Type II injury, amputation or devascularization of all fingers, with the thumb spared.* **C)** *Type III injury, amputation or devascularization of multiple fingers, with the thumb and at least one finger spared.*

injury involves the loss of all digits, including the thumb. **Type II injury** involves the loss of all fingers with preservation of the thumb. **Type III injury**, as described by Maxim, involves the loss of the thumb and one or more fingers on the radial aspect of the hand. Type III injuries have been described more recently as multiple digit injuries in any location but with the preservation of at least one finger and the thumb[19] (Figure 24-2). Type II and type III injuries occur more often than type I injuries, with the thumb injured about half as often as any other digit.[17,19]

Management

Emergency treatment consists of pain control with parenteral narcotics, regional anesthesia, or both. Because there is a high incidence of cultured Gram-positive and Gram-negative organisms from these wounds, prophylaxis with parenteral second-generation cephalosporins has been recommended.[17] Heavy wound contamination mandates thorough surgical débridement and irrigation.[19,23] Primary closure is not usually indicated; revascularization attempts usually fail.[17,19] Delayed closure and reconstruction are referred for later care.

The clinical presentation determines which reconstructive techniques are used. The goal of complex surgical reconstructive procedures is to maintain function of the uninjured thumb as in type II and type III injuries. The goal for type I injuries is to provide prehension with an opposable, mobile, sensible thumb, such as with toe-to-thumb transfer if there is insufficient thumb length.[19]

Snowblower Injuries

Snowblowers were introduced approximately 30 years ago, and their use has become widespread. The first data related to snowblower injuries were published in 1973.[25] With few exceptions, injuries occur to the hand and take place when the operator attempts to dislodge impacted snow while the engine is running.[26] Simple preventive measures would seem to be the solution in reducing the risk of injury.[27] However, despite improved safety features, operator carelessness continues to be a primary risk factor.

Epidemiology

The Centers for Disease Control reported in 1983 that approximately 3,000 snowblower-related injuries occur each year.[28] This number has most likely increased with more prevalent use. The estimated annual injury rate is 5.3 injuries per 1,000 operators.[29]

An increased frequency of injury is noted during early or late winter snowfall.[25,26,28,30] Higher temperatures (at or above 28°F) tend to produce a heavier, wetter snow, which is more likely to obstruct the discharge chute. Frequency of injury also is directly related to the depth of snowfall.[30] Other causative factors include operator inexperience and inadequately functioning machines.[31]

Mechanism of Injury

Snowblowers operate by one of two mechanisms. With a one-stage snowblower, an auger blade both gathers and throws the snow out the exhaust chute. A two-stage snowblower consists of a slowly rotating auger blade that gathers snow plus an impeller blade, located at the base, that quickly propels snow out the exhaust chute[30,31] (Figure 24-3). Most snowblowers have several safety features, including "dead-man switches." The clutch and blades, when depressed, engage simultaneously; when released, the blades cease rotation.

Most hand injuries occur when the victim's fingers are struck by the impeller blade while he or she clears the frequently unguarded clogged exit chute. In nearly all cases, injuries are to the dominant hand.[30,32-34]

Clinical Presentation

Victims sustain injuries to, on average, two digits at or distal to the DIP joints. The index, middle, and ring fingers are most frequently involved; the thumb is almost always spared.[25,30,32-34]

Snowblower injuries are characterized by extensive lacerations and contusions, particularly to the dorsal aspect of the hand and fingers. Concomitant extensor tendon lacerations, comminuted and complicated fractures, and traumatic amputations also occur.[32]

Management

Initial patient evaluation must include an in-depth sensory and motor evaluation and vascular function assessment. Appropriate analgesia can be provided with digital anesthesia. Radiographs are essential because of the high incidence of fractures.

Débridement and repair are reserved for the operating room. Primary closure is thought to be acceptable because the kinetic energy of a snowblower is similar to that of a low-velocity missile.[35] Delayed primary closure is indicated with gross contamination or massive tissue destruction.[32] Prophylaxis with parenteral antibiotics is reserved for complex contaminated wounds or open fractures.

Microvascular repair, tendon repair, and K-wire fixation should be performed as indicated.[30] Replantation of amputated digits is dependent on the level of amputation and on the number and severity of injury to the involved digits.[36]

Followup care is associated with low complication rates.[30,32] The low incidence of infection probably is the result of minimal contamination of the wound at the time of injury. Occasionally, glove or mitten fibers have been found embedded within wounds, and these are easily débrided.[30]

Figure 24-3.

Two-stage snowblower.

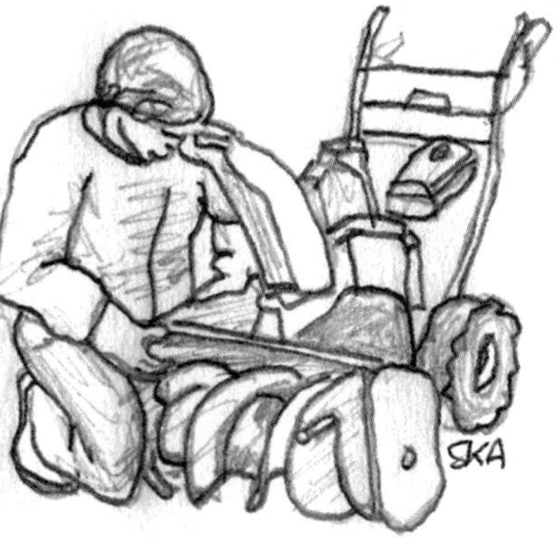

High-Pressure Injection Injuries

High-pressure injection injuries were reported infrequently in the medical literature in the earlier part of the 20th century. They were reported as early as 1925 by Hesse in England and were described in 1937 by Rees.[37,38] Similar injection injuries have become more prevalent due to the multiple industrial uses of high-pressure injection guns[39] for lubrication, cleaning, painting, and mass farm animal vaccination.[40,41] A variety of materials can be injected with these devices, including paint, paint thinners, grease, oil, wax, plastic, water, and cement.

High-pressure injection injuries occur readily because a pressure of only 100 psi is required to breach the skin. Industrial high-pressure injection machines generate much higher pressures and therefore penetrate the skin more readily. Due to the high pressure produced by the spray gun, direct contact with the skin is not necessary to cause significant injury.

Epidemiology

In high-pressure injection injuries, patient characteristics and injury circumstances often are similar. Injection injuries often occur in the workplace. The patient usually presents with a history of coming into close proximity of the jet stream during the cleaning of an obstructed nozzle or operation of the equipment.[42,43] The nondominant hand is involved in 76% of cases; the index finger is the most common injury site, followed by the middle finger and the palm.[44] Victims most often are manual laborers, with an average age of 35 years.[44] Injury most commonly results from operator inexperience.[45]

Mechanism of Injury

Three pieces of industrial equipment (grease guns, spray guns, and diesel injectors) account for most of these injuries.[46] Fifty-seven percent of high-pressure injection injuries are caused by grease guns.[43] Air compression generates the propulsive forces for the grease to reach emission pressures of 5,000 to 10,000 psi. The kinetic energy created has been compared with that of a 450-lb weight falling from a height of 25 cm.[47]

High-pressure spray guns account for 18% of injection injuries.[46] Their use is widespread in the automotive industries. Spray guns deliver material such as paint, lacquer, semifluid cement and sand, hydraulic fluids, and solvents, including paint thinner, turpentine, and gasoline, at pressures between 3,000 and 7,000 psi.[48]

Diesel fuel injectors produce 14% of high-pressure hand injuries. In diesel engines, diesel oil passes into an injector mechanism, which compresses the fuel to very high pressures before it flows through a nozzle into the combustion chamber. Oil pressure is emitted in a range from 2,000 to 12,000 psi. Injuries often occur when the engine is being serviced or the injection apparatus is being tested.[43]

Other sources of injection injuries include defects in pneumatic hoses, ruptures of hydraulic lines in sandblasters, defective valves from the grease boxes of tractors, and defects in oil rig drilling and pipeline equipment.[39,43,46]

Tissue injury from high-pressure injection is dependent on the type and amount of material injected, the anatomic location, and the velocity of the injected material.

Type of Material Injected

The most important prognostic factor is the type of material injected. This influences tissue inflammatory response along with the resultant fibrosis that occurs during healing. Despite having the largest in vivo antibacterial activity, paint (especially oil-based) and paint thinner generate a large and early inflammatory response that leads to severe fibrosis, as well as amputations in 70% of injection injuries.[43,49-53] In contrast, grease gun injuries cause a large inflammatory response only when a bacterial infection develops.[44,51] Morbidity is caused by a high incidence of fibrosis, oleomas, and draining sinuses.[39]

Amount Injected

The amount of material injected determines the degree of mechanical distention that impairs the arteriovenous circulation.[46] An inflammatory response results in edema. Various mechanisms that interfere with vascular supply have been proposed, including massive thrombosis of the blood vessels as oil volatilizes, digital vasospasm, venous obstruction from tissue distention, and digital artery compression from tissue distention. Regardless of the exact mechanism, the resulting chemical inflammatory response and vascular impairment lead to tissue necrosis and the potential for superimposed bacterial infection.

Anatomic Location

Material is dispersed according to the site of tissue penetration. Spread of the substance occurs along fascial planes, within flexor tendon sheaths, and through subcutaneous tissue. The flexor tendon sheath is most easily penetrated at the DIP and PIP flexion creases. The tendon sheaths of the index, middle, and ring fingers end approximately at the MCP joint; hence, injected material is confined to the digits.[40] However, the tendon sheaths of the thumb and little finger extend into the radial and ulnar bursae, allowing retrograde extension of material into the forearm. This has the potential to cause a compartment syndrome or a median or ulnar nerve entrapment at the carpal tunnel. Palmar injection damages deep palmar structures if the aponeurosis is ruptured; however, this is uncommon, and spread usually occurs medially or laterally.[46]

Velocity of Injected Material

The velocity of the injected material does not lead directly to tissue damage.[46,50] Increased velocity, however, leads to greater dispersion of the material and therefore greater tissue damage.

Clinical Presentation

The early presentation of an injured patient may reveal no apparent break in the skin or only a benign-appearing pinhole-sized puncture wound with minimal symptoms. Then, several hours later, the digit may progressively become extremely painful, swollen, and pale. This initial benign presentation may cause physicians to overlook potentially severe injuries that can lead to permanent disability.

Historically, clinical symptoms and signs have been classified into three stages: acute, intermediate, and late.[54]

Acute Phase

Findings in the acute stage include swelling, anesthesia, and vascular insufficiency, which usually occur within 4 to 6 hours. Edema is secondary to the inflammatory response; injected material may be seen draining from the puncture site.[40]

Without proper treatment, tissue ischemia and necrosis occur at 4 to 12 hours. The digit subsequently becomes numb and pale as a result of vascular compromise. Rarely, injected material is absorbed systemically, causing a generalized toxic reaction; this may lead to lymphangitis, lymphadenitis, leukocytosis, or fever.[55]

Intermediate Stage

The intermediate stage is characterized by the development of oleomas at the injection site and throughout the tissue. Because of the foreign body tissue reaction that develops from injected material, these nodular tumors are prone to form.[43] They can remain dormant for many years, but fibrosis often occurs, leading to functional loss.

Late Stage

The late stage is marked by the breakdown of skin overlying the oleoma, which results in ulcers and draining sinuses that may become infected secondarily. As a late complication, squamous epitheliomas may develop within the sinuses.[43]

Management

Outcome is enhanced by the physician's ability to promptly recognize the severity of injury, initiate aggressive treatment, and arrange emergent orthopedic referral.

Patients usually present in the acute stage several hours after injury. A detailed history that focuses on the time of injury and type of material injected is essential. Careful examination of the extremity is necessary to assess neurovascular function.

In addition to initiating pain management and ordering appropriate radiographs, the emergency physician must obtain immediate orthopedic referral for surgical open wound management and start appropriate antibiotic prophylaxis. Mandatory hospitalization should be anticipated.

Radiography

Radiographs of the hand and extremity help determine the extent of dispersion and thus the extent of surgical exploration and débridement required.[39,46,56,57] Lead-based paints appear as radiopaque soft tissue densities not to be confused with a calcification (Figure 24-4). Non–lead-based paints

Figure 24-4.

Extent of radiopaque material dispersed in a digit injured by a high-pressure injection device.

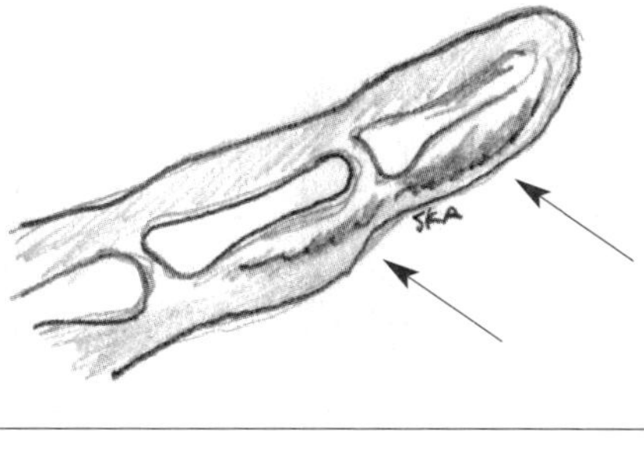

appear as subcutaneous emphysema; grease appears as a lucency. Xeroradiography may show the extent of soft tissue injection from grease more clearly.[46]

Pain Management

Pain usually is severe and should be treated with parenteral analgesics. Brachial plexus or stellate ganglion blocks also may be performed. Digital blocks are contraindicated because of the potential for increased tissue pressure and further compromise of tissue perfusion.[39,43,46,51]

Treatment

Standard surgical incisions are necessary for decompression and wide exploration to expose all areas infiltrated by the injected material. Necrotic tissue and foreign material should be débrided unless neurovascular bundles are involved; their removal may cause unnecessary injury. The wound should be irrigated copiously with normal saline, which also helps reduce fibrosis and scarring. Solvent irrigation is contraindicated because it causes tissue inflammation. Wounds are left open with the use of Penrose drains and can be closed later with split-thickness skin grafts.[46]

The high incidence of gangrene requiring surgical amputation of digits is related both to delayed treatment and injected material.[50,56] If débridement is delayed by more than 6 to 10 hours, the amputation rate increases. High-pressure injection of paint and paint solvent results in the highest incidence of amputation. However, 84% of digits can be salvaged using the open wound technique, with 60% restored to normal function.[58,59]

Prophylactic broad-spectrum antibiotics such as ceftriaxone or chloramphenicol are indicated, although most injected materials exhibit antibacterial activity.[49,58] Other medications such as steroids, heparin, and dextran, remain controversial. Steroids, however, have been recommended for severe inflammatory responses that develop because of a delay in treatment and for systemic symptoms.[45,58]

Nail Gun Injuries

Industrial nail guns, which were introduced in 1959, have increased application and use in both industry and by the general public. Variously described as nail guns, cartridge compression guns, or power-actuated tools, they are used to fire nails into steel, wood, and masonry.[60,61] The nail gun can produce velocities as high as 1,400 feet per second, at which speed a nail can penetrate stressed concrete up to 10 cm.[62]

Epidemiology

Injuries from nail guns often are not reported because victims typically treat themselves, seeking emergency treatment only when a wound is deep or a nail cannot be extracted. Sites of injury include the head, neck, chest, abdomen, vertebral column, spinal cord, and extremities, with fatal injuries reported. The hand is the most common site, accounting for 65% of all nail gun injuries.[63-68] Typically, the nondominant hand of a carpenter or construction worker is injured on the radial aspect due to the position of the hand when the gun is fired.[64-68]

The most common cause of injury is related to improper operator use of the nail gun trigger. The incorrect but common technique is to continuously depress the trigger and activate the firing mechanism by pressing against the material to be nailed. Because the contact pressure required to fire the gun is so low,[67] injuries also occur when a gun misfires in space without being in direct contact with any solid material.

Mechanism of Injury

Nail guns are distinguished by their velocity. High-velocity tools use an explosive cartridge, which detonates and fires the projectile. The more commonly used low-velocity nail guns eject nails indirectly by using an explosive cartridge or compressed air (delivering pressures of 60 to 120 psi) through the use of a captive piston.[68]

The nails have a polymer coating to increase their penetration and adherence to surrounding structures.[68] Nails preloaded into the nail gun also are affixed by copper wire; when fired, copper barbs remain attached to the nail by the adhesive resin.[62,68]

Mechanisms of nail gun injury include direct penetration, shrapnel wounds from exploding cartridges, and high-pressure injection injuries from the compressed air used to activate the gun.[62]

Clinical Presentation

Injuries to the hand can be classified into three general types:

- Soft tissue
- Bone and soft tissue, including phalanges, metacarpals, carpals, radius, and ulna
- Joints, bones, and other structures, including IP and radiocarpal joints

The third type is associated with the poorest prognosis and longest disability. Most injuries involve retained nails, with trauma limited to the surrounding soft tissues. On impact, the nail may cause a circumferential full-thickness avulsion of skin. In the hand, the skin may be driven down into the deep palmar space, possibly serving as a nidus for a deep palmar infection or subsequent inclusion cyst formation. Tendon and neurovascular injuries are rare.[62,65,68]

Management

Knowing what type of nail gun was used is essential to the initial evaluation; thorough sensory, motor, soft tissue, and neurovascular examinations also must be performed. Radiographs, with a minimum of two views (AP and lateral), always should be obtained to determine the presence of associated fractures or joint penetration and to determine the presence of barbs on the nail shaft.[62]

Pain control with either regional or digital anesthesia, as indicated, enhances wound exploration, débridement, and nail extraction, which is the most important aspect of management.[62]

Wound care is guided by the injury type. Soft tissue injuries can be explored locally by extending the entrance and exit wounds. Contaminants such as skin avulsions and clothing fibers must be removed. The adhesive resin from the nail, although a polymer and chemically inert, also should be extracted to further reduce the risk of infection. Barbed nails are extracted by first removing the head of the nail and then pulling the nail out antegrade in the same direction as its introduction. This reduces the potential for a barb-induced injury to neurovascular structures and for the barb to become detached. Barbless nails should be removed in the same manner.[62,64,68] The wound then should be débrided, copiously irrigated with normal saline under high pressure, and left open to heal by secondary intention. Prophylactic first-generation cephalosporins have been advocated.[62,68] Orthopedic followup care is recommended.

Orthopedic consultation for surgical intervention should be initiated for injuries that involve bone or joints or cause neurovascular impairment.[62,64,68] A late complication of adhesions between the flexor and extensor tendons and overlying scar formation that results in digit flexor limitation has been reported and may be more likely when these structures are involved.[61]

References

1. MacCollum DW. Wringer arm: a report of twenty-six cases. *N Engl J Med.* 1938;218:549-554.
2. Allen HS. Wringer injuries of the upper extremity. *Ann Surg.* 1941;113:1101-1102.
3. Hausmann PF, Everett HH. Wringer injury. *Surgery.* 1950;28:71-74.
4. Posch JL, Weller CN. Mangle and severe wringer injuries of the hand in children. *J Bone Joint Surg [Am].* 1954;36:57-63.
5. Jeng SF, Wei FC. Resurfacing a circumferentially degloved hand by using a full-thickness skin graft harvested from an avulsed skin flap. *Ann Plast Surg.* 1997;39:360-365.
6. Cheng SL, Wong SS. Salvage of superficial palmar avulsion. *J Trauma.* 1996;40:22-26.
7. Cabbabe ED, Korock SW. Wringer washer injuries in children. *Ann Plast Surg.* 1983;10:135-142.
8. Lee RW. Special injuries of the hand. *Trauma Q.* 1985;1:88-94.
9. Adams JP, Fowler FD. Observations in wringer injuries. *J Bone Joint Surg [Am].* 1961;42:1179-1186.
10. Thompson HG, Hampole MK. Monkey-hand wringer injury. *Plast Reconstr Surg.* 1970;45:471-479.
11. McCulloch JH, Boswick JA, Roseann J. Household wringer injuries: a three year review. *J Trauma.* 1973;13:1-8.
12. Chamberlain JW, Soltes M. Wringer injuries. *Pediatrics.* 1961;28:96-100.
13. Askins G, Finley R, Parenti J, et al. High-energy roller injuries to the upper extremity. *J Trauma.* 1986;26:1127-1131.
14. Golden G, Fisher JC, Edgerton MT. Wringer arm reevaluated. *Ann Surg.* 1973;177:362-369.
15. Bennett JE, Zook EG, Ashbell TS, et al. The spreading enzymes and localized edema: a study of wringer crush injury in the rabbit. *J Trauma.* 1970;10:240-248.
16. Melvin PM. Corn picker injuries of the hand. *Arch Surg.* 1972;104:26-29.
17. Campbell DC, Bryan RS, Cooney WP, et al. Mechanical cornpicker hand injuries. *J Trauma.* 1979;19:678-681.
18. Nachlas N, Schlenker JD. The mechanical cornpicker. *Ind Med J.* 1981;159:371-374.
19. Gorsche TS, Wood MB. Mutilating corn-picker injuries of the hand. *J Hand Surg.* 1988;13A:423-427.
20. Bruner JM. Corn picker injuries of the hand. *Plast Reconstr Surg.* 1958;21:306-314.

21. Hardin CA, Robinson DW. Compound injuries of the hand due to mechanical corn picker. *J Kans Med Soc.* 1950;51:114-118.
22. Robinson DW, Hardin CA. Corn picker injuries. *Am J Surg.* 1955;89:780-783.
23. Wolfort FG. Special injuries. In: *Acute Hand Injuries: A Multispecialty Approach.* Boston, Mass: Little, Brown; 1980.
24. Maxim ES, Webster FS, Willander DA. The cornpicker hand. *J Bone Joint Surg [Am].* 1954;36:21-29.
25. Lucas GL. Snowblower injuries of the hand. *Wisc Med J.* 1973;72:193-198.
26. Labow SS. Snowblower injuries. *Can Med Assoc J.* 1974;110:1019.
27. Boswick JA. Snow blower injuries to the hand [editorial]. *J Trauma.* 1989;29:267.
28. Centers for Disease Control: Snow-blower injuries—Colorado, New York. *MMWR Morb Mortal Wkly Rep.* 1983;32:77-78.
29. Waller JA. Snowblower injuries. *J Trauma.* 1977;17:122-125.
30. Millea TP, Hansen RH. Snowblower injuries to the hand. *J Trauma.* 1989;29:229-233.
31. Bowen V, Loback D, Tokaryk R. Snowblower injuries to the hand. *Can J Surg.* 1987;30:111.
32. Almdahl SM, Saeboe-Larsen J, Due J. Injuries to the hand inflicted by rotary snowcutters. *J Trauma.* 1989;29:227-228.
33. Drewniang JJ, Palmer AK. Snowblower injuries to the hand. *Orthop Rev.* 1983;12:83-87.
34. Gould LV, Hughes EC, Lehrman A. Snowblower injuries. *N Y State J Med.* 1974;74:887-889.
35. Barry TP, Linton PC. Biophysics of rotary mower and snowblower injuries of the hand: high-vs-low velocity "missile" injury. *J Trauma.* 1977;17:211-214.
36. Schlenker JD. Fingertip injuries and reimplantations. *Trauma Q.* 1985;1:38-45.
37. Rees CE. Penetration of tissue by fuel oil under high pressure from diesel engine. *JAMA.* 1937;109:866-867.
38. Hesse E. Die ehirurgische und gerechtlich-medizinische Bedeutung der Künstlich hervorgerufenen Erkrankungen. *Arch Klin Chir.* 1925;136:277-291.
39. Harter BT, Harter KC. High-pressure injection injuries. *Hand Clin.* 1986;2:547-551.
40. Schnall SB, Mirzayan R. High pressure injection injuries to the hand. *Hand Clin.* 1999;75:245-248.
41. Couzens G, Burke FD. Veterinary high pressure injection injuries with inoculations for large animals. *J Hand Surg [Br].* 1995;20:497-499.
42. Harrison R. Grease-gun injury. *Br J Surg.* 1959;46:514-515.
43. Kaufman HD. The clinicopathological correlation of high-pressure injection injuries. *Br J Surg.* 1968;55:214-218.
44. Shoo MJ, Scott FA, Boswick JA. High-pressure injection injuries to the hand. *South Med J.* 1980;73:896-898.
45. Herrick RT, Godsil RD, Widener JH. High-pressure injection injuries to the hand. *South Med J.* 1980;73:896-898.
46. Sirio CA, Smith JS, Graham WP. High-pressure injection injuries of the hand. *Am Surg.* 1989;55:714-718.
47. Kaufman HD. High pressure injection injuries: the problems, pathogenesis and management. *Hand.* 1978;2:63-73.
48. Parks BJ, Horner FL, Trimblers C. Emergency treatment of high-pressure injection injuries of the hand. *JACEP.* 1975;4:216-217.
49. Gillespie CA, Rodeheaver GT, Smith S, et al. Airless paint gun injuries: definition and management. *Am J Surg.* 1974;128:383-391.
50. Neal NC, Burke FD. High-pressure injection injuries. *Injury.* 1991;22:467-470.
51. Stark HH, Ashworth CR, Boyes JH. Paint-gun injuries of the hand. *J Bone Joint Surg [Am].* 1967;49:637-647.
52. Hayes CW, Pan HC. High pressure injection injuries of the hand. *South Med J.* 1982;75:1491-1498.

53. Geller ER, Gursel E. A unique case of high pressure injection injury of the hand. *J Trauma.* 1986;26:483-485.
54. Mason ML, Queen FB. Grease gun injuries to the hand. *Q Bull Northwest Med Sch.* 1941;15:122-132.
55. Jebson PJ, Sanderson M, Ran VR, et al. High-pressure injuries of the hand. *Wisc Med J.* 1993;92:13-16.
56. Chung-Ho P, Wei DC, Hon SP. High-pressure injection injuries of the hand. *J Trauma.* 1991;31:110-112.
57. Smoot EC, Robson MC. Acute management of foreign body injuries of the hand. *Ann Emerg Med.* 1983;12:434-437.
58. Vasilevski D, Noorbergen M, Depierreux M, et al. High-pressure injection injuries to the hand. *Am J Emerg Med.* 2000;18:820-824.
59. Pinto MR, Turkula-Pinto LD, Cooney WP, et al. High pressure injection injuries of the hand: review of 25 patients managed by open wound technique. *J Hand Surg* [Am]. 1993;18:125-130.
60. Lyons FR. Industrial nail gun injuries. *Med J Aust.* 1983;2:483-487.
61. Edlich RF, Silloway KA, Rodeheaver GT, et al. Industrial nail gun injuries. *Compr Ther.* 1986;12:42-46.
62. Hoffman DR, Jebson PJ, Curtis SM. Nail gun injuries of the hand. *Am Fam Physician.* 1997;53:1643-1646.
63. le Nobel JL, Wing MB. Pneumatic nail gun injuries of the knee. *Clin Orthop.* 1987;217:228-229.
64. al-Qattan MM, Stranc MF. Nail gun injuries of the fingers: a safer method of nail gun removal. *J Hand Surg [Br].* 1993;18:652-653.
65. Braun RM. Nail gun injury of the hand. *J Bone Joint Surg [Am].* 1971;53:383-384.
66. Kenny NW, Kay PR, Haines JF. Nail gun injuries to the hand. *J Hand Surg [Br].* 1992;17:577-578.
67. Kenny N, O'Donaghue D, Hains J. Nail gun injuries. *J Trauma.* 1993;35:943-945.
68. Van Demark RE Jr, Van Demark RE Sr. Nail gun injuries of the hand. *J Orthop Trauma.* 1993;7:506-509.

CHAPTER 25

Risk Management Issues

John P. Rudzinski, MD, FACEP

The specter of medical malpractice litigation threatens emergency physicians in every patient encounter. Unfortunately, the situation appears to be worsening; most emergency physicians are sued at least once during their clinical careers. Recent factors have added to the inherent medical-legal exposure of the emergency department. For example, the widespread use of the Internet and mass media has increased the accessibility and awareness of litigation resources such as specialized attorneys, class action lawsuits, and expert witnesses. A published report by the Institute of Medicine has gained widespread attention for its conclusion that errors are common in medical practice and result in significant morbidity and mortality.[1] Although the accuracy and conclusion of the report have been questioned,[2,3] its widespread dissemination and attendant publicity have made it a significant force in public policy and the media, resulting in heightened public awareness of potential medical errors and malpractice.

The purpose of risk management is to increase physician awareness of potential areas of litigation and to identify specific preventive measures that can improve clinical outcomes and patient satisfaction and reduce liability. In addition to issues related to documentation and communication, this chapter addresses two high-risk clinical topics that are relevant when caring for hand injuries: fractures and wound care.

Risk Issues

Orthopedic injuries are a common basis for allegations of medical malpractice for emergency physicians. Injuries to the hand are an important subset of orthopedic injuries for a number of reasons. First, a person's choice of occupation and ability to work often are related directly to the ability to use the hand. Functional impairment can lead to significant occupational restrictions and resultant monetary awards. Problematic injuries such as tendon disruption frequently lead to obvious deformities, providing visual evidence of a physician's alleged negligence. A jury may wonder how an emergency physician failed to diagnose a defect that is so obvious at a later trial. The inherent complexity of the anatomy and function of the hand, especially combined with the duplicative capabilities of nearby uninjured structures, can make diagnosis difficult. This adds to the inherent risk potential of hand injuries.

History and Physical Examination

The history and physical examination are of the utmost importance in the evaluation of any orthopedic injury and often can be used to predict radiographic and other abnormalities. Whenever possible, the patient's hand dominance, significant past medical history, confounding factors, and, in particular, the mechanism of injury should be routinely sought and documented. A focused but thorough hand examination should be performed routinely and documented appropriately. These simple measures performed routinely are the emergency physician's best protection against later litigation. Failure to diagnose is the most commonly alleged error in medicine.

Fractures

Missed fracture is one of the most common complaints made against emergency physicians, accounting for 17% of all claims and 17% of total dollars paid.[4] Fractures should be sought through the ordering and evaluation of appropriate high-quality radiographs. A **rule of two's** has been suggested for radiograph use[5]: at least *two views* of the area in question; *two occasions*, with imaging repeated at a later date if initial films do not reveal a visible fracture when a high clinical index of suspicion exists; *two limbs* when comparison views of the opposite side may be helpful, as in children with open epiphyses; and *two joints*, with the joint above and below a fracture adequately visualized when indicated.

The treating physician also should consider the limitations of radiography. Careful examination may elicit the rotational deformity of an occult fracture of the metacarpals or phalanges that was not initially visualized on routine radiography. Negative radiographs obviously do not preclude the presence of other injuries and should not evoke complacency; for example, volar plate damage not seen on a normal radiograph, and thus not treated, can later result in a swan-neck deformity.

Finally, each emergency department should have a system to resolve discrepancies in the interpretation of radiographs between emergency physicians and radiologists. For an emergency physician not to diagnose each abnormality on the first interpretation of a radiograph is not in and of itself malpractice. If a patient's injured extremity is immobilized and treated as a potential fracture pending final interpretation, there is no opportunity for that patient to claim any additional harm.

Wound Care

According to a study published in 1996,[4] lawsuits related to wounds represented 19.85% of claims filed against emergency physicians in

Massachusetts from 1975 through 1993, making wound care one of the most significant high-risk aspects of emergency medical practice. In the emergency and primary care of the hand, wound care and laceration management have risk potential, in particular, in the treatment of bites, foreign bodies, and tendon injuries.

Bites

Animal and human bites to the hand pose significant potential risk. Cat bites, in particular, can result in deep tissue penetration and severe infectious complications. Human bites are considered to be even more infective than cat bites (see Chapter 18). A careful history may elicit such exposure, especially for lacerations over the MCP joints of a clenched fist. Such suspected wounds should be examined carefully for tooth fragments and injuries to tendons and joints, and appropriate radiographs should be considered. Consultation with an appropriate specialist and surgical exploration may be indicated.

Foreign Bodies

Claims related to failure to diagnose a retained foreign body also are common in emergency medicine. In general, consideration of a potential retained foreign body should be automatic when a patient presents with an open wound of the hand. Often, a thorough history and physical examination, especially when the wound is carefully explored in a bloodless field obtained through careful tourniquet application, suffice to eliminate this consideration. For other cases, however, additional efforts to diagnose a retained foreign body, including appropriate imaging studies and specialist consultation, often serve the physician and patient well.

Tendon Injuries

Tendon injuries are perhaps the most problematic hand liability issue for emergency physicians, for a number of reasons.

- A tendon injury may not be diagnosed initially because of the duplicative functional capabilities of adjacent structures. Flexion of the PIP joint is still possible despite complete laceration of the FDS tendon. This occurs if the FDP tendon is intact.
- A tendon injury may take time to fully develop and may not even be diagnosable on the initial emergency department visit. This is seen with the boutonnière deformity, which may take weeks to develop after the initial extensor tendon tear.
- The patient may have confounding factors that can limit the initial evaluation. For example, a patient who is uncooperative due to alcohol intoxication or pain may not allow stress testing of the thumb after a skiing accident; if radiographs of the joint are normal, the patient may be inadvertently discharged with an undiagnosed ulnar collateral ligament disruption.
- A partial to near-total tendon laceration may display amazingly intact function, underscoring the importance of testing tendon function against resistance.

Emergency physicians should have a high index of suspicion for occult tendon injuries of the hand. Whenever possible, wounds should be explored fully, in a bloodless field if necessary, and the tendons should be inspected through full range of motion. Tendon function also should be assessed by testing against resistance. Pain and weakness with attempted contraction of a potentially damaged muscle and/or tendon should lead to the consideration of a partially severed tendon.

Controversy exists over the repair of tendon injuries, namely, whether to undertake repair of partially severed tendons, immediate versus delayed repair of tendons, and even the optimal timing of delayed repair. In *Suburban Hospital Association v Mewhinny* (1963),[6] the patient requested that her index finger tendon laceration be repaired immediately upon diagnosis, but the emergency physician sutured the wound and referred the patient to a surgeon within 3 days. An unsuccessful tendon graft was performed by the followup surgeon, and the patient subsequently sued. At trial, defense counsel presented evidence that two schools of thought existed as to the timing of tendon repair: immediate (majority) versus delayed (minority). Although the jury found in favor of the plaintiff, an appellate court ruled that the defendant physician had followed the minority but accepted rule of delayed tendon repair and, thus, had not violated the standard of practice. The jury's verdict was reversed.

Regardless of such concerns, emergency physicians are best served by initial diagnosis or consideration of a tendon injury with appropriate consultation, timely referral, immobilization of the injured appendage, and the appropriate use of antibiotics.

Documentation

It must seem to practicing emergency physicians that most risk management suggestions can be reduced to the practice of good medicine and enhanced documentation. "Good medicine," from a risk management perspective, seems to be the routine practice of obtaining a thorough history and physical examination for each patient with a hand injury, focused by a heightened clinical suspicion for occult injuries. The apparent desire of attorneys to have every detail of every interaction documented must be weighed by the emergency physician against the needs of the next waiting patient and the minimal requirement that the documentation summarize the current encounter and allow the continued care of the patient by the next provider. Nonetheless, enhanced documentation may very well protect emergency physicians from undeserved litigation. When possible, emergency physicians may protect themselves with written documentation of the following items:

- Focused history (mechanism of injury, pertinent medical history)
- Neurovascular examination (two-point discrimination, vascular refill)
- Range of motion testing (all appropriate joints, testing against resistance)
- Wound exploration (with inspection of a tendon throughout its range)

- Consideration of a retained foreign body
- Consultation (as indicated)
- Splinting and referral (position of function)
- Discharge instructions (with recheck and/or return indications)

Despite appropriate initial diagnosis and treatment, adverse outcomes may still occur and result in litigation. In *Todd v Turnbull*,[7] a patient had sustained a thumb injury after being cut by a piece of glass. The tendon injury was repaired, and the thumb was immobilized in a cast. A significant delay in followup care ensued, perhaps due in part to the patient's underlying alcoholism, and the condition of the thumb injury changed dramatically. Despite the ultimate loss of the patient's digit, the court ruled in favor of the defendant physician, undoubtedly influenced by the physician's charting and documentation.

Communication

Enhanced communication may be the physician's best tool to avoid malpractice litigation. Discrepancies between documentation by the emergency department staff (as well as prehospital personnel) and that by the emergency physician should be sought out and addressed. Communication is crucial to managing patient expectations. A patient who understands that his or her initial radiographs will also be interpreted by a radiologist, and even then may not be diagnostic, also understands the limitations of the emergency department visit. A patient who is informed that a followup examination is crucial to detect a potential occult tendon injury or the development of an infection also is informed of the need for continued care. A patient who is told to return immediately for physician care if new symptoms arise or the current condition worsens also shares the responsibility for his or her treatment and outcome.

Finally, despite the emergency physician's best efforts (Figure 25-1), the risk of an adverse outcome and potential lawsuit may be evident; frank discussion with the patient[8] and early consultation with department administrators (guest relations, risk management) or the insurance carrier may prevent a lawsuit.

Figure 25-1.

Techniques to reduce risk exposure.

Establish Patient Rapport
- Sit down when possible
- Be personable and caring

Beware of High-Risk Situations
- Exchange of patients with shift change
- Intoxicated patients
- Return visits
- Undiagnosed fractures
- Retained foreign bodies/laceration management, especially tendons

Follow the Rules
- EMTALA
- JCAHO
- Organizational policies

Enhance Communication
- Manage patient expectations
- Do not criticize other providers
- Respond honestly to patients' concerns and complaints

Documentation
- Make it legible and complete
- Never alter the medical record
- Search out and address inconsistencies from other providers

Followup Care
- Written discharge instructions
- Mechanism to follow up on delayed results (radiologists' reports)
- Splint and refer

Report Problems Early
- Communicate with risk management and administration

References

1. Kohn LT, Corrigan JM, Donaldson MS, eds. *To Err Is Human: Building a Safer Health System.* Washington, DC: National Academy Press; 2000.
2. Hayward RA, Hofer TP. Estimating hospital deaths due to medical errors. Preventability is in the eye of the reviewer. *JAMA.* 2001;286:415-420.
3. Brennan TA. The Institute of Medicine report on medical errors—could it do harm? *N Engl J Med.* 2000;15:1123-1125.
4. Karcz A, Korn R, Burke MC, et al. Malpractice claims against emergency physicians in Massachusetts: 1975-1993. *Am J Emerg Med.* 1996;14:341-345.
5. Moore MN. Orthopedic pitfalls in emergency medicine. *South Med J.* 1988;81(3):371-378.
6. *Suburban Hospital Association, Inc v Mewhinny.* 230 Md 480, 187 A2d 671 (1963).
7. *Todd v Turnbull.* 469 So2d 71 (Miss 1985).
8. Wu AW. Handling hospital errors: is disclosure the best defense? *Ann Intern Med.* 1999;131(12):970-972.

Index

Page numbers followed by "f" represent figures. Page numbers followed by "t" represent tables.

C

D

F

J

M

O

P

R

S

U

V

W

X

Z